Treatment Guidelines
for Medicine and Primary Care

New Practice Parameters

2002 Edition

Paul D. Chan, MD
Margaret T. Johnson, MD

Current Clinical Strategies Publishing

www.ccspublishing.com/ccs

Digital Book and Updates

Purchasers of this book can download the digital version and updates at the Current Clinical Strategies Publishing web site: www.ccspublishing.com/ccs

Current Clinical Strategies Publishing
27071 Cabot Road
Laguna Hills, California 92653

Phone: 800-331-8227 or 949-348-8404
Fax: 800-965-9420 or 949-348-8405
E-mail: info@ccspublishing.com
www.ccspublishing.com/ccs

Printed in USA

ISBN 1929622-00-7

Contents

Cardiovascular Disorders

Myocardial Infarction

Each year 1.5 million people are diagnosed with an acute myocardial infarction. Diagnosis of acute myocardial infarction (AMI) rests upon the triad of chest pain suggestive of cardiac disease, an ECG with characteristic changes suggesting myocardial infarction, and cardiac-specific biochemical markers exceeding the standard reference ranges. Two of the three findings are necessary to diagnose AMI.

I. **Clinical evaluation**
   A. **History.** Chest pain is present in 65-69% of patients with AMI. The pain may be characterized as a constricting or squeezing sensation in the chest. Pain can radiate to the upper abdomen, back, either arm, either shoulder, neck, or jaw. Atypical pain presentations in AMI include pleuritic, sharp, burning or reproducible chest pain, as well as pain referring to the back, abdomen, neck, or arm. Anginal equivalents such as dyspnea, nausea, vomiting, palpitations, syncope, or depressed mental status may be the only complaints.
   B. **Risk factors.** Significant cardiac risk factors include hypertension, hyperlipidemia, diabetes, smoking, and a strong family history (coronary artery disease in early or mid-adulthood in a first-degree relative).
   C. **Physical examination** of the patient with AMI reveals such abnormal signs as a tachy- or bradycardia, other arrhythmias, hyper- or hypotension, and tachypnea. Inspiratory rales and an S3 gallop are associated with left-sided failure. Jugulovenous distentions (JVDs), hepatojugular reflux, and peripheral edema suggest right-sided failure. A systolic murmur may indicate ischemic mitral regurgitation or ventricular septal defect (VSD).

II. **Laboratory evaluation**
   A. **Electrocardiogram (ECG).** Although the ECG is highly specific for diagnosis of AMI, the initial ECG reveals diagnostic ST elevations in only 40% of patients with a confirmed AMI. ST-segment elevation (equal to or greater than 1 mV) in contiguous leads provides strong evidence of thrombotic coronary arterial occlusion and makes the patient a candidate for immediate reperfusion therapy. Symptoms consistent with AMI and new left bundle branch block (LBBB) should be managed like ST-segment elevation.
   B. **Laboratory markers**
      1. **Creatine kinase** (CK) enzyme is found in nearly all tissues. The cardiac-specific dimer, CK-MB, however, is present almost exclusively in myocardium. The most common causes for serum increases in total creatine kinase (TCK) include trauma, rhabdomyolysis, hyperthermia, vigorous physical activity, renal or endocrine disease, systemic infections, or any disease state causing destruction to muscle tissue. However, in the setting of chest pain in the absence of trauma, an elevated TCK level increases the likelihood that myocardial necrosis is present.

Common Markers for Acute Myocardial Infarction			
Marker	Initial Elevation After MI	Mean Time to Peak Elevations	Time to Return to Baseline
Myoglobin	1-4 h	6-7 h	18-24 h
CTnl	3-12 h	10-24 h	3-10 d
CTnT	3-12 h	12-48 h	5-14 d
CKMB	4-12 h	10-24 h	48-72 h
CKMBiso	2-6 h	12 h	38 h
LD	8-12 h	24-48 h	10-14 d

CTnl, CTnT = troponins of cardiac myofibrils; CPK-MB, MM = tissue isoforms of creatine kinase; LD = lactate dehydrogenase.

2. **CK-MB subunits.** Subunits of CK, CK-MB, -MM, and -BB, are markers associated with a slow release into the blood from damaged cells. Although CK-MB is produced almost exclusively in the myocardium, trace mounts of activity are also found in the small intestine, tongue, diaphragm, uterus, and prostate. Elevated CK-MB enzyme levels are observed in the serum 2-6 hours after MI, but may not be detected until up to 12 hours after the onset of symptoms. The mean time to exceed reference standard is about 4.5 hours. Peak CK-MB levels are observed from 12-24 hours after AMI, and the enzyme is cleared from the bloodstream within 48-72 hours.

3. **Cardiac-specific troponin T (cTnT)** is a qualitative assay and cardiac troponin I (cTnl) is a quantitative assay. cTnT remains elevated in serum up to 14 days and cTnl for 3-7 days after infarction.

Treatment Recommendations for AMI	
Supportive Care with Management of Chest Pain • All patients should receive supplemental oxygen, 2 L/min by nasal canula, for a minimum of three hours • Two large-bore IVs should be placed	
Aspirin	
Inclusion Exclusion Recommendation	Clinical symptoms or suspicion of AMI Aspirin allergy, active GI bleeding ASA 160-325 mg chewable. Immediately and every daily

Thrombolytics	
Inclusion	All patients with AHA/ACC criteria for thrombolytic infusion therapy. Up to six hours after chest pain begins
Exclusion	Active internal bleeding; history of cerebrovascular accident; recent intracranial or intraspinal surgery or trauma; intracranial neoplasm, arteriovenous malformation, or aneurysm; known bleeding diathesis; severe, uncontrolled hypertension
Recommendation	Front-loaded t-PA regimen 15 mg IV over 1-2 min, then 0.75 mg/kg IV up to 50 mg IV over 30 min, then 0.5 mg/kg IV up to 35 mg IV over 60 minutes

Beta-Blockade	
Inclusion	All patients with the diagnosis of AMI. Immediate upon diagnosis of AMI
Exclusion	Asthma, hypotension, bradycardia, AV block, pulmonary edema
Recommendation	Atenolol (Tenormin), 5 mg IV, repeated in 5 minutes, followed by 50-100 mg PO qd. Metoprolol (Lopressor), 5 mg IV push every 5 minutes for three doses; followed by 25 mg PO bid. Titrate up to 100 mg PO bid.

Nitrates	
Inclusion	All patients with diagnosis of AMI. Immediate upon diagnosis of MI
Exclusion	Nitrate allergy; sildenafil (Viagra); hypotension; caution in right ventricular infarction
Recommendation	0.4 mg NTG initially q 5 minutes, up to 3 doses. IV infusion of NTG at 10-20 mcg/min, titrating upward by 5-10 mcg/min q 5-10 minutes (max 200 mcg/min). Slow or stop infusion if systolic BP < 90 mmHg

ACE INHIBITORS	
Inclusion	All patients with the diagnosis of AMI. Up to 24 hours to initiate treatment
Exclusion	Severe heart failure, history of renal failure, creatine >2.5 mg/dL, renal artery stenosis, hypotension with SBP <100
Recommendation	Lisinopril (Prinivil) 5 mg po qd up to 10 mg qd as tolerated or lisinopril 2.5 mg po if SBP < 120

Heparin	
Inclusion	Patients receiving t-PA or those patients not receiving ASA. To be given concomitantly with t-PA
Exclusion	Hypersensitivity, active internal bleeding, prolonged CPR, recent head trauma/CNS surgery/known intracranial neoplasm, hemorrhagic ophthalmic condition
Recommendation	With t-PA administration, begin IV heparin to maintain a PTT at 1.5 to 2.0 × control for the next 48 hours

III. Treatment of myocardial infarction non-thrombolytic agents

A. Pain control. Administer morphine sulfate 24 mg IV every 5-10 minutes prn for pain or anxiety.

B. Nitroglycerin. Sublingual nitroglycerin (NTG) may improve ischemic chest pain. Initially, give up to three doses of 0.4 mg sublingual NTG every five minutes. NTG should be used with caution in patients with inferior-wall MI. An infusion of intravenous NTG may be started at 10-20 mcg/min, titrating upward by 5-10 mcg/min every 5-10 minutes (maximum, 200 mcg/min). Titrate to decrease the mean arterial pressure by 10% in normotensive patients and by 30% in those with hypertension. Slow or stop the infusion when the SBP drops below 90.

C. **Aspirin** therapy reduces mortality after MI and with unstable angina, demonstrating a 20% reduction in mortality. In the absence of contraindications (allergy, active GI bleeding, or recent intracranial hemorrhage), aspirin should be administered to all patients presenting with cardiac chest pain. A dose of 160-325 mg should be given on day 1 and continued indefinitely on a daily basis thereafter. For the rare patient with a contraindication to aspirin, another antiplatelet drug, such as ticlopidine, should be administered.

D. **Beta blockade** use during AMI reduces mortality by 11%. Contraindications to beta-blockade include allergy, significant bronchial hyperreactivity, bradycardia, hypotension, PR interval greater than 0.24 s, second- or third-degree AV block, pulmonary edema, insulin-dependent diabetes mellitus, severe peripheral vascular disease, or hypoperfusion.
   1. **Atenolol (Tenormin),** 5 mg IV, repeated in 5 minutes, followed by 50-100 mg PO qd.
   2. **Metoprolol (Lopressor),** 5 mg IV push every 5 minutes for three doses; followed by 25 mg PO bid. Titrate up to 100 mg PO bid.

E. **Heparin.** The AHA/ACC criteria for using heparin are as follows:
   1. Patients undergoing percutaneous or surgical revascularization.
   2. Intravenously in patients undergoing reperfusion therapy with alteplase.
   3. Subcutaneously (7500 U bid) in all patients not treated with thrombolytic therapy who do not have a contraindication to heparin.
   4. Intravenously in patients treated with nonselective thrombolytic agents (streptokinase, anistreplase, urokinase) who are at high risk for systemic emboli (large or anterior MI, AF, previous embolus, or known LV thrombus).

F. **ACE inhibitors** increase survival in patients with AMI. Captopril is given as a 6.25 mg initial dose and titrated up to 50 mg po bid for one month. Lisinopril (Prinivil) may be given as 5-10 mg qd. ACE-inhibitors are recommended within the first 24 hours of AMI.

IV. Thrombolytics
A. **AHA/ACC ECG criteria for thrombolysis**
   1. ST Elevation (greater than 0.1 mV, two or more contiguous leads), time to therapy 12 hours or less, age younger than 75 years.
   2. Bundle branch block (obscuring ST-segment analysis) and history suggesting acute MI.

B. **Streptokinase (SK, Streptase).** The recommended dose of IV SK is 1.5 million units given over 60 minutes. About 5.7% of patients develop allergic reactions and 13% have sustain hypotension. Because of this potential, it is not recommended for use in those with recent streptococcal throat infection or readministration to those who have had previous use in the prior 12 months.

C. **Tissue plasminogen activator (t-PA, alteplase, Activase)**
   1. This agent converts plasminogen to plasmin. t-PA is clot-specific because of its propensity to bind to new thrombus. Activase is superior to streptokinase. Thirty-day mortality rates for accelerated Activase with IV heparin are 6.3%, compared with 7.3% for streptokinase.
   2. **Weight-adjusted dosing of alteplase.** For patients weighing more than 67 kg, the dose is 100 mg as a 15-mg intravenous bolus, followed by 50 mg infused over the next 30 minutes, and then 35 mg infused over the next 60 minutes. For patients weighing less than or equal to 67 kg, the dose is 15-mg intravenous bolus, followed by 0.75 mg/kg infused over the next 30 minutes

not to exceed 50 mg, and then 0.5 mg/kg over the next 60 minutes not to exceed 35 mg. Total dose should not exceed 100 mg.

Contraindications to Thrombolytic Therapy

Contraindications
- Active internal bleeding
- History of cerebrovascular accident
- Recent intracranial or intraspinal surgery to trauma.
- Intracranial neoplasm, arteriovenous malformation, or aneurysm
- Known bleeding diathesis
- Severe uncontrolled hypertension

Warnings
- Recent major surgery (eg, coronary artery bypass graft, obstetrical delivery, organ biopsy, previous puncture of noncompressible vessels)
- Cerebrovascular disease
- Recent gastrointestinal or genitourinary bleeding
- Recent trauma
- Hypertension: systolic BP ≥ 180 mmHg and/or diastolic BP ≥ 110 mmHg
- High likelihood of left heart thrombus (eg, mitral stenosis with atrial fibrillation)
- Acute pericarditis
- Subacute bacterial endocarditis
- Hemostatic defects including those secondary to severe hepatic or renal disease
- Significant hepatic dysfunction
- Pregnancy
- Diabetic hemorrhagic retinopathy or other hemorrhagic ophthalmic conditions
- Septic thrombophlebitis or occluded AV cannula at seriously infected site
- Advanced age (eg, older than 75 years)
- Patients currently receiving oral anticoagulants (eg, warfarin sodium)
- Any other condition in which bleeding constitutes a significant hazard or would be particularly difficult to manage because of its location

---

V. **Percutaneous coronary angioplasty**
   A. The incidence of reinfarction and death is lower in those treated with percutaneous transluminal coronary angioplasty (PTCA) vs. patients treated with thrombolytic therapy. Patients who received PTCA also have a lower incidence of intracranial bleeding (0% vs 2%). However, there is no statistical difference in mortality rates after 30 days.
   B. PTCA is an alternative to thrombolytic therapy if performed in a timely fashion by individuals skilled in the procedure (more than 75 PTCA procedures per year) and supported by the experienced personnel in high-volume centers. It is recommended in patients with cardiogenic shock, at high risk for intracranial bleeding and in individuals who fail to qualify for thrombolytic therapy.

References, see page 268.

Unstable Angina

Unstable angina represents a clinical spectrum of coronary artery disease that lies between stable angina and acute myocardial infarction. Unstable angina typically presents with a prolonged episode of substernal chest pain, or as stable angina that has been increasing in frequency, severity, or duration.

I. **Clinical evaluation of unstable angina**
   A. The diagnosis of unstable angina depends on clinical history, physical examination, and a 12-lead ECG. Compared with patients with stable angina, those with unstable angina are more likely to have multivessel disease and progression of atherosclerosis.
   B. Pain may be accompanied by reversible, horizontal or down-sloping ST-segment depression or deep symmetric T-wave inversion.
   C. **Factors that may precipitate unstable angina:**
      1. Lung disease (chronic obstructive pulmonary disease)
      2. Anemia (occult gastrointestinal bleeding)
      3. Fever or hyperthyroidism
      4. Uncontrolled hypertension or arrhythmias
   D. If no precipitating factors are found, unstable angina is most likely due to significant atherosclerotic coronary artery disease with plaque disruption. Plaque disruption leads to platelet aggregation, thrombus formation, and decreased coronary blood flow.

II. **Treatment**
   A. **Aspirin** is the cornerstone of therapy for unstable angina. It is effective in reducing mortality, nonfatal myocardial infarctions, and cardiac deaths. The mechanism responsible for this benefit in unstable angina is thought to be the irreversible inhibition of the cyclooxygenase pathway in platelets.
   B. **Heparin** is the recommended antithrombotic agent in the inpatient management of unstable angina. Heparin binds to antithrombin III and induces a conformational change that results in rapid inhibition of thrombin, preventing propagation of an established thrombus.
   C. **Nitrates** are used in the management of ischemic heart disease for the relief of anginal pain. The primary action of nitrates is vasodilatation of veins, arteries, and arterioles.
   D. **Beta-blockers** have been shown to reduce mortality and reinfarction in post-myocardial infarction patients. In stable angina patients, beta-blockers have been shown to reduce the frequency of symptoms and increase the anginal threshold.
   E. **Calcium antagonists** reduce myocardial oxygen demand, especially in patients in whom vasospasm may be present. There is no evidence that calcium antagonists reduce mortality or myocardial infarction in patients with unstable angina.

III. **Outpatient management of unstable angina**
   A. Patients with unstable angina who are judged to be at a low risk can be treated as outpatients in most cases. These patients are typically patients with new onset or worsening exertional angina, but who have not had prolonged or rest episodes of angina in the past 2 weeks. Any patient with significant ECG changes suggestive of ischemia should be evaluated and treated as an inpatient.

Commonly Used Nitrates in Angina Pectoris		
Agent	Dosage	Duration of Action
Sublingual nitroglycerin	0.3-0.6 mg q5-10 min	15-20 min
Isosorbide dinitrate Oral Sublingual Chewable	10-60 mg q8h 2.5-10 mg q4-6h 5-10 mg q3-5h	4-6 h 1.5-4 h 2-3 h
2% nitroglycerin ointment	0.50-2 in (1.3-5 cm; 7.5-30 mg) q6-8h	3-6 h
Transdermal nitroglycerin	5-30 cm², 20-120 mg; 0.1-0.6 mg/h; on 12 h/off 12 h	6-8 h

B. All patients with suspected unstable angina should be started on aspirin, 80 to 324 mg/d unless contraindicated. For patients who have aspirin hypersensitivity or recent bleeding, ticlopidine (Ticlid), 250 mg twice a day, or clopidogrel (Plavix), 75 mg qd should be considered.

C. Those patients who are newly diagnosed with unstable angina should also be given sublingual nitroglycerin for treatment of individual episodes and treated with either a beta-blocker or long-acting nitrates as prophylactic therapy. Patients who exhibit evidence of autonomic instability, such as inappropriate tachycardia or hypertension, should be treated with beta-blockers as the initial therapy. Therapy is usually initiated with one major antianginal drug, preferably a long-acting preparation, and a second agent is added if there are recurrent symptoms on optimal doses of the first agent. The first two classes used should be nitrates and beta-blockers followed by calcium antagonists.

D. **Beta-blockers**
   1. Atenolol (Tenormin) 50-100 mg qd
   2. Metoprolol (Lopressor) 50 mg qd-100 mg bid
   3. Pindolol (Visken) 40-240 mg qd
   4. Nadolol (Corgard) 5 mg bid-20 mg tid
   5. Propranolol LA (Inderal LA) 10-320 mg qd
   6. Timolol (Blocadren) 10-320 mg

IV. **Inpatient medical management**

A. Patients who are assessed as being moderate or high risk, as well as those patients who have had rest angina in the last 48 hours, should be admitted and treated as inpatients. Patients with recent rest angina, but who no longer are experiencing chest pain, should be treated with aspirin, oral or topical nitrates, or beta-blockers while further evaluation is undertaken as inpatients.

B. Patients with ongoing angina should be admitted to an ECG-monitored unit. All patients who do not have a contraindication to aspirin therapy should be given an aspirin in the emergency room.

C. **Heparin** should be initiated with initial bolus dose of 80 units/kg, followed by a continuous infusion of 18 units/kg/h, titrated as needed to achieve an activated partial thromboplastin time of 1.5 to 2.5 times the control. Intravenous heparin is usually continued for 3 to 5 days or 48 hours after the last episode of angina.

D. Sublingual nitroglycerin should also be given in the emergency room. If the pain episode is controlled with this therapy, the patient should then be converted to longer-acting oral forms of nitrates with the addition of a beta-blocker if possible. If the pain persists despite sublingual nitrate therapy intravenous nitrates should be started. An initial nitroglycerin infusion rate of 10 to 30 mcg/min is recommended with upward adjustments at intervals of 10 to 30 minutes until the ischemic symptoms disappear. A maximum dose level of 40 mcg/min is advised. The systolic blood pressure should not fall below 90 mm Hg or 30% below the starting mean arterial pressure if significant hypertension is present.

Drugs Commonly Used in Intensive Medical Management of Patients with Unstable Angina

Nitrates

Nitroglycerin 10-30 mcg/min infusion (50 mg in 250-500 mL D5W, 100-200 mcg/mL). Titrate every 3-5 minutes to control symptoms in 5-10 mcg/min steps, up to 200-300 mcg/min; maintain systolic blood pressure >90 mm hg.

Nitroglycerin sublingual, 1-3 tabs SL prn chest pain may also be used.

Antiplatelet Agents

Aspirin should be given upon presentation, 160 mg chewed and swallowed immediately, then take 160-325 mg daily.

Clopidogrel (Plavix), 75 mg qd, or **ticlopidine (Ticlid)**, 250 mg bid ,are alternative if aspirin is contraindicated; may cause neutropenia, skin rash, diarrhea.

Beta-Blockers

Metoprolol (Lopressor), cardioselective beta1-blocker; 1-5 mg doses by slow IV infusion over 1-2 min. q5min to 15 mg total; 100 mg PO bid; reduces the risk of recurrent ischemia or myocardial infarction within 48 hours.

Atenolol (Tenormin), cardioselective beta1-blocker; 5 mg IV q5min to 10 mg total; 50-100 mg PO qd.

Esmolol (Brevibloc). 2 mg/min IV infusion, increase up to 24 mg/min. The dose is increased at 5-minute intervals to achieve a 25% reduction in heart rate. May be immediately withdrawn if bradycardia, heart block, hypotension, bronchospasm, or heart failure occur.

Heparin. 80 U/kg IV bolus, then IV infusion at 18 U/kg/h titrated to a activated partial thromboplastin time (aPTT) 1.5-2.5 times control.

E. Nitrate tolerance is a major concern when continuous administration of any form of nitrate is given. Oral nitrates should be given in an intermittent dosing regimen that allows a drug-free interval. Isosorbide dinitrate appears to be more effective if given as a three-times-daily regimen. An asymmetric dosing regimen of isosorbide mononitrate at 8 AM and 3 PM has also been shown to prevent the development of tolerance. Nitrate patches should be removed for a period of 12 to 14 hours daily to prevent tolerance. Despite the concerns over nitrate tolerance, however, patients with unstable angina should not be given nitrates intermittently until their condition has stabilized because of the potential for rebound symptoms with abrupt discontinuation of therapy. Intravenous nitrates should not be stopped suddenly. Rather, oral or transdermal nitrate preparations should be gradually substituted with intravenous therapy during a period of 24 to 48 hours.

    F. Beta-blockers should be considered as the next line of therapy in those patients with evidence of increased sympathetic tone such as inappropriate tachycardia or hypertension. Beta-blockers are very effective anti-ischemic agents and an intravenous bolus of beta-blockers may result in stabilization of evolving or recurrent ischemic symptoms.

V. Management of stabilized patients

    A. Discontinuation of intravenous therapy
1. **Heparin.** Discontinue heparin after 2-5 days.
2. **Aspirin.** Continue at 160 mg per day.
3. **Convert to oral beta blockers** after the initial intravenous beta blocker:
   a. Metoprolol (Lopressor) 100 mg PO bid **OR**
   b. Propranolol LA (Inderal-LA), 80-120 mg PO qd [60, 80, 120, 160 mg] **OR**
   c. Atenolol (Tenormin) 50-100 mg PO qd.
4. Change to oral nitrate therapy when the patient has been pain-free for 24 hours.
   a. Isosorbide mononitrate (ISMO) 10-20 mg bid, with doses at 8 am and 3 pm **OR** Isosorbide mononitrate sustained release (Imdur) 60-120 mg qd.
   b. Isosorbide dinitrate (Isordil Titradose) 10-40 mg PO bid, with doses of 8 am and 3 pm [5,10,20, 30,40 mg].
   c. Isosorbide sustained release (Isordil Tembids) 80-120 mg qd, or 40-80 mg bid, at 8 am and 3 pm.
   d. Nitroglycerin sublingual, 1-3 tabs SL prn chest pain should also be used.

VI. Indications for cardiac catheterization in stabilized patients

    A. Early conservative strategy. Unless contraindicated, cardiac catheterization is done if one or more of the following high-risk indicators are present: Prior revascularization; congestive heart failure or depressed left ventricular function (ejection fraction <0.50); ventricular arrhythmia; persistent or recurrent pain/ischemia; functional study indicating high risk.

    B. Patients with one or more recurrent, severe, prolonged (>20 minutes) ischemic episodes, should be considered for early cardiac catheterization.

VII. Progression to nonintensive medical therapy

    A. Most patients with unstable angina stabilize and become pain-free with intensive medical management.

    B. Requirements for transfer from intensive to nonintensive medical management
1. Hemodynamically stable (no uncompensated heart failure) for 24 hours or longer.
2. Ischemia has been suppressed for 24 hours or longer.

    C. Twelve-lead ECG. Repeat 24 hours after admission or whenever the patient has recurrent symptoms or a change in clinical status.

    D. Two-dimensional echocardiogram. Resting left ventricular function should be measured in patients who do not have early cardiac catheterization.

    E. Recurrent ischemic episodes should prompt an assessment and ECG. Patients who have pain or ECG evidence of ischemia lasting 20 minutes or longer, which is unresponsive to sublingual nitroglycerin, should be transferred back to the intensive medical management.

VIII. Noninvasive testing

    A. Noninvasive testing is used in recently stabilized patients to estimate prognosis, especially for the next 3-6 months, and to make adjustments in therapy. Noninvasive testing may be considered within 72 hours of presentation in low-risk patients. Noninvasive testing should be delayed until after the patient has been free of angina and congestive heart failure for a minimum of 48 hours.

B. **Choice of noninvasive test**
   1. Selection of stress testing method is based on an evaluation of the patient's resting ECG and ability to perform exercise.
   2. **Exercise treadmill testing** is the standard method of stress testing in male patients with a normal ECG who are not taking digoxin. In women, the stress echocardiogram is superior to exercise ECG for initial diagnostic testing. Exclusions from exercise treadmill testing include S3 gallop, rales, hypertension, chest pain, and an unstable ECG.
   3. **A stress echocardiogram** should be used for patients with an abnormal ECG, including widespread resting ST-segment depression, ST-segment changes secondary to digoxin, left ventricular hypertrophy, left bundle branch block or significant intraventricular conduction deficit.
   4. **Pharmacologic stress testing with an imaging modality** is used if physical limitations prevent exercise. Pharmacologic studies include dipyridamole and dobutamine.

References, see page 268.

Chronic Stable Angina

Chronic stable angina includes patients with prior myocardial infarction, prior revascularization, coronary atherosclerosis, or noninvasive evidence of myocardial ischemia. Typical symptoms include chest pressure, heaviness, and/or pain, with or without radiation of the pain and/or shortness of breath.

I. **Clinical evaluation**
   A. History taking and physical examination are important to confirm the diagnosis, assist in risk stratification, and develop a treatment plan. Important points include the following:
      1. History of previous heart disease
      2. Possible non-atheromatous causes of angina (eg, aortic stenosis)
      3. Symptoms of systemic atherosclerosis
      4. Severity and pattern of symptoms of angina
      5. Risk factors for coronary heart disease include smoking, inappropriate activity level, stress, hyperlipidemia, obesity, hypertension, and diabetes mellitus. Comorbid conditions that could affect myocardial ischemia include hypertension, anemia, thyroid disease, and hypoxemia.
   B. **Physical examination** should include a cardiovascular examination as well as evaluation for evidence of hyperlipidemia, hypertension, peripheral vascular disease, congestive heart failure, anemia, and thyroid disease.
   C. **Laboratory studies** should include an electrocardiogram and a fasting lipid profile. Further studies may include chest films, hemoglobin, and tests for diabetes, thyroid function, and renal function.
   D. **Exercise electrocardiography**
      1. Sensitivity of exercise electrocardiography may be reduced for patients unable to reach the level of exercise required for near maximal effort, such as:
      2. Patients taking beta blockers
      3. Patients in whom fatigue, dyspnea, or claudication symptoms develop
      4. Patients with vascular, orthopedic, or neurologic conditions who cannot perform leg exercises
      5. Reduced specificity may be seen in patients with abnormalities on baseline

electrocardiograms, such as those taking digitalis medications, and in patients with left ventricular hypertrophy or left bundle branch block.

E. Noninvasive imaging, such as myocardial perfusion scintigraphy or stress echocardiography may be indicated in patients unable to complete exercise electrocardiography.

II. Medical therapy

A. Combination Therapy. Monotherapy with a beta blocker or a nitrate is the first choice for patients with stable angina if there are no contraindications. If monotherapy fails to produce improvement, the combination of a beta blocker and a nitrate may relieve symptoms and mitigate ischemia. If combination therapy fails to relieve symptoms, invasive approaches to treatment should be considered.

B. Nitrates

1. Nitrates are potent venodilators and, at higher doses, they are also arterial dilators. Tolerance loss of antianginal effect develops with long-term use of any form of nitrate. It is therefore important to assure a 10- to 12-hour nitrate-free interval.

2. **Immediate-release nitroglycerin**
   a. Nitroglycerin, sublingually or in spray form, is the only agent that is effective for rapid relief of an established angina attack. Patients should carry nitroglycerin tablets or spray at all times and use it as needed.
   b. Nitroglycerin SL (Nitrostat), 0.3-0.6 mg SL q5min prn pain [0.15, 0.3, 0.4, 0.6 mg].
   c. Nitroglycerin oral spray (Nitrolingual) 1-2 sprays prn pain.

3. **Nitroglycerin patches:** Tolerance may be avoided by removing the patch at 2 p.m. for 8 hours each day. Nitroglycerin patch (Transderm-Nitro) 0.6-0.8 mg/h applied for 16 hours each day [0.4, 0.6, 0.8 mg/h patches].
   a. **Isosorbide mononitrate immediate release (ISMO, Monoket),** 10 to 20 mg bid in the morning and again 7 hours later [10, 20 mg].
   b. **Isosorbide dinitrate**
      (1) Isosorbide dinitrate slow-release, (Dilatrate-SR, Isordil Tembids) one tab bid-tid.
      (2) Isosorbide sustained release (Isordil SR) 40-80 mg PO bid in AM and 7 hours later [40 mg].
   c. **Isosorbide mononitrate extended-release (Imdur):** Start with 30 mg, and increase the dose to 120 mg once daily [30, 60,120 mg].
   d. **Adverse effects.** Nitrates are well tolerated. The most common adverse effect is headache (30-60%). Symptomatic postural hypotension or syncope may rarely occur.

C. Beta-adrenergic blockers

1. Beta-adrenergic blockers have been shown to be effective in reducing the frequency of symptomatic and silent episodes of ischemia and the rate of cardiac events in patients with stable ischemia. They exert their actions by blocking beta$_1$ and beta$_2$ receptors on myocardial and smooth muscle cells.

2. Initial titration of the beta-blocker dose should achieve a resting heart rate of 50 to 60 beats per minute. Further modification of the dose to eliminate symptoms is the goal in the treatment of angina. Beta-blocker therapy must be discontinued gradually over five to 10 days to avoid rebound angina or hypertension.

3. Cardioselective formulations, such as acebutolol (Sectral), atenolol (Tenormin), betaxolol (Kerlone) and metoprolol (Lopressor), mainly block beta$_1$ cardiac receptors and are advantageous in patients with reactive airways disease or peripheral vascular disease. All beta blockers, however,

become nonselective at higher dosages. Beta blockers with intrinsic sympathomimetic activity, such as acebutolol and pindolol (Visken), may be useful if sinus bradycardia is a problem.

4. **Non-cardioselective beta-blockers**
   a. **Propranolol sustained-release (Inderal LA)**, 60-160-mg qd [60, 80, 120, 160 mg].
   b. **Nadolol (Corgard)**, 40-80 mg qd [20, 40, 80, 120, 160 mg].
5. **Cardioselective beta-blockers**
   a. **Metoprolol (Lopressor)**, 100 mg bid [25, 50, 100 mg] or metoprolol XL (Toprol XL) 100-200 mg qd [50, 100, 200 mg tab ER].
   b. **Atenolol (Tenormin)**, 100 mg qd [25, 50, 100 mg].
   c. **Bisoprolol (Zebeta)** 5-20 mg qd [5, 10 mg].
6. **Adverse Effects**. Beta blockers are usually well tolerated. Symptomatic bradycardia, hypotension, fatigue, heart failure, dyspnea, cold extremities, and bronchospasm may occur. Impotence, constipation, and vivid dreams may occasionally occur.

D. **Calcium Channel Blockers**
1. The calcium channel blockers block calcium entry into the myocardial muscle cells, causing muscular relaxation and vascular dilatation. Some of the calcium channel blockers also exert an inhibitory effect on the sinus and atrioventricular nodes, causing the heart rate to slow.
2. Caution needs to be exercised when prescribing any negative inotropic agent to patients with impaired left ventricular function. The dihydropyridines have the least effect on contractility and appear to be safer in such situations. Calcium channel blockers should be withdrawn gradually to avoid rebound effects. Calcium channel blockers play an important role in the management of angina in patients with contraindications to beta blockers.
3. **Nifedipine XL (Procardia XL)** 30-120 mg qd [30, 60, 90 mg].
4. **Diltiazem SR (Cardizem SR)** 60-120 mg bid [60, 90, 120 mg].
5. **Diltiazem CD (Cardizem CD)** 120-300 mg qd [120, 180, 240, 300 mg]
6. **Verapamil SR (Calan SR, Isoptin SR)**, 120-240 mg qd [120, 180, 240 mg].

Coexisting Medical or Cardiovascular Conditions That May Influence the Selection of Antianginal Drugs		
Condition	**Use recommended**	**Use with caution or avoid**
Hypertension	Beta blocker, calcium channel blocker	---
Left ventricular impairment or congestive heart failure	Nitrate, beta blocker	Calcium channel blocker
Postmyocardial infarction	Beta blocker without ISA	Nondihydropyridine calcium channel blocker
Hyperlipidemia	--	Beta blocker
Supraventricular or ventricular arrhythmia	Beta blocker, nondihydropyridine calcium channel blocker	--

Condition	Use recommended	Use with caution or avoid
Chronic obstructive pulmonary disease or asthma	--	Beta blocker
Raynaud's phenomenon	--	Beta blocker

E. Aspirin
1. Aspirin inhibits the synthesis of prostaglandins, notably thromboxane A_2, a potent vasoconstrictor and platelet activator. Aspirin improves short- and long-term mortality and reduces the rate of cardiac events, stroke myocardial infarction and unstable angina
2. As a primary preventive measure, aspirin decreases fatal and nonfatal cardiac events. Aspirin, in the absence of contraindications, is recommended as secondary prevention in all patients with heart disease. Aspirin therapy may also play a role in primary prevention in otherwise healthy men with cardiac risk factors. While the most common dosage of aspirin for primary and secondary prevention is 325 mg daily, a dosage as low as 75 mg per day results in a similar reduction in cardiac events and mortality rate, and may be associated with fewer side effects.

F. Lipid-Lowering Therapy. A reduction in elevated serum low-density lipoprotein (LDL) level decreases the risk of fatal and nonfatal cardiac events. A reduction in the LDL cholesterol level to 100 mg per dL in men and women with known coronary artery disease significantly reduces the risk of fatal and nonfatal coronary events.

References, see page 268.

Heart Failure

Congestive heart failure (CHF) is defined as the inability of the heart to meet the metabolic and nutritional demands of the body. Approximately 75% of patients with heart failure are older than 65-70 years of age. Approximately 8% of patients between the ages of 75 and 86 have heart failure.

I. Etiology
   A. The most common causes of CHF are coronary artery disease, hypertension, and alcoholic cardiomyopathy. Valvular diseases such as aortic stenosis and mitral regurgitation, are also very common etiologies.
   B. Coronary artery disease is the etiology of heart failure in two-thirds of patients with left ventricular dysfunction. Heart failure should be presumed to be of ischemic origin until proven otherwise.

II. Clinical presentation
   A. Left heart failure produces dyspnea and fatigue. Right heart failure leads to lower extremity edema, ascites, congestive hepatomegaly, and jugular venous distension. Symptoms of pulmonary congestion include dyspnea, orthopnea, and paroxysmal nocturnal dyspnea. Clinical impairment is caused by left ventricular systolic dysfunction (ejection fraction of less than 40%) in 80-90% of patients with CHF.
   B. Patients should be evaluated for coronary artery disease, hypertension, or

valvular dysfunction. Use of alcohol, chemotherapeutic agents (daunorubicin), negative inotropic agents, and symptoms suggestive of a recent viral syndrome should be assessed. Pulmonary embolism, myocardial infarction (MI), and underlying pulmonary disease should be considered.

C. CHF can present with shortness of breath, dyspnea on exertion, paroxysmal nocturnal dyspnea, orthopnea, nocturia, and cough. Exertional dyspnea is extremely common in patients with heart failure. Atypical symptoms include chronic cough, fatigue, and insomnia. Patients can also present with ascites, right upper quadrant pain (from hepatic congestion), and weakness.

Precipitants of Congestive Heart Failure	
• Myocardial ischemia or infarction • Atrial fibrillation • Worsening valvular disease – mitral regurgitation • Pulmonary embolism • Hypoxia • Severe, uncontrolled hypertension • Thyroid disease	• Pregnancy • Anemia • Infection • Tachycardia or bradycardia • Alcohol abuse • Medication or dietary noncompliance

D. **Physical examination.** Lid lag, goiter, medication use, murmurs, abnormal heart rhythms may suggest a treatable underlying disease. Patients with CHF may present with resting tachycardia, jugular venous distension, a third heart sound, rales, lower extremity edema, or a laterally displaced apical impulse. Poor capillary refill, cool extremities, or an altered level of consciousness may also be present. A third heart sound is one of the most reliable indicators of CHF.

New York Heart Association Criteria for Heart Failure	
Class I	Asymptomatic
Class II	Symptoms with moderate activity
Class III	Symptoms with minimal activity
Class IV	Symptoms at rest

E. **Laboratory assessment.** Every patient with symptoms suggestive of CHF should have a 12-lead ECG and should be placed on a cardiac monitor. A chest x-ray should be performed to identify pleural effusions, pneumothorax, pulmonary edema, or infiltrates. Patients in whom a diagnosis of cardiac ischemia or infarction is suspected should have cardiac enzymes drawn. A complete blood count, electrolytes, and digoxin level, if applicable, also are mandatory. Patients with suspected hyperthyroidism should have thyroid function studies drawn.

F. Echocardiography is recommended to evaluate for the presence of pericardial effusion, tamponade, valvular regurgitation, or wall motion abnormalities.

Laboratory Workup for Suspected Heart Failure	
Blood urea nitrogen	Magnesium
Cardiac enzymes (CK-MB, troponin, or both)	Thyroid-stimulating hormone
	Urinalysis
Complete blood cell count	Echocardiogram
Creatinine	Electrocardiography
Electrolytes	
Liver function tests	

III. Management of chronic heart failure

A. Patients should also be placed on oxygen to maintain adequate oxygen saturation. In patients with severe symptoms (ie, pulmonary edema), other continuous positive airway pressure (CPAP) and endotracheal intubation (ETI) may be employed.

B. Angiotensin-converting enzyme inhibitors significantly reduce morbidity and mortality in CHF. Side effects include cough, worsening renal function, hyperkalemia, hypotension, and the risk of angioedema. ACEIs should be started at a very low dose and titrated up gradually over several weeks to relieve fatigue or shortness of breath. Renal function and electrolytes should be monitored.

ACE Inhibitors used in the treatment of heart failure

Captopril (Capoten) – start 6.25-12.5 mg po tid, usual dose 50-100 mg tid
Enalapril (Vasotec) – start 2.5 mg po qd/bid, usual 2.5-10 mg tid
Lisinopril (Prinivil, Zestril) – start 5 mg po qd, usual 5-20 mg/d
Quinapril (Accupril) – start 5 mg po bid, usual 20-40 mg/d
Fosinopril (Monopril) – start 10 mg po qd, usual 20-40 mg/d
Ramipril (Altace) – start 2.5 mg po bid, usual 10 mg/d

C. Angiotensin II receptor blockers (ARBs). In patients who cannot tolerate or have contraindications to ACE inhibitors, ARBs should be considered. ARBs offer advantages of the ACE inhibitors, but side effects such as cough and angioedema are rare.

D. Diuretics induce peripheral vasodilation, reduce cardiac filling pressures, and prevent fluid retention. Diuretics in severe CHF, the most commonly used agents are loop diuretics, including furosemide (Lasix). Diuretics should be prescribed for patients with heart failure who have volume overload. These agents should be used in conjunction with ACEIs.

Diuretic Therapy in Congestive Heart Failure

Loop diuretics
- Furosemide (Lasix)--20-200 mg daily or bid
- Bumetanide (Bumex)--0.5-4.0 mg daily or bid
- Torsemide (Demadex)--5-100 mg daily

Long-acting thiazide diuretics
- Metolazone (Zaroxolyn) 2.5-10.0 mg qd bid
- Hydrochlorothiazide 25 mg qd

E. Beta-Blockers. Atenolol and propranolol provide a 27% reduction in recurrent MI. Beta-blockers appear to be beneficial in heart failure and may prevent adverse remodeling of the left ventricle, as well as improve survival. Beta-blockers improve survival post-MI. Beta-blockers should not be used in acute pulmonary edema or decompensated heart failure. Beta-blockers should only be initiated in the hemodynamically stable patient. Beta-blockers should be considered add-on or adjunctive therapy in patients already being treated with ACE inhibitors.

Carvedilol, Metoprolol, and Bisoprolol – Dosages and Side Effects

- Carvedilol (Coreg) --start at 3.125 mg bid; target dose 6.25-25 mg bid
- Metoprolol (Lopressor) --start at 12.5 mg bid; target dose 200 mg qd
- Bisoprolol (Zebeta) --start at 1.25 mg qd; target dose 10 mg qd

Caution should be exercised in patients with clinical decompensation. Do not start beta-blocker therapy unless patient is near euvolemic.

F. Digoxin. Digoxin does not demonstrate improved survival rates in CHF (as do ACEIs). Digoxin may be added to a regimen of ACEIs and diuretics if symptoms of heart failure persist. Digoxin can increase exercise tolerance, improve symptoms of CHF, and decrease the risk of hospitalization.

Digoxin Dosing

- Start at 0.250 mg/d with near normal renal function; start at 0.125 mg/d if renal function impaired.
- Toxicity exacerbated by hypokalemia.
- Frequent drug levels.

G. Nonpharmacologic treatments include salt restriction (a diet with 2 g sodium or less), alcohol restriction, water restriction for patients with severe renal impairment, and regular aerobic exercise as tolerated.

H. Inotropic Support
1. Parenterally administered positive inotropic therapy increases cardiac output and decreases symptoms of congestion.
2. Parenteral inotropic agents can be administered continuously to patients admitted to the hospital with exacerbations of heart failure. These agents can be administered in the hospital or continuously at home with an infusion pump.

Inotropic Agents for Cardiogenic Shock

- Dopamine--start at 2-5 mcg/kg/min and titrate upward
- Dobutamine--start at 2-3 mcg/kg/min and titrate upward
- Norepinephrine--start at 2-4 mcg/min and titrate upward

Treatment of Acute Heart Failure/Pulmonary Edema

- Oxygen therapy, 2 L/min by nasal canula
- Lasix 20-80 mg IV (patients already on outpatient dose may require more)
- Nitroglycerine start at 10-20 mcg/min and titrate to BP (use with caution if inferior/right ventricular infarction suspected)
- Sublingual nitroglycerin 0.4 mg
- Captopril: 25 mg SL
- Morphine sulfate 2-4 mg IV. Avoid if inferior wall MI suspected or if hypotensive or presence of tenuous airway

References, see page 268.

Atrial Fibrillation

Atrial fibrillation (AF) is the most common arrhythmia seen in clinical practice. The median age of onset is 75, and the incidence and prevalence increase dramatically with age. For those between the ages of 50-59, the incidence is 0.5%, for patients older than 80 years, the incidence of AF is 9%. The incidence of thromboembolism also increases with age. For patients aged 80-90, nearly one-third of strokes that occur are related to AF.

I. **Pathophysiology.** The cardiac conditions most commonly associated with AF are hypertension, atherosclerotic cardiovascular disease, rheumatic heart disease, mitral valve disease, and cardiomyopathies. Hypertension and coronary artery disease are the most frequent risk factors and accounting for 65% of AF cases. The most common noncardiac conditions associated with AF are pulmonary diseases (including COPD), systemic illnesses, and thyrotoxicosis.

II. **Clinical evaluation**
   A. Patients with AF are often asymptomatic. The arrhythmia may be found during a routine physical examination by either the presence of an irregular pulse or an abnormal electrocardiogram. AF may be associated with palpitations, dizziness, dyspnea, chest pain, syncope, fatigue, or confusion.

Causes of Atrial Fibrillation	
Structural Heart Disease	**Absence of Structural Heart Disease**

Hypertension
Ischemic heart disease
Valvular heart disease
   Rheumatic: mitral stenosis
   Nonrheumatic: aortic stenosis, mitral
   regurgitation
Pericarditis
Cardiac tumors
Sick sinus syndrome
Cardiomyopathies
Congenital heart disease
Wolf-Parkinson-White syndrome
	Pulmonary diseases
	   COPD
	   Pneumonia
	   Pulmonary embolus
	Metabolic disorders
	   Thyrotoxicosis
	   Electrolyte imbalance
	Acute ethanol intoxication
	Methylxanthine derivatives
	   Theophylline
	   Caffeine
	Systemic illness
	   Sepsis
	   Malignancy
	Lone atrial fibrillation

   B. The most common physical sign of AF is an irregular pulse. Other physical exam findings include a pulse deficit, absent "a" wave in the jugular venous pulse, and a variable intensity of the first heart sound.

III. Diagnostic studies

   A. Laboratory studies should include chemistries, CBC, PT/PTT, and a TSH. A chest x-ray may uncover COPD, pneumonia, CHF, or cardiomegaly.

   B. Ambulatory 24-hour (Holter) ECG monitoring can be performed to determine both the frequency and duration of AF.

   C. Echocardiogram provides information on cardiac dimensions, particularly left atrial size, LV systolic function, presence and severity of valvular disease, and the presence of LV hypertrophy.

IV. Initial management

   A. AF is classified as occurring less than 48 hours or more than 48 hours. If the duration of AF is less than 48 hours, the initial goals are either cardioversion or ventricular rate control and observation. If the patient is not hemodynamically compromised and the AF is of new onset, an initial period of observation using both medications for rate control and anticoagulation with heparin are initiated. If AF persists despite rate control, restoration of sinus rhythm is the usual goal if the patient is symptomatic during AF, requires AV synchrony for improved cardiac output, or wants to avoid lifelong anticoagulation. Sinus rhythm can be achieved with either external cardioversion and/or pharmacological agents.

   B. Initial treatment of atrial fibrillation

      1. Anticoagulation in patients with nonvalvular AF reduces the incidence of embolic strokes. Warfarin is more efficacious than aspirin in reducing the incidence of stroke in patients with AF.

      2. Oral anticoagulation therapy with warfarin with a goal of an INR between 2.0-3.0 should be considered in all AF patients with rheumatic heart disease younger than 75 years old.

      3. In patients without rheumatic heart disease who are younger than 75 years of age, warfarin therapy should be initiated if risk factors are present, including previous transient ischemic attack or stroke, hypertension, heart failure, diabetes, clinical coronary artery disease, mitral stenosis, prosthetic heart valves, or thyrotoxicosis. In patients younger than 65 and without these risk factors (lone AF), aspirin alone may be appropriate for stroke prevention. Patients between the ages of 65 and 75 with none of these risk factors could be treated with either warfarin or aspirin. In patients older than 75 with AF, oral anticoagulation with warfarin is recommended. In patients with major contraindications to warfarin (intracranial hemorrhage, unstable gait, falls, syncope, or poor compliance), a daily aspirin is a reasonable alternative.

4. If the duration of AF is unknown or more than 48 hours, then rate control and anticoagulation therapy should be initiated first. The patient should be to evaluated for the presence of an intracardiac thrombus with a transesophageal echocardiography (TEE). If the TEE demonstrates a clot, the patient is anticoagulated for three weeks before a scheduled cardioversion. If no left atrial thrombus is identified by TEE, heparin is started and the patient is cardioverted. Following successful cardioversion, the patient is placed on warfarin for an additional three to four weeks.

C. **Rate control**
1. Patients with AF of greater than one year duration or a left atrial size greater than 50 mm may have difficulty in converting to sinus rhythm. In these patients, rate control rather than conversion to sinus rhythm may be as beneficial in terms of controlling symptoms and optimizing hemodynamics. A controlled ventricular rate in AF is less than 90 bpm at rest. The pharmacological agents primarily used for rate control are digoxin, beta blockers, and calcium channel blockers.

2. **Beta-blockers** slow AV nodal and sinoatrial nodal conduction. The most commonly used beta-blockers are metoprolol and atenolol. For acute rate control, intravenous esmolol is available. Esmolol is a beta-1 selective blocking agent, administered by intravenous infusion.

Agents Used for Heart Rate Control in Atrial Fibrillation

Agent	Loading Dose	Onset of Action	Maintenance Dosage	Major Side Effects
Esmolol (Brevibloc)	0.5 mg per kg IV over one minute	5 minutes	0.05 to 0.2 mg/kg/minute IV	Hypotension, heart block, bradycardia, asthma, heart failure
Metoprolol (Lopressor)	2.5 to 5 mg IV bolus over 2 minutes, up to 3 doses	5 minutes	50 to 200 mg PO every day in divided doses	Hypotension, heart block, bradycardia, asthma, heart failure
Propranolol (Inderal)	0.15 mg per kg	5 minutes	40 to 320 mg PO every day in divided doses	Hypotension, heart block, bradycardia, asthma, heart failure

Diltiazem (Cardizem)	0.25 mg per kg IV over 2 minutes	2 to 7 minutes	10 to 15 mg per hour IV or 120 to 360 mg PO every day in divided doses	Hypotension, heart block, heart failure
Verapamil (Calan, Isoptin)	0.075 to 0.15 mg per kg IV over 2 minutes	3 to 5 minutes	240 to 360 mg PO every day in divided doses	Hypotension, heart block, heart failure
Digoxin (Lanoxin)	0.25 mg IV or PO every 2 hours, up to 1.5 mg	5 to 30 minutes for IV therapy or 30 minutes to 2 hours	0.125 to 0.25 mg every day (oral or IV) for oral therapy	Digitalis toxicity, heart block, bradycardia

3. **Calcium channel blockers** can slow AV node conduction and be used as rate-controlling agents. Calcium channel blockers are the first line for rate control therapy in patients who cannot tolerate beta blockers, such as those with asthma or COPD.
4. **Digoxin** has numerous drug interactions, an unpredictable dose response curve, and a potentially lethal toxicity. Digoxin works by slowing AV node conduction and increasing AV node refractoriness. Its use is limited to patients with systolic dysfunction.
   D. **Antiarrhythmics.** Restoration of sinus rhythm is the optimal goal, as it may relieve symptoms and improve cardiac output.
   1. **Class Ia.** These medications act by blocking the fast sodium channel, reducing the impulse conduction through the myocardium. The class includes quinidine, procainamide, and disopyramide.
      a. **Quinidine** can be used to convert as well as to maintain sinus. Quinidine predisposes to torsade de pointes arrhythmia.

Commonly Used Antiarrhythmics					
Class	Drug	Action	ECG	Dose	Adverse Reaction
Ia	Quinidine	Decrease Na influx Reduce upstroke velocity, Prolong repolarization	QRS widens QT lengthens	Sulfate 300-600 mg po q 6-8 hrs Quinaglute 324-628 mg po q 8-12 hrs	GI, cinchonism VT/VF/Torsade de pointes
	Procainamide			Load: IV 13-17 mcj/kg over 30-60 min Maintenance: IV 2-8 mg/min Procan SR 750-1500 mg po q 6 hr	SLE-like syndrome, confusion

Ic	Flecainide	Reduction in upstroke velocity	QRS widens	Start 50-100 mg po q 12 hr; max. 400 mg/day	Dizziness, headaches
	Propafenone			Start 150 mg po q 8 hrs; max. 300 mg po q 8 hrs	Dry mouth, GI, dizziness
III	Amiodarone	Block K efflux, Prolong Repolarization	QT lengthens	Load 400 mg po tid x 5d, then 400 mg po qd x 1 month; Maintenance: 100-400 mg/day	Ataxia, pulmonary fibrosis, pneumonitis/alveolitis, skin discoloration, thyroid and LFT abnormalities
	Sotalol			80 mg po bid; max. 240 mg po bid	Bradycerdia, torsade de pointes
	Ibutilide			1 mg IV push over 10 min, may repeat once after 10 min	Heart block and heart failure, 3-8% torsade

    b. Procainamide can also be used for both acute conversion and maintenance. It is not as effective as the other Ia agents but can be given intravenously. It can result in life-threatening arrhythmias including torsade de pointes.

    c. Disopyramide has negative inotropic properties. Torsade de pointes can occur. Disopyramide is no longer used in the treatment of AF due to poor efficacy and frequent side effects.

2. Class Ic. This class of medications acts by prolonging intraventricular conduction. The most prescribed members of the class are flecainide and propafenone.

    a. Flecainide can result in acute conversion to sinus rhythm in 75%. Due to its negative inotropic action, flecainide should be used cautiously in patients with AF and hypertrophic cardiomyopathy. It should not be used in patients with structural heart disease. It is reserved for patients with normal LV function and refractory AF.

    b. Propafenone may have fewer side effects and better tolerability than the Ia agents. It is available only in an oral form and can also be given as a single bolus dose for AF of less than 24 hours. Proarrhythmia can occur but is reported less frequently than with the other Ic medications. Propafenone is advocated in patients who are hypertensive and have a structurally normal heart with AF. Propafenone should also be avoided in patients with structural heart disease.

3. Class III. The medications in this class act by blocking outward potassium currents, resulting in increased myocardial refractoriness.

    a. Amiodarone has sodium, calcium, and beta-blocking effects. Amiodarone has a low proarrhythmia profile. It has been shown to be safe and efficacious in patients with AF and CHF. Side effects include: pulmonary fibrosis, pneumonitis, skin discoloration, and thyroid and liver abnormalities.

   b. **Sotalol** has a beta-blocking effect. It is less effective than quinidine. It is most effective for sinus maintenance in patients with AF and coronary artery disease or LV hypertrophy. Sotalol should be avoided in patients with severe LV dysfunction and COPD.

   c. **Ibutilide** is effective for the conversion of recent onset AF. There is an 8.3% incidence of polymorphic ventricular tachycardia.

   d. **Dofetilide** is a class III oral agent. A recent multicenter placebo-controlled trial showed its efficacy in acute conversion of AF.

E. **Nonpharmacologic strategies.** Due to drug intolerance, possible proarrhythmic effects, and disappointing long-term efficacy of the antiarrhythmic agents, nonpharmacological therapies have an important role in the management of AF.

   1. **Electrical cardioversion** has proved to be both rapid and highly effective, with success rates greater than 80%. The success rate is dependent on left atrial size, duration of AF, presence of mitral stenosis, and the patient's age.

   2. **Radiofrequency catheter ablation/atrial defibrillators.** The delivery of radiofrequency current through a catheter tip advanced to the atrium via femoral vein access has been demonstrated to be both highly effective and safe in the treatment of arrhythmias. For AF refractory to drug therapy, AV node ablation with permanent pacemaker implantation can relieve symptoms and improve exercise and performance.

   3. **A surgical technique, the "Maze" procedure,** has also been used for patients who cannot be medically managed. In this method, the right and left atria are divided by multiple surgical incisions. The procedure is effective in 98% of patients with medically refractory AF.

References, see page 268.

Hypertension

High blood pressure is defined as a systolic blood pressure of 140 mm Hg or greater or a diastolic pressure of 90 mm Hg or greater. Hypertension is a major risk factor for coronary artery disease (CAD), heart failure, stroke, and renal failure. Approximately 50 million Americans have hypertension.

I. **Clinical evaluation of the hypertensive patient**

A. Evaluation of hypertension should include an assessment of missed doses of maintenance antihypertensive therapy, use of nonsteroidal anti-inflammatory drugs, decongestants, diet medications, cocaine, or amphetamines.

B. History should assess the presence of coronary heart disease (chest pain), hyperlipidemia, diabetes, or smoking.

C. **Physical examination**. The diagnosis of hypertension requires three separate readings of at least 140/90. The physical exam should search for retina hemorrhages, carotid bruits, left ventricular enlargement, coarctation of the aorta, aortic aneurysm, and absence of a peripheral pulse in an extremity.

Classification of blood pressure for adults		
Category	**Systolic (mm Hg)**	**Diastolic (mm Hg)**
Optimal	<120	<80
Normal	<130	<85
High-normal	130-139	85-89
Hypertension		
Stage 1	140-159	90-99
Stage 2	160-179	100-109
Stage 3	>180	>110

The sixth report of the Joint National Committee on Prevention, Detection, Evaluation, and Treatment of High Blood Pressure.

Target organ damage associated with hypertension

Heart disease
    Left ventricular hypertrophy
    Coronary artery disease, myocardial infarction
    Heart failure
Cerebrovascular disease
    Stroke
    Transient ischemic attack
Peripheral vascular disease
    Aortic aneurysm
    Peripheral occlusive disease
Nephropathy, renal failure
Retinopathy

II. **Initial diagnostic evaluation of hypertension**
   A. **12 lead electrocardiography** may document evidence of ischemic heart disease, rhythm and conduction disturbances, or left ventricular hypertrophy.
   B. **Screening labs** include a complete blood count, glucose, potassium, calcium, creatinine, BUN, and a fasting lipid panel.
   C. **Urinalysis.** Dipstick testing should include glucose, protein, and hemoglobin.
   D. Selected patients may require plasma renin activity, 24 hour urine catecholamines, or renal function testing (glomerular filtration rate and blood flow).

III. **Secondary hypertension**
   A. Only 1-2% of all hypertensive patients will prove to have a secondary cause of hypertension. Age of onset greater than 60 years, age of onset less than 20 in African-American patients, or less than 30 in white patients suggests a secondary cause. Blood pressure that is does not respond to a three-drug regimen or a sudden acceleration of blood pressure suggests secondary hypertension.
   B. **Hypokalemia** (potassium <3.5 mEq/L) suggests primary aldosteronism.

Cushingoid features suggests Cushing's disease. Spells of anxiety, sweating, or headache suggests pheochromocytoma.

C. **Aortic coarctation** is suggested by a femoral pulse delayed later than the radial pulse, or by posterior systolic bruits below the ribs. Renovascular stenosis is suggested by paraumbilical abdominal bruits.

D. **Pyelonephritis** is suggested by persistent urinary tract infections or costovertebral angle tenderness. Renal parenchymal disease is suggested by an increased serum creatinine ≥1.5 mg/dL and proteinuria.

Evaluation of Secondary Hypertension	
Renovascular Hypertension	Captopril test: Plasma renin level before and 1 hr after captopril 25 mg. A greater than 150% increase in renin is positive Captopril renography: Renal scan before and after 25 mg MRI angiography Arteriography (DSA)
Hyperaldosteronism	Serum potassium Serum aldosterone and plasma renin activity CT scan of adrenals
Pheochromocytoma	24 hr urine catecholamines CT scan Nuclear MIBG scan
Cushing's Syndrome	Plasma cortisol Dexamethasone suppression test
Hyperparathyroidism	Serum calcium Serum parathyroid hormone

IV. **Treatment of hypertension**
   A. Treatment should begin with an aggressive lifestyle modification program. Some patients can bring blood pressure down to normal with lifestyle modification alone.

Lifestyle modifications for prevention and management of hypertension
Lose weight if over ideal body weight Limit alcohol intake to no more than 1 oz of ethanol per day Increase aerobic physical activity Reduce sodium intake to no more than 2.4 g sodium per day Maintain adequate intake of dietary potassium, calcium, and magnesium Stop smoking Reduce intake of saturated fat and cholesterol

B. **Diuretics**
   1. Diuretics are recommended as the initial treatment for patients with uncomplicated hypertension. Hydrochlorothiazide is the most widely used diuretic; it is easy to use, effective, and inexpensive.
   2. Most of the blood-pressure-lowering effect of diuretics is achieved at low doses (ie, 12.5 mg of hydrochlorothiazide). Little further benefit accrues at higher doses. A number of drugs combine hydrochlorothiazide with other

agents.

3. Side effects of diuretics include dehydration and orthostatic hypotension, which may lead to falls. Hypokalemia and hypomagnesemia are also possible side effects of diuretics, which can precipitate life-threatening arrhythmias. Gout and leg cramps are common.

Thiazide Diuretics	
Drug	Usual dose
Hydrochlorothiazide (HCTZ, Hydrodiuril)	12.5-50 mg qd
Chlorthalidone (Hygroton)	12.5-25 mg qd
Chlorothiazide (Diuril)	125-500 mg qd
Indapamide (Lozol)	1.25 mg qd
Metolazone (Zaroxolyn)	1.25-5 mg qd

C. Beta-blockers

1. Beta-blockers are effective at reducing the incidence of fatal and nonfatal stroke. The Joint National Committee recommends beta blockers as first-line therapy for treatment of hypertension if no contraindications are evident.

2. These drugs should be the first choice for hypertension in myocardial infarction survivors. Even patients with lung disease tolerate beta blockers well if no active bronchospasm is present.

3. Beta-blockers may provide substantial benefit for patients with systolic heart failure. Carvedilol (Coreg), a nonselective beta blocker with alpha-blocking activity, reduces the risk of death in patients with heart failure.

Beta-blockers		
Drug	Usual dose	Maximum dose
Acebutolol (Sectral)	200-800 mg/d (qd or bid)	1.2 g/d (bid)
Atenolol (Tenormin)	50-100 mg qd	100 mg qd
Betaxolol (Kerlone)	10 mg qd	20 mg qd
Bisoprolol (Zebeta)	5 mg qd	20 mg qd
Carteolol (Cartrol)	2.5 mg qd	10 mg qd
Carvedilol (Coreg)	6.26-25 mg bid	100 mg/d
Labetalol (Normodyne, Trandate)	100-600 mg bid	1200 mg/d
Metoprolol succinate (Toprol XL)	100-200 mg qd	400 mg qd

Drug	Usual dose	Maximum dose
Metoprolol tartrate (Lopressor)	100-200 mg/d (qd or bid)	450 mg/d (qd or bid)
Nadolol (Corgard)	40 mg qd	320 mg/d
Penbutolol sulfate (Levatol)	20 mg qd	NA
Pindolol (Visken)	5 mg bid	60 mg/d
Propranolol (Inderal, Inderal LA)	120-160 mg qd (LA 640 mg/d)	
Timolol (Blocadren)	10-20 mg bid	60 mg/d (bid)

D. **Angiotensinogen-converting enzyme inhibitors**
1. ACE inhibitors are the drugs of choice for treating heart failure. The ACE inhibitor enalapril maleate (Vasotec) improves overall survival and quality of life for patients with severe heart failure. Patients with asymptomatic left ventricular dysfunction also benefit from ACE inhibition.
2. ACE inhibitors are also beneficial after myocardial infarction. Overall mortality and the incidence of fatal and nonfatal myocardial infarction are significantly reduced.
3. Patients with diabetes-induced renal disease may also benefit from treatment with ACE inhibitors because these drugs prevent progression from microalbuminuria to proteinuria and offer protection against deterioration of renal function. Serum potassium levels should be monitored in patients with chronic renal failure treated with ACE inhibitors, and the drugs should be stopped if potassium levels increase to 6 mEq/L.

Angiotensin-converting enzyme inhibitors		
Drug	Usual doses	Maximum dose
Benazepril (Lotensin)	10-40 mg qd or divided bid	80 mg/d
Captopril (Capoten)	50 mg bid-qid	450 mg/d
Enalapril (Vasotec, Vasotec IV)	10-40 mg qd or divided bid	40 mg/d
Fosinopril (Monopril)	20-40 mg qd or divided bid	80 mg/d
Lisinopril (Prinivil, Zestril)	20-40 mg qd	40 mg/d
Moexipril (Univasc)	15-30 mg qd	30 mg/d
Quinapril (Accupril)	20-80 mg qd or divided bid	80 mg/d
Ramipril (Altace)	5-20 mg qd or divided bid	20 mg/d
Trandolapril (Mavik)	1-4 mg qd	8 mg/d

E. Angiotensin II receptor blockers

1. These antihypertensive agents block the action of angiotensin II. They effectively lower blood pressure and bring about the same hemodynamic changes that occur with ACE inhibitors. Patients are less likely to have the dry cough that sometimes occurs with use of ACE inhibitors.

2. The angiotensin II receptor blockers used for treatment of hypertension are losartan (Cozaar), valsartan (Diovan), irbesartan (Avapro), and candesartan (Atacand). Angiotensin II receptor blockers are often substituted for ACE inhibitors in patients who experience chronic cough.

Angiotensin II Receptor Blockers		
Drug	**Usual dose**	**Maximum dose**
Candesartan (Atacand)	4-8 mg qd	16 mg/d
Irbesartan (Avapro)	150-300 mg qd	300 mg/d
Losartan (Cozaar)	50 mg qd	100 mg/d
Telmisartan (Micardis)	40-80 mg qd	80 mg/d
Valsartan (Diovan)	80 mg qd	320 mg/d

F. Calcium channel blockers

1. Calcium channel blockers are very effective antianginal agents and are often used in combination with beta blockers and nitrates for treatment of ischemic heart disease. The dihydropyridine calcium channel blockers are often used in difficult cases.

2. The first-generation calcium channel blockers are all negative inotropic drugs and can worsen heart failure. New long-acting calcium channel blockers are safer to use in patients with left ventricular dysfunction.

3. **Alpha blockers,** such as terazosin (Hytrin) and doxazosin mesylate (Cardura), are often used to alleviate symptoms associated with prostatic hypertrophy and are also effective in lowering blood pressure. A major side effect is orthostatic hypotension.

Alpha-1-blockers		
Drug	**Initial dose**	**Maximum dose**
Terazosin (Hytrin)	1 mg qhs; titrate slow Usual: 1-5 mg qhs	20 mg/d
Doxazosin (Cardura)	1 mg qd; titrate slowly every 2 weeks	16 mg/d

Combination Agents for Hypertension

Drug	Initial dose	Comments
Beta-Blocker/Diuretic		
Atenolol/chlorthalidone (Tenoretic)	50 mg/25 mg, 1 tab qd	Additive vasodilation
Bisoprolol/HCTZ (Ziac)	2.5 mg/6.25 mg, 1 tab qd	
Metoprolol/HCTZ (Lopressor HCTZ)	100 mg/25 mg, 1 tab qd	
Nadolol/HCTZ (Corzide)	40 mg/5 mg, 1 tab qd	
Propranolol/HCTZ (Inderide LA)	80 mg/50 mg, 1 tab qd	
Timolol/HCTZ (Timolide)	10 mg/25 mg, 1 tab qd	
ACE inhibitor/Diuretic		
Benazepril/HCTZ (Lotensin HCT)	5 mg/6.25 mg, 1 tab qd	ACE inhibitor conserves potassium and magnesium; combination beneficial for CHF patients with HTN
Captopril/HCTZ (Capozide)	25 mg/15 mg, 1 tab qd	
Enalapril/HCTZ (Vaseretic)	5 mg/12.5 mg, 1 tab qd	
Lisinopril/HCTZ (Zestoretic, Prinzide)	10 mg/12.5 mg, 1 tab qd	
Moexipril/HCTZ (Uniretic)	7.5 mg/12.5 mg, 1 tab qd	
ACE inhibitor/Calcium-channel blocker		
Benazepril/amlodipine (Lotrel)	2.5 mg/10 mg, 1 tab qd	
Enalapril/felodipine (Lexxel)	5 mg/5 mg, 1 tab qd	
Enalapril/diltiazem (Teczem)	5 mg/180 mg, 1 tab qd	
Trandolapril/verapamil (Tarka)	2 mg/180 mg, 1 tab qd	
Angiotensin II receptor blocker/Diuretic		
Losartan/HCTZ (Hyzaar)	50 mg/12.5 mg, 1 tab qd	
Valsartan/HCTZ (Diovan HCT)	80 mg/12.5 mg, 1 tab qd	
Alpha-1-Blocker/Diuretic		
Prazosin/polythiazide (Minizide)	1 mg/0.5 mg, 1 cap bid	Synergistic vasodilation

Drug	Initial dose	Comments
K⁺-sparing diuretic/Thiazide		
Amiloride/HCTZ (Moduretic)	5 mg/50 mg, 1 tab qd	Electrolyte-sparing effect
Triamterene/HCTZ (Dyazide, Maxzide)	37.5 mg/25 mg, ½ tab qd	

Consideration of Concomitant Conditions in the Treatment of Hypertension	
Compelling indications	
Heart failure	ACE inhibitor, diuretic
Isolated systolic hypertension	Diuretic (first choice), long-acting calcium-channel blocker (second choice)
Post acute myocardial infarction	β-blocker (non-ISA); ACE inhibitor (in systolic dysfunction)
Type 1 diabetes mellitus	ACE inhibitor
Likely to be beneficial to patients with comorbidity	
Angina	β-blocker, calcium-channel blocker
Atrial fibrillation	β-blocker, calcium-channel blocker
Benign prostatic hyperplasia	α₁-blocker
Heart failure	Carvedilol, angiotensin II receptor blocker
Diabetes mellitus	ACE inhibitor (first choice); calcium-channel blocker

References, see page 268.

Hypertensive Emergency

Hypertensive crises are severe elevations in blood pressure (BP) characterized by a diastolic blood pressure (BP) is usually higher than 120-130 mmHg.

I. Clinical evaluation of hypertensive crises
  A. Hypertensive emergency is defined by a diastolic blood pressure >120 mmHg associated with ongoing vascular damage. Symptoms or signs of neurologic, cardiac, renal, or retinal dysfunction are present. Hypertensive emergencies include severe hypertension in the following settings:
  1. Aortic dissection
  2. Acute left ventricular failure and pulmonary edema
  3. Acute renal failure or worsening of chronic renal failure
  4. Hypertensive encephalopathy
  5. Focal neurologic damage indicating thrombotic or hemorrhagic stroke
  6. Pheochromocytoma, cocaine overdose, or other hyperadrenergic states

7. Unstable angina or myocardial infarction
8. Eclampsia

B. **Hypertensive urgency** is defined as diastolic blood pressure >120 mmHg without evidence of vascular damage; the disorder is asymptomatic and no retinal lesions are present.

C. **Causes of secondary hypertension** include renovascular hypertension, pheochromocytoma, cocaine use, withdrawal from alpha-2 stimulants, clonidine, beta blockers or alcohol, and noncompliance with antihypertensive medications.

II. Initial assessment of severe hypertension

A. When severe hypertension is noted, the measurement should be repeated in both arms to detect any significant differences.

B. Peripheral pulses should be assessed for absence or delay, which suggests a dissecting aortic aneurysm. Evidence of pulmonary edema should be sought.

C. Target organ damage is suggested by chest pain, neurologic signs, altered mental status, profound headache, dyspnea, abdominal pain, hematuria, focal neurologic signs (paralysis or paresthesia), or hypertensive retinopathy.

D. Prescription drug use should be assessed, including missed doses of antihypertensives. History of recent cocaine or amphetamine use should be sought.

E. If focal neurologic signs are present, a CT scan may be required to differentiate hypertensive encephalopathy from a stroke syndrome. In stroke syndromes, hypertension may be secondary to the neurologic event; the neurologic deficits are fixed and follow a predictable neuroanatomic pattern. By contrast, in hypertensive encephalopathy, the neurologic signs follow no anatomic pattern, and there is diffuse alteration in mental function.

III. Laboratory evaluation

A. Complete blood cell count, urinalysis for protein, glucose, and blood; urine sediment examination; chemistry panel (SMA-18).

B. If chest pain is present, cardiac enzymes are obtained.

C. If the history suggests a hyperadrenergic state, the possibility of a pheochromocytoma should be excluded with a 24-hour urine for catecholamines. A urine drug screen may be necessary to exclude illicit drug use.

D. Electrocardiogram should be completed.

E. Suspected primary aldosteronism can be excluded with a 24 hour urine potassium and an assessment of plasma renin activity. Renal artery stenosis can be excluded with captopril renography and intravenous pyelography.

Screening Tests for Secondary Hypertension	
Renovascular Hypertension	Captopril renography: Renal scan before and after 25 mg PO Intravenous pyelography MRI angiography
Hyperaldosteronism	Serum potassium 24-hr urine potassium Plasma renin activity CT scan of adrenals
Pheochromocytoma	24-hr urine catecholamines CT scan Nuclear MIBG scan

Cushing's Syndrome	Plasma ACTH Dexamethasone suppression test
Hyperparathyroidism	Serum calcium Serum parathyroid hormone

IV. Management of hypertensive emergencies

A. The patient should be hospitalized for intravenous access, continuous intra-arterial blood pressure monitoring, and electrocardiographic monitoring. Volume status and urinary output should be monitored.

B. Rapid, uncontrolled reductions in blood pressure should be avoided because coma, stroke, myocardial infarction, acute renal failure, or death may result.

C. The goal of initial therapy is to terminate ongoing target organ damage. The mean arterial pressure should be lowered not more than 20-25%, or to a diastolic blood pressure of 100 mmHg over 15 to 30 minutes.

V. Parenteral antihypertensive agents

A. Nitroprusside (Nipride)

1. Nitroprusside is the drug of choice in almost all hypertensive emergencies (except myocardial ischemia or renal impairment). It dilates both arteries and veins, and it reduces afterload and preload.

2. Onset of action is nearly instantaneous, and the effects disappear 1-10 minutes after discontinuation.

3. The starting dosage is 0.25-1.0 mcg/kg/min by continuous infusion with a range of 0.25-8.0 mcg/kg/min. Titrate dose to gradually reduce blood pressure over minutes to hours.

4. When treatment is prolonged or when renal insufficiency is present, the risk of cyanide and thiocyanate toxicity is increased. Signs of thiocyanate toxicity include anorexia, disorientation, fatigue, hallucinations, nausea, toxic psychosis, and seizures. Clinical deterioration with cyanosis, metabolic acidosis and arrhythmias indicates cyanide toxicity.

B. Nitroglycerin

1. Nitroglycerin is the drug of choice for hypertensive emergencies with coronary ischemia. It should not be used with hypertensive encephalopathy because it increases intracranial pressure.

2. Nitroglycerin increases venous capacitance, decreases venous return and left ventricular filling pressure. It has a rapid onset of action of 2-5 minutes. Tolerance may occur within 24-48 hours.

3. The starting dose is 15 mcg IV bolus, then 5-10 mcg/min (50 mg in 250 mL D5W). Titrate by increasing the dose at 3-5-minute intervals up to max 1.0 mcg/kg/min.

C. Labetalol IV (Normodyne)

1. Labetalol is a good choice if BP elevation is associated with hyperadrenergic activity, aortic dissection, or postoperative hypertension. It is also an excellent choice for patients with aortic or abdominal aneurysm.

2. It is administered as 20 mg slow IV over 2 min. Additional doses of 20-80 mg may be administered q5-10min, then q3-4h prn or 0.5-2.0 mg/min IV infusion.

3. Labetalol is contraindicated in obstructive pulmonary disease, decompensated CHF, or heart block greater than first degree.

D. Enalaprilat IV (Vasotec)

1. Enalaprilat is an ACE-inhibitor with a rapid onset of action (15 min) and long duration of action (11 hours). It is ideal for patients with heart failure or accelerated-malignant hypertension.

  2. Initial dose 1.25 mg IVP (over 2-5 min) q6h, then increase up to 5 mg q6h. Reduce dose in azotemic patients. Contraindicated in renal artery stenosis.
  E. **Phentolamine (Regitine)** is an intravenous alpha-adrenergic antagonist used in excess catecholamine states, such as pheochromocytomas, rebound hypertension due to withdrawal of clonidine, and drug ingestions. The dose is 2-5 mg IV every 5 to 10 minutes.
  F. **Trimethaphan (Arfonad)** is a ganglionic-blocking agent that blocks both adrenergic and cholinergic ganglia. It is useful in dissecting aortic aneurysm when beta blockers are contraindicated; however, it is rarely used. The dose is 0.3-3 mg/min IV infusion.

References, see page 268.

Syncope

Syncope is defined as a sudden, transient loss of consciousness characterized by unresponsiveness and loss of postural tone. The prognosis for most persons with syncopal episodes is good; however, persons with syncope caused by a cardiac disorder have a one-year mortality rate of 20-30%. Hospitalization is generally not necessary, unless a cardiac etiology or a significant injury during the syncopal event is suspected.

I. **Pathophysiology**
  A. Vasovagal attacks, cardiac disorders and pulmonary outflow obstruction produce syncope because of a reduction of cerebral blood flow. Hypoxia, hyperventilation and hypoglycemia, increased intracranial pressure, seizures and hysteria can cause syncope.
  B. Cardiac syncope is caused by inadequate output from the left ventricle. Mechanical causes of cardiac syncope include aortic stenosis, hypertrophic cardiomyopathy, myocardial infarction and pulmonary embolus. Tachyarrhythmias, especially ventricular tachycardia, account for most of the arrhythmias that result in cardiac syncope. Syncope of cardiac origin results in markedly increased rates of mortality and sudden death. The cause of syncope can not be determined in 38-47% of patients.
II. **Clinical evaluation**
  A. The history and physical examination can identify potential causes of syncope in 50-85% of cases in which a successful diagnosis is made. A young, healthy patient with a history compatible with vasovagal syncope probably needs no further diagnostic testing.
  B. A complete description of the syncopal episode, prodromal circumstances and symptoms following the syncopal episode should be obtained. The relationship of fainting to micturition, defecation, cough, swallowing or postural change may reveal a cause.
  C. Vasovagal syncope is usually preceded by nausea, diaphoresis, pallor and light-headedness, commonly occurring after a stressful or frightful situation.
  D. Syncope that has an abrupt onset, without warning, suggests a cardiac arrhythmia, especially in a person known to have cardiac disease.
  E. Syncope that occurs with exertion is indicative of aortic stenosis, hypertrophic cardiomyopathy, left ventricular dysfunction, or a cardiac arrhythmia.
  F. Activities that involve stretching the neck, such as shaving or looking back over one's shoulder, can cause carotid sinus syncope. The relationship of syncope

to meals or alcohol or drug ingestion should be determined.
G. Rapid return to alertness usually follows a syncopal episode; however, a period of postictal confusion usually follows a seizure (Todd's paralysis). Prodromal auras and fecal and urinary incontinence are suggestive of a seizure.

Medications Associated with Syncope

Antihypertensives/anti-anginals
    Adrenergic antagonists
    Calcium channel blockers
    Diuretics
    Nitrates
    Vasodilators
Antidepressants
    Tricyclic antidepressants
    Phenothiazines

Antiarrhythmics
    Digoxin
    Quinidine
Insulin
Drugs of abuse
    Alcohol
    Cocaine
    Marijuana

Differential Diagnosis of Syncope

Non-cardiovascular	Cardiovascular

Metabolic
   Hyperventilation
   Hypoglycemia
   Hypoxia
Neurologic
   Cerebrovascular insufficiency
   Normal pressure hydrocephalus
   Seizure
   Subclavian steal syndrome
   Increased intracranial pressure
Psychiatric
   Hysteria
   Major depression
	Reflex syncope (heart structurally normal)
	   Vasovagal
	   Situational
	   Cough
	   Defecation
	   Micturition
	   Postprandial
	   Sneeze
	   Swallow
	   Carotid sinus syncope
	Orthostatic hypotension
	Drug-induced
	Cardiac
	   Obstructive
	   Aortic dissection
	   Aortic stenosis
	   Cardiac tamponade
	   Hypertrophic cardiomyopathy
	   Left ventricular dysfunction
	   Myocardial infarction
	   Myxoma
	   Pulmonary embolism
	   Pulmonary hypertension
	   Pulmonary stenosis
	   Arrhythmias
	      Bradyarrhythmias
	         Sick sinus syndrome
	         Pacemaker failure
	      Supraventricular and ventricular
	         tachyarrhythmias

Clues to the Etiology of Syncope	
Associated Feature	**Etiology**
Cough Micturition Defecation Swallowing	Situational syncope
Post-syncopal disorientation Urinary or fecal incontinence	Seizure
Syncope with arm exercise	Subclavian steal syndrome
Syncope with shaving	Carotid sinus syncope
Prodromal symptoms (nausea, diaphoresis)	Vasovagal syncope
Abrupt onset	Cardiac syncope
Syncope with exertion	Aortic stenosis, hypertrophic cardiomyopathy, arrhythmias
Syncope with change of position	Orthostatic hypotension
Blood pressure/pulse differential	Aortic dissection, subclavian steal syndrome
Abnormal postural vital signs	Orthostatic hypotension
Cardiac murmurs/rhythms	Aortic stenosis, hypertrophic cardiomyopathy, arrhythmias, pulmonary hypertension
Carotid bruit	Cerebrovascular insufficiency

III. **Physical examination**
   A. **Orthostatic blood pressure and pulse measurements**, taken with the patient standing for two minutes after a supine period of at least five minutes, can be used to detect orthostatic hypotension.
   B. **A difference in pulse intensity or blood pressure** of more than 20 mm Hg between the two arms may indicate aortic dissection or subclavian steal syndrome.
   C. **Carotid or subclavian bruits** can be indicators of vascular disease.
   D. **Cardiac examination** may reveal aortic stenosis, idiopathic hypertrophic subaortic stenosis, mitral valve prolapse, or pulmonary hypertension.
   E. **Carotid sinus pressure** can be applied during electrocardiographic monitoring to assess potential vascular flow abnormalities. Because ventricular fibrillation and prolonged asystole are potential complications, intravenous access should be established before carotid massage is performed. Severe cerebrovascular disease is a relative contraindication to carotid massage.
   F. **Neurologic examination** should then be performed to exclude focal deficits, and stool should be tested for occult blood.
IV. **Laboratory tests**
   A. **Blood tests** may be helpful in confirming anemia, hypoglycemia, hypoxia, electrolyte abnormality or renal failure. An associated seizure disorder may explain a low bicarbonate level obtained soon after a syncopal event. Cardiac

enzyme determinations can be of value if myocardial infarction is suspected.
B. **Computed tomographic (CT) scans** of the head are unlikely to reveal useful information unless focal neurologic findings or a head injury are present.
C. **Electroencephalogram (EEG)** should be obtained if a seizure disorder is suspected.
D. **Noninvasive cardiac evaluation**
   1. **Electrocardiography** is the most useful test when a cardiac source of syncope is suspected. The likelihood is low that arrhythmias are a cause of syncope in persons with a normal ECG.
   2. **Echocardiography** may be valuable in the evaluation of patients with suspected structural heart disease.
   3. **Ambulatory electrocardiographic monitoring** frequently shows arrhythmia. Only 2 percent of patients developed arrhythmia-related symptoms during monitoring.
E. **Electrophysiologic studies** are sometimes helpful in the evaluation of patients with syncope. Use in the evaluation of patients with syncope should be limited to patients with significant structural heart disease and recurrent syncope.
F. **Tilt table test** can be used in the evaluation of recurrent syncope. The table is tilted in an effort to induce a vasovagal-like reaction.

References, see page 268.

Dyslipidemia

Dyslipidemias are characterized by elevation of the serum total cholesterol, low-density lipoprotein (LDL) cholesterol and triglycerides, and a decrease in the high-density lipoprotein (HDL) cholesterol. Elevated serum cholesterol levels are associated with coronary heart disease, and cholesterol reduction results in coronary artery plaque regression.

I. **Diagnosis and classification**
A. Secondary causes of dyslipidemia include hypothyroidism and autosomal dominant familial hypercholesterolemia. Triglyceride elevation may occur in association with diabetes mellitus, alcoholism, obesity and hypothyroidism.
B. The National Cholesterol Education Program (NCEP) guidelines are based on clinical cut points that indicate relative risk for coronary heart disease. Total cholesterol and HDL cholesterol levels should be measured every five years beginning at age 20 in patients who do not have coronary heart disease or other atherosclerotic disease. Both of these measurements may be obtained in the nonfasting state. The results of these measurements and the presence of other risk factors for coronary heart disease may demand a lipoprotein analysis.

Coronary Heart Disease Risk Based on Risk Factors Other Than the LDL Level

Positive risk factors
  Male ≥45 years
  Female ≥55 years or postmenopausal without estrogen replacement therapy
  Family history of premature coronary heart disease (definite myocardial infarction or sudden death before age 55 in father or other male first-degree relative or before age 65 in mother or other female first-degree relative)
  Current cigarette smoking
  Hypertension (blood pressure ≥140/90 mm Hg or patient is receiving antihypertensive drug therapy)
  HDL cholesterol level <35 mg/dL
  Diabetes mellitus
Negative risk factor*
  High HDL cholesterol level

*--Subtract one positive risk factor if negative risk factor is present.
The LDL cholesterol level can be calculated (mg/dL)=total cholesterol - HDL - (triglyceride/5)

II. Management

A. **The target LDL cholesterol in patients with coronary heart disease** or other atherosclerotic disease is 100 mg/dL or lower. If the LDL level does not exceed 100 mg/dL in a patient with coronary heart disease, the patient should begin the step I diet, regularly participate in physical activity and stop smoking. Annual lipoprotein analysis is indicated for this group. Premenopausal women and men 35 years of age or younger with dyslipidemia, but without other risk factors for coronary heart disease or a genetic predisposition, are considered at low risk.

B. The NCEP guidelines recommend that patients at higher risk of coronary heart disease receive more intensive interventions for dyslipidemia than patients at lower risk. Persons at highest risk for future coronary events have a history of coronary heart disease or extracoronary atherosclerotic disease.

Risk Classification of Hypercholesterolemia in Patients Without Coronary Heart Disease

Classification	Total cholesterol level	LDL cholesterol level	HDL cholesterol level
Desirable	200 mg/dL	<130 mg/dL	≥60 mg/dL
Borderline high risk	200 to 239 mg/dL	130 to 159 mg/dL	35 to 59 mg/dL
High risk	≥240 mg/dL	≥160 mg/dL	<35 mg/dL

III. Lifestyle modifications

A. The NCEP guidelines recommend dietary modification, exercise and weight control as the foundation of treatment of dyslipidemia. These interventions may provide sufficient treatment for up to 90 percent of persons with dyslipidemia.

B. **Exercise and weight reduction** lowers total cholesterol and its LDL and VLDL fractions, lowers triglycerides and raises HDL cholesterol. Most patients benefit from aerobic exercise, performed for 30 minutes four or more times a week.

C. Step I and step II diets

1. Dietary therapy should be initiated in patients who have borderline-high LDL cholesterol levels (130 to 159 mg/dL) and two or more risk factors for coronary heart disease and in patients who have LDL levels of 160 mg/dL or greater. The objective of dietary therapy in primary prevention is to decrease the LDL cholesterol level to 160 mg/dL if only one risk factor for coronary heart disease is present and to less than 130 mg/dL if two or more risk factors are identified. In the presence of documented coronary heart disease, dietary therapy is indicated in patients who have LDL values exceeding 100 mg/dL, with the aim of lowering the LDL level to 100 mg/dL or less.

2. **Step I diets** limit calories derived from saturated fats to 8 to 10 percent of total calories and cholesterol to less than 300 mg/day.

3. **Step II diets** further restrict calories from saturated fats to less than 7 percent of total calories and restrict cholesterol to less than 200 mg/day.

4. In primary prevention of coronary heart disease (without evidence of coronary heart disease), dietary therapy should be maintained for six months before drug therapy is initiated. In patients with coronary heart disease and an LDL cholesterol value above 100 mg/dL, therapy should begin with the step II diet.

IV. Drug therapy

A. Because dietary modification rarely reduces LDL cholesterol levels by more than 10 to 20 percent, consideration be given to the use of cholesterol-lowering agents if lipid levels remain elevated after six months of intensive dietary therapy.

B. **A patient with a very high LDL cholesterol level** may need to start drug therapy sooner, because it is unlikely that a patient with an LDL level of 130 mg/dL or greater will be able to achieve the goal of 100 mg/dL with diet alone.

C. **HMG-CoA reductase inhibitors** are the drugs of choice for most patients with hypercholesterolemia because they reduce LDL cholesterol most effectively. Gemfibrozil (Lopid) or nicotinic acid may be better choices in patients with significant hypertriglyceridemia.

Cholesterol-Lowering Agents, Their Dosages and Cost	
Agent	**Maintenance dosage**
HMG-CoA reductase inhibitors (statins)	
Atorvastatin (Lipitor)	10 mg, 20 mg, 40 mg, or 80 mg/day anytime [10, 20, 40 mg]
Cerivastatin (Baycol)	0.3 mg in the evening
Fluvastatin (Lescol)	20 mg or 40 mg at bedtime, or 20 mg twice daily
Lovastatin (Mevacor)	20 mg, 40 mg or 80 mg with evening meal
Pravastatin (Pravachol)	10 mg, 20 mg or 40 mg at bedtime
Simvastatin (Zocor)	5 mg, 10 mg, 20 mg or 40 mg at bedtime
Bile acid—binding resins	
Cholestyramine (Questran, Questran Lite)	4 g, 8 g , 12 g or 16 g twice daily
Colestipol (Colestid)	5 g twice daily or 30 g/day, in divided doses
Fibric acid analogs	
Clofibrate (Atromid-5)	500 mg four times daily
Gemfibrozil (Lopid)	600 mg twice daily

Agent	Maintenance dosage
Nicotinic acid	1.5 to 6 g daily in divided doses

Changes in Serum Lipid Values with Different Classes of Cholesterol-Lowering Drugs and Some of Their Side Effects

Drug class	Total cholesterol levels	LDL levels	HDL levels	Triglycerides	Side effects
HMG-CoA reductase inhibitors	↓ 15% to 30%	↓ 20% to 60%	↑ 5% to 15%	↓ 10% to 40%	Myositis, myalgia, elevated hepatic transaminases
Bile acid-binding resins	↓ 20%	↓ 10% to 20%	↑ 3% to 5%	Neutral or ↑	Unpalatability, bloating, constipation, heartburn
Nicotinic acid	↓ 25%	↓ 10% to 25%	↑ 15% to 35%	↓ 20% to 50%	Flushing, nausea, glucose intolerance, abnormal liver function test
Fibric acid analogs	↓ 15%	↓ 5% to 15%	↑ 14% to 20%	↓ 20% to 50%	Nausea, skin rash

D. HMG-CoA reductase inhibitors

1. Lovastatin (Mevacor), pravastatin (Pravachol), simvastatin (Zocor), fluvastatin (Lescol), atorvastatin (Lipitor) and cerivastatin (Baycol) are HMG-CoA reductase inhibitors, or statins, that inhibit cholesterol synthesis. These agents lower total cholesterol, LDL cholesterol and triglycerides and slightly raise the HDL fraction. While these agents are generally well tolerated; 1% may develop elevated hepatic transaminase levels. Other adverse effects include myopathy (0.1%) and gastrointestinal complaints. Statins should generally be taken in a single dose with the evening meal or at bedtime.
2. **Atorvastatin (Lipitor)** may exert a greater effect on lowering LDL cholesterol, total cholesterol and triglycerides.

E. Bile acid-binding resins

1. The anion exchange resins cholestyramine (Questran) and colestipol (Colestid) bind cholesterol-containing bile acids in the intestines. These agents decrease LDL cholesterol levels by up to 20 percent. They may be a good choice in patients with hepatic disease because they do not affect hepatic metabolism. They are also a good choice in very young patients and women of childbearing age.
2. Bile acid-binding resins may cause an increase in triglyceride levels. Side effects include constipation, abdominal discomfort, flatulence, nausea, bloating and heartburn.
3. Bile acid sequestrants can bind with warfarin, digitalis, thyroxine, thiazides, furosemide, tetracycline, penicillin G, phenobarbital, iron, propranolol, acetaminophen, nonsteroidal anti-inflammatory agents, oral phosphate, and hydrocortisone.

F. Nicotinic acid

1. Nicotinic acid, or niacin, decreases the synthesis of LDL cholesterol. This agent increases the HDL level by 15 to 35 percent, reduces total and LDL cholesterol levels by 10 to 25 percent, and decreases the triglyceride level by 20 to 50 percent.

2. Side effects of nicotinic acid include flushing, pruritus, gastrointestinal discomfort, hyperuricemia, gout, elevated liver function tests and glucose intolerance. Taking 325 mg of aspirin 30 minutes before the drug may minimize flushing. It should be avoided in diabetes because it tends to worsen glycemic control.

G. Fibric acid derivatives

1. Fibric acid derivatives, or fibrates, increase the clearance of VLDL cholesterol by enhancing lipolysis and reducing hepatic cholesterol synthesis. These agents lower triglyceride levels by 20 to 50 percent, raise HDL levels by up to 20 percent, and reduce LDL levels by 5 to 15 percent. Gemfibrozil (Lopid) is useful in patients with diabetes and familial dysbetalipoproteinemia.

2. Side effects of gemfibrozil include nausea, bloating, flatulence, abdominal distress and mild liver-function abnormalities. Myositis, gallstones and elevation of the LDL cholesterol level have also been reported. Fibrates should generally not be used with HMG-CoA reductase inhibitors because of the risk of severe myopathy.

H. Multiple drug therapy.
The NCEP guidelines define a target LDL cholesterol level of 100 mg/dL as a goal for high-risk patients with established coronary heart disease.

Combination Therapies If Single-Agent Therapy Is Not Effective in Reducing Lipid Levels	
Lipid levels	**First drug → drug to add**
Elevated LDL level and triglyceride level <200 mg/dL	Statin → bile acid-binding resin Nicotinic acid* → statin* Bile acid-binding resin → nicotinic acid
Elevated LDL level and triglyceride level 200 to 400 mg/dL	Statin* → nicotinic acid* Statin* → gemfibrozil (Lopid)††

LDL=low-density lipoprotein.
*--Possible increased risk of myopathy and hepatitis.
††--Increased risk of severe myopathy.

I. Estrogen replacement therapy.
The NCEP recommends that consideration be given to estrogen replacement therapy as a means of decreasing (by about 15 percent) LDL cholesterol levels and increasing HDL cholesterol levels in postmenopausal women.

References, see page 268.

Pulmonary Disorders

Asthma

Asthma is the most common chronic disease among children. Asthma triggers include viral infections; environmental pollutants, such as tobacco smoke; certain medications, (aspirin, nonsteroidal anti-inflammatory drugs), and sustained exercise, particularly in cold environments.

I. **Diagnosis**
   A. **History**
      1. Symptoms of asthma may include episodic complaints of breathing difficulties, seasonal or nighttime cough, prolonged shortness of breath after a respiratory infection, or difficulty sustaining exercise.
      2. Wheezing does not always represent asthma. Wheezing may persist for weeks after an acute bronchitis episode. Patients with chronic obstructive pulmonary disease may have a reversible component superimposed on their fixed obstruction. Etiologic clues include a personal history of allergic disease, such as rhinitis or atopic dermatitis, and a family history of allergic disease.
      3. The frequency of daytime and nighttime symptoms, duration of exacerbations and asthma triggers should be assessed.
   B. **Physical examination.** Hyperventilation, use of accessory muscles of respiration, audible wheezing, and a prolonged expiratory phase are common. Increased nasal secretions or congestion, polyps, and eczema may be present.
   C. **Measurement of lung function.** An increase in the forced expiratory volume in one second (FEV_1) of 12 percent after treatment with an inhaled beta$_2$ agonist is sufficient to make the diagnosis of asthma. A similar change in peak expiratory flow rate (PEFR) measured on a peak flow meter is also diagnostic.

Asthma Classification			
Symptoms			
Classification	**Daytime**	**Nighttime**	**Lung function**
Mild intermittent	Symptoms occur up to 2 times/week; exacerbations are brief (hours to days), with normal PEFR and no symptoms between exacerbations	Symptoms occur up to 2 times/month	PEFR or FEV_1 ≥80% of predicted; <20% variability in PEFR
Mild persistent	Symptoms occur more than 2 times/week but less than one time/day; exacerbations may affect normal activity	Symptoms occur more than 2 times/month	PEFR or FEV_1 ≥80% of predicted; PEFR variability 20-30%

Classifica-tion	Daytime	Nighttime	Lung function
Moderate persistent	Symptoms occur daily; daily need for inhaled short-acting beta$_2$ agonist; exacerbations affect normal activity; exacerbations occur more than 2 times/week and may last for days	Symptoms occur more than one time/week	PEFR or FEV$_1$ >60 but <80% of predicted; PEFR variability >30%
Severe persistent	Symptoms are continual; physical activity is limited; exacerbations are frequent	Symptoms are frequent	PEFR or FEV$_1$ <60% of predicted; PEFR variability >30%

II. Treatment of asthma

A. Beta$_2$ agonists

1. Inhaled short-acting beta$_2$-adrenergic agonists are the most effective drugs available for treatment of acute bronchospasm and for prevention of exercise-induced asthma. Regular use of short-acting beta$_2$ agonists offers no advantage over "as needed" use. Levalbuterol, the R-isomer of racemic albuterol, offers no clinically significant advantage over racemic albuterol.

2. Salmeterol, a long-acting beta$_2$ agonist, has a relatively slow onset of action and a prolonged effect; it is not recommended for treatment of acute bronchospasm. Patients taking salmeterol regularly should use a short-acting beta$_2$ agonist PRN to control acute symptoms. Twice-daily inhalation of salmeterol has been effective for maintenance treatment in combination with inhaled corticosteroids and may be especially useful in patients with nocturnal symptoms.

3. **Adverse Effects.** Tachycardia, palpitations, tremor and paradoxical bronchospasm can occur, and high doses can cause hypokalemia.

Drugs for Asthma			
Drug	Formulation	Adult Dosage	Pediatric Dosage
Inhaled beta2-adrenergic agonists, short-acting			
Albuterol *Proventil* *Proventil-HFA* *Ventolin* *Ventolin Rotacaps*	metered-dose inhaler (90 µg/puff)	2 puffs q4-6h PRN	2 puffs q4-6h PRN
	dry-powder inhaler (200 µg/inhalation)	1-2 capsules q4-6h PRN	1-2 capsules q4-6h PRN
Albuterol *Proventil* multi-dose vials *Ventolin Nebules* *Ventolin*	nebulized	2.5 mg q4-6h PRN	0.1-0.15mg/kg q4-6h PRN

Levalbuterol - *Xopenex*	nebulized	0.63 mg q6-8h PRN	not approved
Inhaled beta2-adrenergic agonist, long-acting			
Salmeterol *Serevent* *Serevent Diskus*	metered-dose inhaler (21 µg/puff) dry-powder inhaler (50 µg/inhalation)	2 puffs q12h 1 inhalation q12h	1-2 puffs q12h 1 inhalation q12h
Inhaled Corticosteroids			
Beclomethasone dipropionate *Beclovent* *Vanceril* *Vanceril Double-Strength*	metered-dose inhaler (42 µg/puff) (84 µg/puff)	4-8 puffs bid 2-4 puffs bid	2-4 puffs bid 1-2 puffs bid
Budesonide *Pulmicort Turbuhaler*	dry-powder inhaler (200 µg/inhalation)	1-2 inhalations bid	1-2 inhalations bid
Flunisolide - *Aerobid*	metered-dose inhaler (250 µg/puff)	2-4 puffs bid	2 puffs bid
Fluticasone *Flovent* *Flovent Rotadisk*	metered-dose inhaler (44, 110 or 220 µg/puff) dry-powder inhaler (50, 100 or 250 µg/inhalation)	2-4 puffs bid (44 µg/puff) 1 inhalation bid (100 µg/inhalation)	1-2 puffs bid (44 µg/puff) 1 inhalation bid (50 µg/inhalation)
Triamcinolone acetonide *Azmacort*	metered-dose inhaler (100 µg/puff)	2 puffs tid-qid or 4 puffs bid	1-2 puffs tid-qid or 2-4 puffs bid
Leukotriene Modifiers			
Montelukast - *Singulair*	tablets	10 mg once/day	5 mg once/day
Zafirlukast - *Accolate*	tablets	20 mg bid	10 mg bid
Zileuton - *Zyflo*	tablets	600 mg qid	Not approved
Mast Cell Stabilizers			
Cromolyn *Intal*	metered-dose inhaler (800 µg/puff)	2-4 puffs tid-qid	2-4 puffs tid-qid

| Nedocromil Tilade | metered-dose inhaler (1.75 mg/puff) | 2-4 puffs bid-qid | 2-4 puffs bid or 2 puffs qid |
| Theophylline Slo-Bid Gyrocaps, Theo-Dur, Unidur | extended-release capsules or tablets | 300-600 mg/day | 10 mg/kg/day |

B. Inhaled corticosteroids

1. Regular use of an inhaled corticosteroid can suppress inflammation, decrease bronchial hyperresponsiveness and decrease symptoms. Inhaled corticosteroids are recommended for treatment of patients with mild or moderate persistent asthma as well as those with severe disease.

2. **Adverse effects.** Recommended doses of inhaled corticosteroids are usually free of toxicity. Dose-dependent slowing of linear growth may occur within six to 12 weeks in some children. Decreased bone density, glaucoma and cataract formation have been reported. Churg-Strauss vasculitis has been reported rarely. Dysphonia and oral candidiasis can occur. The use of a spacer device and rinsing the mouth after inhalation decreases the incidence of candidiasis.

C. Leukotriene modifiers

1. Leukotrienes increase migration of eosinophils, production of mucus and edema of the airway wall, and cause bronchoconstriction. Montelukast and zafirlukast are leukotriene receptor antagonists. Zileuton inhibits synthesis of leukotrienes.

2. **Montelukast (Singulair)** is modestly effective for maintenance treatment of intermittent or persistent asthma. It is taken once daily in the evening. As monotherapy it is less effective than inhaled corticosteroids, but addition of montelukast may permit a reduction in corticosteroid dosage. Montelukast added to oral or inhaled corticosteroids can improve symptoms.

3. **Zafirlukast (Accolate)** is modestly effective for maintenance treatment of mild-to-moderate asthma It is less effective than inhaled corticosteroids. Taking zafirlukast with food markedly decreases its bioavailability. Theophylline given concurrently can decrease its effect. Zafirlukast increases serum concentrations of oral anticoagulants and may cause bleeding. Infrequent adverse effects include mild headache, gastrointestinal disturbances and increased serum aminotransferase activity. Drug-induced lupus and Churg-Strauss vasculitis have been reported.

4. **Zileuton (Zyflo)** is modestly effective for maintenance treatment, but it is taken four times a day and patients must be monitored for hepatic toxicity.

D. Cromolyn (Intal) and Nedocromil (Tilade)

1. Cromolyn sodium, an inhibitor of mast cell degranulation, can decrease airway hyperresponsiveness in some patients with asthma. The drug has no bronchodilating activity and is useful only for prophylaxis. Cromolyn has virtually no systemic toxicity.

2. Nedocromil has similar effects. Both cromolyn and nedocromil are much less effective than inhaled corticosteroids.

E. Theophylline

1. Oral theophylline has a slower onset of action than inhaled beta$_2$ agonists and has limited usefulness for treatment of acute symptoms. It can, however, reduce the frequency and severity of symptoms, especially in

nocturnal asthma, and can decrease inhaled corticosteroid requirements.
2. When theophylline is used alone, serum concentrations between 5 and 15 µg/mL are most likely to produce therapeutic results with minimal adverse effects.

F. **Oral Corticosteroids** are the most effective drugs available for acute exacerbations of asthma unresponsive to bronchodilators.

1. Oral corticosteroids decrease symptoms and may prevent an early relapse. Chronic daily use of oral corticosteroids can cause glucose intolerance, weight gain, increased blood pressure, bone demineralization leading to osteoporosis, cataracts, immunosuppression and decreased growth in children. Alternate-day use of corticosteroids can decrease the incidence of adverse effects, but not of osteoporosis.

2. **Prednisone, prednisolone or methylprednisolone** (Solu-Medrol), 40 to 60 mg qd; for children, 1 to 2 mg/kg/day to a maximum of 60 mg/day. Therapy is continued for 3-10 days. The oral steroid dosage does not have to be tapered after short-course "burst" therapy if the patient is receiving inhaled steroid therapy.

G. **Choice of Drugs**

1. Both children and adults with infrequent mild symptoms of asthma may require only intermittent use, as needed, of a short-acting inhaled beta$_2$-adrenergic agonist. Overuse of inhaled short-acting beta$_2$ agonists or more than twice a week indicates that an inhaled corticosteroid should be added to the treatment regimen.

Pharmacotherapy for Asthma Based on Disease Classification		
Classification	**Long-term control medications**	**Quick-relief medications**
Mild intermittent		Short-acting beta$_2$ agonist as needed
Mild persistent	Low-dose inhaled corticosteroid or cromolyn sodium (Intal) or nedocromil (Tilade)	Short-acting beta$_2$ agonist as needed
Moderate persistent	Medium-dose inhaled corticosteroid plus a long-acting bronchodilator (long-acting beta$_2$ agonist) if needed	Short-acting beta$_2$ agonist as needed
Severe persistent	High-dose inhaled corticosteroid plus a long-acting bronchodilator and systemic corticosteroid if needed	Short-acting beta$_2$ agonist as needed

III. **Management of acute exacerbations**

A. High-dose, short-acting beta$_2$ agonists delivered by a metered-dose inhaler with a volume spacer or via a nebulizer remain the mainstays of urgent treatment.

B. Most patients require therapy with systemic corticosteroids to resolve symptoms and prevent relapse.

C. Hospitalization should be considered if the PEFR remains less than 70% of predicted. Patients with a PEFR less than 50% of predicted who exhibit an increasing pCO_2 level and declining mental status are candidates for intubation.

References, see page 268.

Chronic Obstructive Pulmonary Disease

Chronic obstructive pulmonary disease affects more than 20 million Americans. This condition is composed of three distinct entities: 1) chronic bronchitis; 2) emphysema; and 3) peripheral airways disease. The greatest percentage of patients with COPD have chronic bronchitis.

I. Patient assessment

   A. The majority of patients with COPD will have either a history of cigarette smoking or exposure to second-hand cigarette smoke. Occasionally, patients will develop COPD from occupational exposure. A minority of patients develop emphysema as a result of alpha-1-protease inhibitor deficiency or intravenous drug abuse. These patients develop emphysema early in life.

   B. The patient with acute exacerbations of COPD (AECOPD) usually will complain of either cough, sputum production, and/or dyspnea. Acute exacerbations may be precipitated by an infectious process, exposure to noxious stimuli, or environmental changes. It is important to compare the current illness with the severity of previous episodes and to be aware of previous intubation or admissions to the ICU.

   C. Cyanosis is a late and uncommon finding. The patient who is confused, combative, or agitated is probably severely hypoxemic. Intercostal retractions, accessory muscle use, and an increase in the pulsus paradoxus usually suggest significant airway obstruction. Wheezing is variably associated with airway obstruction. Emphysema is manifested by an elongated, hyperresonant chest. Diaphragmatic flattening and increased radiolucency is seen on the chest x-ray.

II. Infectious precipitants of acute exacerbations of COPD

   A. About 32% of patients with an acute exacerbation have a viral infection. The most common agents identified include influenza virus, parainfluenzae, and respiratory syncytial (RSV) virus.

   B. Bacterial precipitants play an important etiologic role in AECOPD. H. influenzae is the most common pathogen, occurring in 19%, followed by Streptococcus pneumoniae in 12% and Moraxella catarrhalis in 8%. Patients with COPD have chronic colonization of the respiratory tree with Streptococcus pneumoniae, Hemophilus influenzae, and Hemophilus parainfluenzae.

III. Diagnostic testing

   A. **Pulse oximetry** is an inexpensive, noninvasive procedure for assessing oxygen saturation.

   B. **Arterial blood gases.** Both hypercarbia and hypoxemia occur when pulmonary function falls below 25-30% of the predicted normal value. ABGs should be obtained for all patients with acute exacerbation of COPD. Comparison of ABG values during an acute exacerbation with baseline values can help establish the severity of an exacerbation and risk-stratify the patient.

   C. **Pulmonary function testing** is a useful means for assessing ventilatory function. Peak flow meters are available that can provide a quick assessment of expiratory function.

   D. **Chest radiography** will permit identification of patients with COPD with pneumonia, pneumothorax, and decompensated CHF.

   E. **An ECG** may be useful, particularly in patients who have a history of chest pain, syncope, palpitations, and when the differential diagnosis includes CHF.

F. The complete blood count (CBC) is useful in patients with acute exacerbation of COPD if pneumonia is suspected. The hematocrit is frequently elevated as a result of chronic hypoxemia. Serum electrolytes may reveal hypokalemia from aggressive use of beta-agonists, corticosteroids, and thiazide diuretics. A serum theophylline level should be obtained in patients who are taking theophylline. Each milligram per kilogram of aminophylline raises the serum theophylline level by 2 mcg/mL.

IV. Pharmacotherapy for patient stabilization

A. Oxygen. Patients in respiratory distress should receive supplemental oxygen therapy. Oxygen therapy usually is initiated by nasal cannula to maintain an O_2 saturation greater than 90%. Patients with hypercarbia may require controlled oxygen therapy using a Venturi mask in order to achieve more precise control of the FiO_2.

B. Beta-agonists are first-line therapy for AECOPD. Albuterol is the most widely used agent.

Beta-Agonist Dosages		
Agent	MDI	Aerosol
Albuterol (Proventil, Ventolin)	2-4 puffs q4h	0.5 cc (2.5 mg) in 2.5 cc NS
Pirbuterol (Maxair)	2 puffs q4-6h	
Salmeterol (Serevent)	2 puffs q12h	

C. Anticholinergic agents. Anticholinergic drugs produce preferential dilatation of the larger central airways, in contrast to beta-agonists, which affect the peripheral airways. Ipratropium is a first-line therapeutic option for chronic, outpatient management of stable patients with COPD. The usual dose is 2-4 puffs every six hours. Ipratropium is available as a metered dose inhaler and as a solution for inhalation.

D. Corticosteroids. Rapidly tapering courses of corticosteroids, in combination with bronchodilators and antibiotics, are effective in preventing relapses and maintaining longer symptom-free intervals in patients who have had AECOPD. Patients with an acute exacerbation of COPD should receive steroids as a mainstay of outpatient therapy. There is no role for inhaled corticosteroids in the treatment of acute exacerbations.

1. Corticosteroids produce a favorable response during acute COPD exacerbations, improving symptoms and reducing the length of hospitalization.
2. Oral steroids are warranted in severe COPD. Prednisone 0.5-1.0 mg/kg or 40 mg qAM. The dose should be tapered over 1-2 weeks following clinical improvement.
3. Aerosolized corticosteroids provide the benefits of oral corticosteroids with fewer side effects.
   Triamcinolone (Azmacort) MDI 2-4 puffs bid.
   Flunisolide (Aerobid, Aerobid-M) MDI 2-4 puffs bid.
   Beclomethasone (Beclovent) MDI 2-4 puffs bid.
   Budesonide (Pulmicort) MDI 2 puffs bid.
4. **Side effects of corticosteroids.** Cataracts, osteoporosis, sodium and water retention, hypokalemia, muscle weakness, aseptic necrosis of femoral and

humeral heads, peptic ulcer disease, pancreatitis, endocrine and skin abnormalities, muscle wasting.

E. **Theophylline** has a relatively narrow therapeutic index with side effects that range from nausea, vomiting, and tremor to more serious side effects, including seizures and ventricular arrhythmias. Dosage of long-acting theophylline (Slo-bid, Theo-Dur). 200-300 mg bid. Theophylline preparations with 24 hour action may be administered once a day in the early evening. Theo-24, 100-400 mg qd [100, 200, 300, 400 mg].

F. **Magnesium** acts by opposing calcium-induced bronchoconstriction. A significant improvement in pulmonary function results in patients given magnesium during an acute exacerbation of COPD. Given at a dose of 1-2 gm over 20 minutes, magnesium significantly improves peak expiratory flow.

G. **Summary of therapeutic approaches.** Albuterol, by nebulizer or meter dose inhaler with spacer, should be initiated promptly as 2.5 mg every 20 minutes prn. In patients who are not responding to these pharmacological maneuvers, consideration may be given to adding ipratropium to the aerosolization. In those individuals who still fail to respond, administration of intravenous theophylline (after measuring the theophylline level) or magnesium at a dose of 2 gm over 20 minutes may be considered. Oral or parenteral steroids can be administered to patients who are deteriorating in spite of adequate beta-agonist therapy.

H. **Antibiotics.** Amoxicillin-resistant, beta-lactamase-producing H. influenzae are common. Azithromycin has an appropriate spectrum of coverage. Levofloxacin also is advantageous when gram-negative bacteria predominate. Amoxicillin-clavulanate also has in vitro activity against beta-lactamase-producing H. influenzae and M. catarrhalis.

Recommended Dosing and Duration of Antibiotic Therapy for Acute Exacerbations of COPD

Mild-to-moderate acute exacerbations of COPD
- Azithromycin (Zithromax): 500 mg on 1st day, 250 mg qd × 4 days. Five-day total course of therapy
- Amoxicillin/clavulanate (Augmentin): 500 mg tid × 10 days (875 mg bid therapy is also an option)

Severe acute exacerbations of COPD
- Levofloxacin (Levaquin): 500 mg qd x 7-14 days

Alternative agents (Generic preparations) for treatment of uncomplicated, acute exacerbations of chronic bronchitis

- Trimethoprim/sulfamethoxazole (Bactrim, Septra): 1 DS tab po bid 7-14 days
- Amoxicillin (Amoxil, Wymox): 500 mg tid x 7-14 days
- Tetracycline: 500 mg qid x 7-14 days
- Doxycycline (Vibramycin): 100 mg bid x 7-14 days

V. **Ventilatory assistance**

A. Patients with extreme dyspnea, discordant breathing, fatigue, inability to speak, or deteriorating mental status in the face of adequate therapy may require ventilatory assistance. Hypoxemia that does not respond to oxygen therapy or worsening of acid-base status in spite of controlled oxygen therapy may also

require ventilatory assistance.
   B. Noninvasive, nasal, or bilevel positive airway pressure (BiPAP) may result in improvement in respiratory rate, tidal volume, and minute ventilation. Patients successfully treated with noninvasive ventilation have a lower incidence of pneumonia and sinusitis.
VI. Surgical treatment. Lung volume reduction surgery (LVRS) consists of surgical removal of an emphysematous bulla. This procedure can ameliorate symptoms and improve pulmonary function. Lung transplantation is reserved for those patients deemed unsuitable or too ill for LVRS.
VII. Hypoxemia adversely affects function and increases risk of the death, and oxygen therapy is the only treatment documented to improve survival in patients with COPD. Oxygen is usually delivered by nasal cannula at a flow rate sufficient to maintain an optimal oxygen saturation level.

References, see page 268.

Acute Bronchitis

Acute bronchitis is one of the most common diagnoses made by primary care physicians. Viruses are the most common cause of acute bronchitis in otherwise healthy adults. Only a small portion of acute bronchitis infections are caused by nonviral agents, with the most common organisms being *Mycoplasma pneumoniae* and *Chlamydia pneumoniae*.

I. Diagnosis
   A. The cough in acute bronchitis may produce either clear or purulent sputum. This cough generally lasts seven to 10 days. Approximately 50 percent of patients with acute bronchitis have a cough that lasts up to three weeks, and 25 percent of patients have a cough that persists for over a month.
   B. Physical examination. Wheezing, rhonchi, or a prolonged expiratory phase may be present.
   C. Diagnostic studies
      1. The appearance of sputum is not predictive of whether a bacterial infection is present. Purulent sputum is most often caused by viral infections. Microscopic examination or culture of sputum generally is not helpful. Since most cases of acute bronchitis are caused by viruses, cultures are usually negative or exhibit normal respiratory flora. M. pneumoniae or C. pneumoniae infection are not detectable on routine sputum culture.
      2. Acute bronchitis can cause transient pulmonary function abnormalities which resemble asthma. Therefore, to diagnose asthma, changes that persist after the acute phase of the illness must be documented. When pneumonia is suspected, chest radiographs and pulse oximetry may be helpful.
II. Differential diagnosis
   A. Acute bronchitis or pneumonia can present with fever, constitutional symptoms and a productive cough. Patients with pneumonia often have rales. When pneumonia is suspected on the basis of the presence of a high fever, constitutional symptoms or severe dyspnea, a chest radiograph should be obtained.

Differential Diagnosis of Acute Bronchitis	
Disease process	**Signs and symptoms**
Asthma	Evidence of reversible airway obstruction even when not infected
Allergic aspergillosis	Transient pulmonary infiltrates Eosinophilia in sputum and peripheral blood smear
Occupational exposures	Symptoms worse during the work week but tend to improve during weekends, holidays and vacations
Chronic bronchitis	Chronic cough with sputum production on a daily basis for a minimum of three months Typically occurs in smokers
Sinusitis	Tenderness over the sinuses, postnasal drainage
Common cold	Upper airway inflammation and no evidence of bronchial wheezing
Pneumonia	Evidence of infiltrate on the chest radiograph
Congestive heart failure	Basilar rales Orthopnea Cardiomegaly Evidence of increased interstitial or alveolar fluid on the chest radiograph S_3 gallop Tachycardia
Reflux esophagitis	Intermittent symptoms worse when lying down Heartburn
Bronchogenic tumor	Constitutional signs often present Cough chronic, sometimes with hemoptysis
Aspiration syndromes	Usually related to a precipitating event, such as smoke inhalation Vomiting Decreased level of consciousness

  B. Asthma should be considered in patients with repetitive episodes of acute bronchitis. Patients who repeatedly present with cough and wheezing can be given spirometric testing with bronchodilation to help differentiate asthma from recurrent bronchitis.
  C. Congestive heart failure may cause cough, shortness of breath and wheezing in older patients. Reflux esophagitis with chronic aspiration can cause bronchial inflammation with cough and wheezing. Bronchogenic tumors may produce a cough and obstructive symptoms.
III. Treatment
  A. Antibiotics. Physicians often treat acute bronchitis with antibiotics, even though scant evidence exists that antibiotics offer any significant advantage over placebo. Antibiotic therapy is beneficial in patients with exacerbations of chronic bronchitis.

Oral Antibiotic Regimens for Bronchitis

Drug	Recommended regimen
Azithromycin (Zithromax)	500 mg; then 250 mg qd
Erythromycin	250-500 mg q6h
Clarithromycin (Biaxin)	500 mg bid
Levofloxacin (Levaquin)	500 mg qd
Sparfloxacin (Zagam)	Day 1,400 mg; then 200 mg qd
Trovafloxacin (Trovan)	200 mg qd
Grepafloxacin (Raxar)	600 mg qd
Trimethoprim/sulfamethoxazole (Bactrim, Septra)	1 DS tablet bid
Doxycycline	100 mg bid

B. Bronchodilators. Significant relief of symptoms occurs with inhaled albuterol (two puffs four times daily). When productive cough and wheezing are present, bronchodilator therapy may be useful.

References, see page 268.

Infectious Disorders

Pneumonia

Community-acquired pneumonia is the leading infectious cause of death and is the sixth-leading cause of death overall.

I. **Clinical diagnosis**
   A. **Symptoms** of pneumonia may include fever, chills, malaise and cough. Patients also may have pleurisy, dyspnea, or hemoptysis. Eighty percent of patients are febrile.
   B. **Physical exam findings** may include tachypnea, tachycardia, rales, rhonchi, bronchial breath sounds, and dullness to percussion over the involved area of lung.
   C. **Chest radiograph** usually shows infiltrates. The chest radiograph may reveal signs of complicated pneumonia, such as multilobar infiltrates, volume loss, or pleural effusion. The chest radiograph may be negative very early in the illness because of dehydration or severe neutropenia.
   D. **Further testing** is required if there are severe signs and symptoms (heart rate >140 beats per minute, altered mental status, respiratory rate >30 breaths per minute) or underlying diseases, such as diabetes mellitus or heart disease. Additional tests may include a complete blood count, pulse oximetry or arterial blood gas analysis.

II. **Laboratory evaluation**
   A. **Sputum for Gram stain and culture** should be obtained in hospitalized patients. In a patient who has had no prior antibiotic therapy, a high-quality specimen (>25 white blood cells and <5 epithelial cells/hpf) may help to direct initial therapy.
   B. **Blood cultures** are positive in 11% of cases, and they may identify a specific etiologic agent.
   C. **Serologic testing for HIV** is recommended in hospitalized patients between the ages of 15 and 54 years. **Urine antigen testing** for legionella is indicated in endemic areas for patients with serious pneumonia.

III. **Indications for hospitalization**
   A. Age >65 years
   B. Unstable vital signs (heart rate >140 beats per minute, systolic blood pressure <90 mm Hg, respiratory rate >30 beats per minute)
   C. Altered mental status
   D. Hypoxemia (PO_2 <60 mm Hg)
   E. Severe underlying disease (lung disease, diabetes mellitus, liver disease, heart failure, renal failure)
   F. Immune compromise (HIV infection, cancer, corticosteroid use)
   G. Complicated pneumonia (extrapulmonary infection, meningitis, cavitation, multilobar involvement, sepsis, abscess, empyema, pleural effusion)
   H. Severe electrolyte, hematologic or metabolic abnormality (ie, sodium <130 mEq/L, hematocrit <30%, absolute neutrophil count <1,000/mm^3, serum creatinine > 2.5 mg/dL)
   I. Failure to respond to outpatient treatment within 48 to 72 hours.

Pathogens Causing Community-Acquired Pneumonia

More Common	Less Common
Streptococcus pneumoniae Haemophilus influenzae Moraxella catarrhalis Mycoplasma pneumoniae Chlamydia pneumoniae Legionella species Viruses Anaerobes (especially with aspiration)	Staphylococcus aureus Gram-negative bacilli Pneumocystis carinii Mycobacterium tuberculosis

IV. Treatment of community-acquired pneumonia

Recommended Drug Therapy for Patients with Community-Acquired Pneumonia

Clinical Situation	Primary Treatment	Alternative(s)
Empiric Outpatient Therapy		
Younger (<60 yr) outpatients without underlying disease	Erythromycin	Clarithromycin [Biaxin], azithromycin [Zithromax], or dirithromycin (Dynabac) (if intolerant of erythromycin or in smokers to treat Haemophilus influenzae) or Tetracycline (doxycycline) or levofloxacin (Levoquin) or sparfloxacin (Zagam)
Older (>60 yr) outpatients with underlying disease	Second-generation cephalosporin (Cefuroxime) or Trimethoprim-sulfamethoxazole	Beta-lactamase inhibitor (with macrolide if legionella infection suspected)
Gross aspiration suspected	Clindamycin (Cleocin)	Amoxicillin-clavulanate

Clinical Situation	Primary Treatment	Alternative(s)
Empiric Inpatient Therapy		
Moderately ill	Second- or third-genera-tion cephalosporin cefuroxime, ceftriaxone [Rocephin], cefotaxime [Claforan]	Beta-lactam/beta-lactamase in-hibitor (Ampicillin-sulbactam [Unasyn], Ticarcillin-clavulanate [Timentin]). A macrolide is added if legionella infection is suspected
Critically ill	Erythromycin (±rifampin if *Legionella* organisms documented) plus Third-generation cephalosporin with *anti-Pseudomonas aeruginosa* activity or another anti-pseudomonal agent (eg, imipenem-cilastatin [Primaxin] or ciprofloxacin [Cipro]) plus Aminoglycoside (pending culture results)	

A. Younger, otherwise healthy outpatients

1. The most commonly identified organisms in this group are *S pneumoniae, M pneumoniae, C pneumoniae,* and respiratory viruses.
2. Erythromycin has excellent activity against most of the causal organisms in this group except H *influenzae.*
3. The newer macrolides, active against H *influenzae* (azithromycin [Zithromax] and clarithromycin [Biaxin]), are effective as empirical monotherapy for younger adults without underlying disease.

B. Older outpatients with underlying disease

1. The most common pathogens in this group are S *pneumoniae,* H *influenzae,* respiratory viruses, aerobic gram-negative bacilli, and S *aureus.* Agents such as *M pneumoniae* and C *pneumoniae* are not usually found in this group. *Pseudomonas aeruginosa* is rarely identified.
2. A second-generation cephalosporin (eg, cefuroxime [Ceftin]) is recommended for initial empirical treatment. Trimethoprim-sulfamethoxazole is an inexpen-sive alternative where pneumococcal resistance to not prevalent.
3. When legionella infection is suspected, initial therapy should include treatment with a macrolide antibiotic in addition to a beta-lactam/beta-lactamase inhibitor (amoxicillin clavulanate).

C. Moderately Ill, Hospitalized Patients

1. In addition to S *pneumoniae* and H *influenzae,* more virulent pathogens, such as S *aureus, Legionella* species, aerobic gram-negative bacilli (including P *aeruginosa,* and anaerobes), should be considered in patients requiring hospitalization.
2. Hospitalized patients should receive an intravenous cephalosporin active against S *pneumoniae* and anaerobes (eg, cefuroxime, ceftriaxone [Ro-cephin], cefotaxime [Claforan]), or a beta-lactam/beta-lactamase inhibitor.
3. When P *aeruginosa* infection is suspected (recent hospitalization, debilitated patient from a nursing home), only antipseudomonal cephalosporins with activity against this organism should be used (eg, ceftazidime [Fortaz], cefepime [Maxipime], cefoperazone [Cefobid]) along with an aminoglycoside or a quinolone (ciprofloxacin). Two agents should be used when Pseudomo-nas aeruginosa is suspected.
4. When legionella is suspected (in endemic areas, cardiopulmonary disease, immune compromise), a macrolide should be added to the regimen. If

legionella pneumonia is confirmed, rifampin (Rifadin) should be added to the macrolide.

D. Critically ill patients

1. S *pneumoniae* and *Legionella* species are the most commonly isolated pathogens, and aerobic gram-negative bacilli are identified with increasing frequency. M pneumoniae, respiratory viruses and H *influenzae* are less commonly identified.

2. Erythromycin should be used along with an antipseudomonal agent (ceftazidime, imipenem-cilastatin [Primaxin], or ciprofloxacin [Cipro]). An aminoglycoside should be added for additional antipseudomonal activity until culture results are known.

Common Antimicrobial Agents for Community-Acquired Pneumonia in Adults

Type	Agent	Dosage
Oral therapy		
Macrolides	Erythromycin Clarithromycin (Biaxin) Azithromycin (Zithromax)	500 mg PO qid 500 mg PO bid 500 mg PO on day 1, then 250 mg qd x 4 days
Beta-lactam/beta-lactamase inhibitor	Amoxicillin-clavulanate (Augmentin)	500 mg tid or 875 mg PO bid
Quinolones	Ciprofloxacin (Cipro) Levofloxacin (Levaquin) Ofloxacin (Floxin) Trovafloxacin (Trovan)	500 mg PO bid 500 mg PO qd 400 mg PO bid 200 mg PO qd
Tetracycline	Doxycycline	100 m g PO bid
Sulfonamide	Trimethoprim-sulfamethoxazole	160 mg/800 mg (DS) PO bid
Intravenous Therapy		
Cephalosporins Second-generation	Cefuroxime (Kefurox, Zinacef)	0.75-1.5 g IV q8h
Third-generation (anti-Pseudomonas aeruginosa)	Ceftizoxime (Cefizox) Ceftazidime (Fortaz)	1-2 g IV q8h 1-2 g IV q8h
Beta-lactam/beta-lactamase inhibitors	Ampicillin-sulbactam (Unasyn) Ticarcillin-clavulanate (Timentin)	1.5 g IV q6h 3.1 g IV q6h
Quinolones	Ciprofloxacin (Cipro) Levofloxacin (Levaquin) Ofloxacin (Floxin) Trovafloxacin (Trovan)	400 mg IV q12h 500 mg IV q24h 400 mg IV q12h 200 mg IV q24h

E. **Antibiotic resistance**
   1. Twenty-five percent of S. pneumoniae isolates in some areas of the United States are no longer susceptible to penicillin, and 9% are no longer susceptible to extended-spectrum cephalosporins. Patients with more severe pneumonia or recurrent pneumonia are more likely to harbor resistant S. pneumoniae.
   2. Pneumonia caused by penicillin-resistant strains of S. pneumoniae should be treated with high-dose penicillin (penicillin G 2-3 MU IV q4h), or cefotaxime (2 gm IV q8h), or ceftriaxone (2 gm IV q12h), or meropenem (Merrem) (500-1000 mg IV q8h), or vancomycin (Vancocin) (1 gm IV q12h).
   3. H. influenzae and Moraxella catarrhalis often produce beta-lactamase enzymes, making these organisms resistant to penicillin and ampicillin. Infection with these pathogens is treated with a second-generation cephalosporin, beta-lactam/beta-lactamase inhibitor combination such as amoxicillin-clavulanate, azithromycin, or trimethoprim-sulfamethoxazole.

. **Clinical course**
   A. In about 50% of patients, a specific pathogen will be identified, and empirical therapy can be changed to a more specific antibiotic.
   B. In hospitalized patients, intravenous therapy can be changed to oral therapy once the clinical condition has stabilized, and fever and leukocytosis have resolved.
   C. Most bacterial infections can be adequately treated with 10-14 days of antibiotic therapy. A shorter treatment course of three to five days is possible with azithromycin because of its long half-life. M pneumoniae and C pneumoniae infections require treatment for up to 14 days. Legionella infections should be treated for a minimum of 14 days; immunocompromised patients require 21 days of therapy.

References, see page 268.

Tuberculosis

ne-third of the world population is infected with tuberculosis. The tuberculosis case te in the United States is 9.4 cases per 100,000 population.

Pathophysiology

A. In most individuals infected with mycobacterium tuberculosis (by respiratory aerosols), the primary pulmonary infection occurs early in life, and the organism is contained by host defenses. The primary infection usually resembles pneumonia or bronchitis, and the infection usually resolves without treatment.
B. After the immune system limits spread of the bacilli during the primary infection, patients are asymptomatic, although the organisms may remain viable and dormant for many years. In these individuals, the only indication of primary infection is conversion to a positive reaction to the purified protein derivative (PPD) skin test. Acid-fast bacilli are not present in the sputum.
C. Later in life, the organism may cause reactivation disease, usually pulmonary, but it may affect the genitourinary system, bones, joints, meninges, brain, peritoneum, and pericardium. Reactivation of tuberculosis is the most common form of disease. Immunocompetent individuals with tuberculosis infection have a 10% chance of developing reactivation disease during their lifetimes.

II. Diagnosis of active pulmonary tuberculosis

A. Chronic cough with scant sputum production and blood streaking of sputum a the most common symptoms of pulmonary disease. Pulmonary tuberculo should be considered in any patient with the following characteristics:

1. Cough for more than 3 weeks
2. Night sweats
3. Bloody sputum or hemoptysis
4. Weight loss
5. Fever
6. Anorexia
7. History of exposure to tuberculosis, institutionalization, HIV infection, o positive PPD test.

B. Diagnosis of active pulmonary tuberculosis rests upon sputum examination acid fast bacilli and subsequent culture and sensitivities. This process requi 4-6 weeks for identification and another 4-6 weeks for sensitivity testing. Smea and cultures should be performed on three different days in patients at high r for infection.

C. **DNA probes** that use polymerase chain reactions (PCR) are available for mo rapid identification of tuberculosis. They are useful for making an early diagno of Tb while awaiting culture results.

D. **Chest radiographs**

1. **Reactivation pulmonary tuberculosis** is characterized by infiltrates in apical and posterior segments of the upper lobes or in the superior segmen of the lower lobes.
2. **Cavitation** is frequently present in regions of substantial infiltration. Lordo views, taken in an anterior-posterior fashion with the patient lean backward, allow better visualization of the lung apices.

E. **Skin testing for tuberculosis**

1. The purified protein derivative (PPD) test is a reliable method of recogniz prior infection; however, it is neither sensitive nor specific. It is useful detecting patients who are harboring latent tuberculosis who may ne "prophylactic" therapy. The test is read at 48-72 hrs.
2. False-positive reactions are possible as a result of exposure to non-patholo cal mycobacterial disease (eg, M. avium complex). False-negative reactio are seen with advancing age and immunosuppression. Twenty-five perce of all individuals with active tuberculosis have a negative skin test. A histo of vaccination with bacille Calmette-Guerin (BCG) should be ignored wh interpreting the results of tuberculin skin testing because skin test reactiv from the vaccine wanes after 2 years.

Interpretation of PPD Results

1. **Induration ≥5 mm is considered positive in:**
   - HIV-positive individuals
   - persons with recent close contact with individual with active tuberculosis
   - persons with chest x-ray consistent with healed tuberculosis

2. **Induration ≥10 mm is considered positive in:**
   High-Risk Groups
   - intravenous drug users who are HIV negative
   - patients with chronic illness at risk for reactivation (silicosis, chronic renal failure, diabetes mellitus, chronic steroid use, hematologic disorders, malignancy)
   - children younger than 4 years of age
   High-Prevalence Groups
   - immigrants from endemic regions (Asia, Africa, Latin America, Caribbean)
   - residents of long-term care facilities (nursing homes, prisons)
   - persons from medically underserved, low-income populations

3. **Induration ≥15 mm is considered positive in all persons.**

4. **Recent conversion criteria:**
   - increase ≥10 mm within two years in individuals younger than 35 years of age
   - increase ≥15 mm within two years in individuals 35 years of age or older

5. **Interpretation of PPD testing in health care workers:**
   - follow guidelines 1-3
   - facilities with a high prevalence of tuberculosis patients may consider induration 10 mm in individuals without other risk factors as a positive reaction
   - recent conversion is an increase in induration of 10 mm in a two-year period in high-prevalence facilities, 15 mm in low-prevalence facilities

F. Tuberculosis is often the initial manifestation of HIV infection; therefore, serologic testing for HIV is recommended in all tuberculosis patients.

III. Chemoprophylaxis for patients with a positive PPD

A. Chemoprophylaxis with isoniazid (INH) greatly decreases the likelihood of progression of latent tuberculous infection to active disease. Before administration of chemoprophylaxis, active tuberculosis must be excluded clinically and by chest x-ray.

Preventive Therapy Considerations

General Population
- Individuals <35 years of age with positive reaction to PPD (including children)
- HIV-positive patients with positive PPD reactions
- Anergic individuals with recent known contact to person(s) with active tuberculosis
- Children with known TB exposure, even if PPD negative

Health Care Workers
(in addition to above recommendations)
- Recent PPD conversion
- Close contact of individual with active tuberculosis
- HIV-positive, regardless of PPD reaction
- Intravenous drug users
- Medical condition that increases risk of progression to active disease

Preventative Therapy Recommendations

Isoniazid
300 mg po daily in adults
10 mg/kg po daily in children

Duration
6-12 months in otherwise healthy adults
9 months in children
12 months in HIV-positive individuals

If exposure to INH resistant organisms has been documented, prophylaxis should be attempted with rifampin and ethambutol for 12 months.

IV. Treatment of active tuberculosis
   A. Suspected TB should be treated empirically with a four-drug combination. The four-drug regimen consists of isoniazid, rifampin, pyrazinamide, and ethambutol. Patients should be treated for 8 weeks with the four-drug regimen, followed by 16 weeks of INH and rifampin daily or 2-3 times weekly.
   B. If multi-drug resistant TB (resistant to both INH and RIF) is encountered, therapy should be more prolonged and guided by antibiotic sensitivities. Directly observed therapy, on a twice-per-week basis, should be instituted when compliance is questioned.

Dosage Recommendations for Treatment of Tuberculosis

Drug	Daily Dose	Two Times/week Dose	Three Times/week Dose
Isoniazid (INH)	5 mg/kg, max 300 mg	15 mg/kg, max 900 mg	15 mg/kg, max 900 mg
Rifampin (RIF)	10 mg/kg, max 600 mg	10 mg/kg, max 600 mg	10 mg/kg, max 600 mg
Pyrazinamide (PZA)	15-30 mg/kg, max 2 g	50-70 mg/kg, max 4 g	50-70 mg/kg, max 3 g
Ethambutol (EMB)	5-25 mg/kg, max 2.5 g	50 mg/kg, max 2.5 g	25-30 mg/kg, max 2.5 g
Streptomycin (SM)	15 mg/kg, max 1 g	25-30 mg/kg, max 1.5 g	25-30 mg/kg, max 1 g

Initial Treatment of Tuberculosis
HIV Negative
INH + RIF + PZA + (EMB) daily for eight weeks followed by INH + RIF daily or 2-3 times weekly for 16 weeks.   Regimen may be tailored following results of susceptibility testing.
HIV Positive
Continue above regimen for a total of nine months and at least six months following culture conversion to negative.

   C. Symptoms should improve within 4 weeks, and sputum cultures should become negative within 3 months in patients receiving effective antituberculosis therapy.

   D. Sputum cultures should be obtained monthly until they are negative, and cultures should be obtained after completion of therapy. A chest x-ray should be obtained after 2-3 months and after completion of treatment to assess efficacy.

References, see page 268.

Tonsillopharyngitis

In about a quarter of patients with a sore throat, the disorder is caused by group A beta-hemolytic streptococcus. Treatment of streptococcal tonsillopharyngitis reduces the occurrence of subsequent rheumatic fever, an inflammatory disease that affects the joints and heart, skin, central nervous system, and subcutaneous tissues.

I. Prevalence of pharyngitis
   A. Group A beta-hemolytic streptococcus (GABHS) typically occurs in patients 5-11 years of age, and it is uncommon in children under 3 years old. Most cases of GABHS occur in late winter and early spring.
   B. Etiologic causes of sore throat
      1. Viral. Rhinoviruses, influenza, Epstein-Barr virus
      2. Bacterial. GABHS (Streptococcus pyogenes), Streptococcus pneumoniae, Haemophilus influenzae, Moraxella catarrhalis, Staphylococcus aureus, anaerobes, Mycoplasma pneumoniae, Candida albicans
   C. In patients who present with pharyngitis, the major goal is to detect GABHS infection because rheumatic fever may result. Severe GABHS infections may also cause a toxic-shock-like illness (toxic strep syndrome), bacteremia, streptococcal deep tissue infections (necrotizing fascitis), and streptococcal cellulitis.

II. Clinical evaluation of sore throat
   A. GABHS infection is characterized by sudden onset of sore throat, fever and tender swollen anterior cervical lymph nodes, typically in a child 5-11 years of age. Headache, nausea and vomiting may occur.
   B. Cough, rhinorrhea and hoarseness are generally absent.

III. Physical examination
   A. Streptococcal infection is suggested by erythema and swelling of the pharynx, enlarged and erythematous tonsils, tonsillar exudate, or palatal petechiae. The clinical diagnosis of GABHS infection is correct in only 50-75% of cases when based on clinical criteria alone.

B. Unilateral inflammation and swelling of the pharynx suggests peritonsillar abscess. Distortion of the posterior pharyngeal wall suggests a retropharyngeal abscess. Corynebacterium diphtheriae is indicated by a dull membrane which bleeds on manipulation. Viral infections may cause oral vesicular eruptions.

C. The tympanic membranes should be examined for erythema or a middle ear effusion.

D. The lungs should be auscultated because viral infection occasionally causes pneumonia.

IV. Diagnostic testing

A. Rapid streptococcal testing has a specificity of 90% and a sensitivity of 80%. A dry swab should be used to sample both the posterior wall and the tonsillar fossae, especially erythematous or exudative areas.

B. Throat culture is the most accurate test available for the diagnosis of GABHS pharyngitis.

C. Diagnostic approach

1. Patients presenting with an acute episode of pharyngitis should receive a rapid streptococcal antigen test. If the rapid test is negative, a culture should be done.

2. If the rapid test is positive, treatment with an antibiotic should be initiated for 10 days. The presence of physical and historical findings suggesting GABHS infection may also prompt the initiation of antibiotic therapy despite a negative rapid strep test.

3. After throat culture, presumptive therapy should be initiated. If the culture is positive for GABHS, a 10-day course of therapy should be completed. If the culture is negative, antibiotics may be discontinued.

V. Antibiotic therapy

A. Starting antibiotic therapy within the first 24-48 hours of illness decreases the duration of sore throat, fever and adenopathy by 12-24 hours. Treatment also minimizes risk of transmission and of rheumatic fever.

B. Penicillin VK is the antibiotic of choice for GABHS; 250 mg PO qid or 500 mg PO bid x 10 days [250, 500 mg]. A 10-day regimen is recommended. Penicillin G benzathine (Bicillin LA) may be used as one-time therapy when compliance is a concern; 1.2 million units IM x 1 dose.

C. Azithromycin (Zithromax) offers the advantage of once-a-day dosing for just 5 days; 500 mg x 1, then 250 mg qd x 4 days [6 pack].

D. Clarithromycin (Biaxin), 500 mg PO bid; bacteriologic efficacy is similar to that of penicillin VK, and it may be taken twice a day.

E. Erythromycin is also effective; 250 mg PO qid; or enteric coated delayed release tablet (PCE) 333 mg PO tid or 500 mg PO bid [250, 333, 500 mg]. **Erythromycin ethyl succinate (EES)** 400 PO qid or 800 mg PO bid [400 mg]. Gastrointestinal upset is common.

VI. Treatment of recurrent GABHS pharyngitis

A. When patient compliance is an issue, an injection of penicillin G benzathine may be appropriate. When patient compliance is not an issue, therapy should be changed to a broader spectrum agent.

1. **Cephalexin (Keflex)** 250-500 mg tid x 5 days [250, 500 mg]
2. **Cefadroxil (Duricef)** 500 mg bid x 5 days [500 mg]
3. **Loracarbef (Lorabid)** 200-400 mg bid x 5 days [200, 400 mg]
4. **Cefixime (Suprax)** 400 mg qd x 5 days [200, 400 mg]
5. **Ceftibuten (Cedax)** 400 mg qd x 5 days [400 mg]
6. **Cefuroxime axetil (Ceftin)** 250-500 mg bid x 5 days [125, 250, 500 mg]

B. Amoxicillin/clavulanate (Augmentin) has demonstrated superior results in comparison with penicillin; 250-500 mg tid or 875 mg bid [250, 500, 875 mg].

C. Sulfonamides, trimethoprim, and the tetracyclines are not effective for the treatment of GABHS pharyngitis.

References, see page 268.

Sinusitis

Sinusitis affects 12% of adults and complicates 0.5% of viral upper respiratory infections. Symptoms that have been present for less than 1 month are indicative of acute sinusitis, while symptoms of longer duration reflect chronic sinusitis.

I. **Pathophysiology**
   A. Factors that predispose to sinus infection include anatomic abnormalities, viral URIs, allergies, overuse of topical decongestants, asthma, and immune deficiencies.
   B. **Acute sinusitis** is associated with the same bacteria as otitis media. Streptococcus pneumoniae, Hemophilus influenzae, and Moraxella catarrhalis are the most commonly encountered pathogens. Thirty-five percent of H influenzae and 75% of M catarrhalis strains produce beta-lactamases, making them resistant to penicillin antibiotics.
   C. **Chronic sinusitis** is associated with Staphylococcus aureus and anaerobes.
II. **Clinical evaluation**
   A. Symptoms of acute sinusitis include facial pain or tenderness, nasal congestion, purulent nasal and postnasal discharge, headache, maxillary tooth pain, malodorous breath, fever, and eye swelling. Pain or pressure in the cheeks and deep nasal recesses is common.
   B. If symptoms have lasted for less than 7 to 10 days and the patient is recovering, a self-limited viral URI is the most likely cause. However, worsening symptoms or symptoms that persist for more than 7 days are more likely to be caused by sinusitis.
   C. High fever and signs of acute toxicity are unusual except in the most severe cases. Purulent drainage in the patient's nose or throat may sometimes be seen.
   D. The nasal mucosa is often erythematous and swollen. The presence of mucopus in the external nares or posterior pharynx is highly suggestive of sinusitis. Facial tenderness, elicited by percussion, is an unreliable sign of sinusitis.
III. **Laboratory evaluation**
   A. **Imaging.** Plain films are usually unnecessary for evaluating acute sinusitis because of the high cost and relative insensitivity.
   B. **CT scanning** is useful if the diagnosis remains uncertain or if orbital or intracranial complications are suspected. CT scanning is nonspecific and may demonstrate sinus abnormalities in 87% of patients with colds.
   C. **MRI** is useful when fungal infections or tumors are a possibility.
   D. **Sinus aspiration** is an invasive procedure, and is only indicated for complicated sinusitis, immunocompromise, failure to respond to multiple courses of empiric antibiotic therapy, or severe symptoms.
   E. Cultures of nasal secretions correlate poorly with results of sinus aspiration.

IV. Management of sinusitis
A. Antibiotic therapy for sinusitis
1. **First-line agents**
   a. Amoxicillin (Amoxil): Adults, 500 mg tid PO for 14 days. Children, 40 mg/kg/d in 3 divided doses.
   b. Trimethoprim/sulfamethoxazole (Bactrim, Septra): Adults, 1 DS tab (160/800 mg) bid. Children, 8/40 mg/kg/d bid.
   c. Erythromycin/sulfisoxazole (Pediazole): Children, 50/150 mg/kg/d qid.
2. A 10- to 14-day course of therapy is recommended; however, if the patient is improved but still symptomatic at the end of the course, the medication should be continued for an additional 5 to 7 days after symptoms subside.
3. **Broader-spectrum agents**
   a. If the initial response to antibiotics is unsatisfactory, beta-lactamase-producing bacteria are likely to be present, and broad-spectrum therapy is required.
   b. Amoxicillin/clavulanate (Augmentin): adults, 250 mg tid or 875 mg bid; children, 40 mg/kg/d in 3 divided doses.
   c. Azithromycin (Zithromax): 500 mg as a single dose on day 1, then 250 mg qd.
   d. Clarithromycin (Biaxin): 500 mg bid.
   e. Cefuroxime axetil (Ceftin): adults, 250 mg bid; children, 125 mg bid.
   f. Cefixime (Suprax): adults, 200 mg bid; children, 8 mg/kg/d bid.
   g. Cefpodoxime (Vantin) 200 mg bid
   h. Cefprozil (Cefzil) 250-500 mg qd-bid
   i. Loracarbef (Lorabid): 400 mg bid.
   j. Levofloxacin (Floxin)
4. **Penicillin-resistant S. Pneumoniae** result from bacterial alterations in penicillin-binding proteins. Highly resistant strains are resistant to penicillin, trimethoprim/sulfamethoxazole (TMP/SMX), and third-generation cephalosporins. The prevalence of multiple-drug resistant S. pneumoniae is 20-35%. High dose amoxicillin (80 mg/kg/d), or amoxicillin plus amoxicillin/clavulanate, or clindamycin are options.
B. Chronic sinusitis is commonly caused by anaerobic organisms. 3-4 weeks of therapy or longer is required.
C. Ancillary treatments
1. **Steam and saline** improves drainage of mucus. Spray saline (NaSal) or a bulb syringe with a saline solution (1 tsp of salt in 1 qt of warm water) may be used.
2. **Decongestants**
   a. Topical or systemic decongestants may be used in acute or chronic sinusitis. Phenylephrine (Neo-Synephrine) or oxymetazoline (Afrin) nasal drops or sprays are commonly used.
   b. Oral decongestants, such as phenylephrine or pseudoephedrine, are active in areas not reached by topical agents.

References, see page 268.

Infectious Conjunctivitis

Infectious conjunctivitis is one of the most common causes of red eye. The clinical term "red eye" is applied to a variety of infectious or inflammatory diseases of the eye. Conjunctivitis is most frequently caused by a bacterial or viral infection. Sexually transmitted diseases such as chlamydial and gonorrhea are less common causes of conjunctivitis. Ocular allergy is a major cause of chronic conjunctivitis.

I. **Clinical evaluation of conjunctivitis**
   A. The history should establish whether the condition is acute, subacute, chronic or recurrent, and whether it is unilateral or bilateral.
   B. **Discharge**
      1. **Serous discharge (watery)** is most commonly associated with viral or allergic ocular conditions.
      2. **Mucoid discharge (stringy or ropy)** is highly characteristic of allergy or dry eyes.
      3. **Mucopurulent or purulent discharge,** often associated with morning crusting and difficulty opening the eyelids, strongly suggests a bacterial infection. The possibility of *Neisseria gonorrhoeae* infection should be considered when the discharge is copiously purulent.

Differential Diagnosis of Red Eye	

Conjunctivitis
  Infectious
    Viral
    Bacterial (eg, staphylococcus,
    Chlamydia)
  Noninfectious
    Allergic conjunctivitis
    Dry eye
    Toxic or chemical reaction
    Contact lens use
    Foreign body
    Factitious conjunctivitis
	Keratitis
	  Infectious. Bacterial, viral, fungal
	  Noninfectious. Recurrent epithelial
	  erosion, foreign body
	Uveitis
	Episcleritis/scleritis
	Acute glaucoma
	Eyelid abnormalities
	Orbital disorders
	  Preseptal and orbital cellulitis
	  Idiopathic orbital inflammation (pseudo-
	  tumor)

   C. **Itching** is highly suggestive of allergic conjunctivitis. A history of recurrent itching or a personal or family history of hay fever, allergic rhinitis, asthma or atopic dermatitis is also consistent with ocular allergy.
   D. **Bilateral conjunctivitis** suggests allergic conjunctivitis. Unilateral conjunctivitis suggests infections caused by viruses and bacteria.
   E. **Pain and photophobia** do not usually occur with conjunctivitis, and these findings suggest an ocular or orbital disease processes, including uveitis, keratitis, acute glaucoma or orbital cellulitis. Blurred vision is not characteristic of conjunctivitis and is indicative of corneal or intraocular pathology.
   F. **Recent contact with an individual with an upper respiratory tract infection** suggests adenoviral conjunctivitis. Chlamydial or gonococcal infection may be suggested by the sexual history, including a history of urethral discharge.

II. **Examination of the eye**
   A. Visual acuity should be tested before the examination. Regional lymphadenopathy should be sought and the face and eyelids examined. Viral or chlamydial inclusion conjunctivitis typically presents with a tender, preauricular or submandibular lymph node. Palpable adenopathy is rare in acute bacterial

conjunctivitis. Herpes labialis or a dermatomal vesicular eruption (shingles) is indicative of a herpetic conjunctivitis.

B. Purulent discharge suggests a bacterial infection. Stringy mucoid discharge suggests allergy. Clear watery discharge suggests viral infection.

III. Cultures and Gram stain usually are not required in patients with mild conjunctivitis of suspected viral, bacterial or allergic origin. However, bacterial cultures should be obtained in patients who have severe conjunctivitis.

IV. Treatment of bacterial conjunctivitis

A. Acute bacterial conjunctivitis typically presents with burning, irritation, tearing and a mucopurulent or purulent discharge. The three most common pathogens in bacterial conjunctivitis are *Streptococcus pneumoniae, Haemophilus influenzae* and *Staphylococcus aureus*.

B. Topical broad-spectrum antibiotics such as erythromycin ointment and bacitracin-polymyxin B ointment as well as combination solutions such as trimethoprim-polymyxin B provide excellent coverage for most pathogens. Ointments are better tolerated by young children. Solutions are preferred by adults.

   1. **Erythromycin ophthalmic ointment**, apply to affected eye(s) q3-4h.
   2. **Bacitracin-polymyxin B (Polysporin)** ophthalmic ointment or solution, apply to affected eye(s) q3-4h.
   3. **Trimethoprim-polymyxin B (Polytrim)**, ointment or solution, apply to affected eye(s) q3-4h.

C. Conjunctivitis due to H. influenzae, N. gonorrhoeae, and N. meningitidis requires systemic antibiotic therapy in addition to topical treatment. Gonococcal conjunctivitis may be treated with ceftriaxone (Rocephin) 1 g IM and topical erythromycin.

D. Chlamydial conjunctivitis can be present in newborns, sexually active teenagers, and adults. Diagnosis is by antibody staining of ocular samples. Treatment includes oral tetracycline, doxycycline (Vibramycin) or erythromycin for two weeks.

V. Viral conjunctivitis

A. Adenovirus is the most common cause of viral conjunctivitis. Viral conjunctivitis often occurs in epidemics, typically presenting with an acutely red eye, watery discharge, conjunctival swelling, a tender preauricular node, photophobia and a foreign-body sensation. Some patients have an associated upper respiratory tract infection.

B. Treatment consists of cold compresses and topical vasoconstrictors (Vasocon-A, Naphcon-A). Patients should avoid direct contact with other persons for at least one week after the onset of symptoms.

C. Ocular herpes simplex and herpes zoster is managed with topical agents, including trifluridine (Viroptic) and systemic acyclovir, famciclovir or valacyclovir.

References, see page 268.

Bacterial Meningitis

Meningitis is a life-threatening emergency that may be associated with devastating neurologic sequelae or death. The age group at greatest risk for acute bacterial meningitis (ABM) includes children between 1 and 24 months of age. Adults older than 60 years old account for 50% of all deaths related to meningitis.

I. Clinical presentation
   A. Eighty-five percent of patients with bacterial meningitis present with fever, headache, meningismus or nuchal rigidity, and altered mental status. Other common signs and symptoms include photophobia, vomiting, back pain, myalgias, diaphoresis, and malaise. Generalized seizures can occur in up to 40% of patients with ABM.
   B. Kernig's sign (resistance to extension of the leg while the hip is flexed) and Brudzinski's sign (involuntary flexion of the hip and knee when the patient's neck is abruptly flexed while laying supine) are observed in up to 50% of patients. However, their presence or absence does not rule in or rule out meningitis.
   C. About 50% of patients with N. meningitidis may present with an erythematous macular rash, which progresses to petechiae and purpura.

II. Patient evaluation
   A. Computerized tomography (CT). Patients who require CT prior to LP include those with focal neurologic findings, papilledema, focal seizures, or abnormalities on exam that suggest increased intracranial pressure. If bacterial meningitis is a strong consideration, and the decision is made to perform a CT prior to LP, two sets of blood cultures should be obtained and antibiotics should be administered before sending the patient for neuroimaging. Urine cultures may be helpful in the very young and very old.
   B. Blood cultures followed by antibiotic administration within 30 minutes of presentation is mandatory in all patients suspected of having bacterial meningitis.
   C. Interpretation of lumbar puncture. Examination of the CSF is mandatory for evaluation of meningitis. The following findings have certainty of higher than 99% for the diagnosis of ABM:
   1. CSF glucose <34 mg/dL
   2. CSF: blood glucose ratio <0.23
   3. CSF protein >220 mg/dL
   4. Total CSF leukocyte count >2 x10^6/L
   5. Total CSF neutrophil count >1180 x 10^6/L

Cerebrospinal Fluid Parameters in Meningitis						
	Normal	Bacterial	Viral	Fungal	TB	Parameningeal Focus or Abscess
WBC count (WBC/µL)	0-5	>1000	100-1000	100-500	100-500	10-1000
% PMN	0-15	90	<50	<50	<50	<50
% lymph		>50	>50	>80		
Glucose (mg/dL)	45-65	<40	45-65	30-45	30-45	45-65

	Normal	Bacterial	Viral	Fungal	TB	Parameningeal Focus or Abscess
CSF: blood glucose ratio	0.6	<0.4	0.6	<0.4	<0.4	0.6
Protein (mg/dL)	20-45	>150	50-100	100-500	100-500	>50
Opening pressure (cm H$_2$0)	6-20	>180 mm H$_2$0	NL or +	>180 mm H$_2$0	>180 mm H$_2$0	N/A

Typical CSF Findings in Patients with Bacterial Meningitis

CSF Parameter	Typical Findings
Opening pressure	>180 mm H$_2$0
White blood cell count	1000-5000/mcL (range, <100 to >10,000)
Percentage of neutrophils	>80%
Protein	100-500 mg/dL
Glucose	<40 mg/dL
Lactate	>35 mg/dL
Gram's stain	Positive in 60-90%
Culture	Positive in 70-85%
Bacterial antigen detection	Positive in 50-100%

D. Obtaining two sets of blood cultures prior to antibiotic administration is imperative.

E. If the CSF parameters are nondiagnostic, or the patient has been treated with prior oral antibiotics, and, therefore, the Gram's stain and/or culture are likely to be negative, then latex agglutination (LA) may be helpful. The test has a variable sensitivity rate, ranging between 50-100%, and high specificity. Latex agglutination tests are available for Hib, Streptococcus pneumoniae, N. meningitidis, Escherichia cell K1, and S. agalactiae (Group B strep). CSF Cryptococcal antigen and India ink stain should be considered in patients who have HIV disease or HIV risk factors.

III. Treatment of acute bacterial meningitis

Antibiotic Choice Based on Age and Comorbid Medical Illness

Age	Organism	Antibiotic
Neonate	E. coil, Group B strep, Listeria monocytogenes	Ampicillin and third-generation cephalosporin
1-3 months	S. pneumoniae, N. meningitidis, H. influenzae, S. agalactiae, Listeria, E. coli	Ampicillin and third-generation cephalosporin
3 months to 18 years	N. meningitidis, S. pneumoniae, H. influenzae	Third-generation cephalosporin
18-50 years	S. pneumoniae, N. meningitidis	Third-generation cephalosporin
Older than 50 years	N. meningitidis, S. pneumoniae Gram negative bacilli, Listeria, Group B strep	Ampicillin and third-generation cephalosporin
Neurosurgery/head injury	S. aureus, S. epidermidis Diphtheroids, Gram neg. bacilli	Vancomycin and Ceftazidime
Immunosuppression	Listeria, Gram negative bacilli, S. pneumoniae, N. meningitidis (consider adding Vancomycin)	Ampicillin and Ceftazidime
CSF shunt	S. aureus, Gram negative bacilli	Vancomycin and Ceftazidime

Antibiotic Choice Based on Gram's Stain

Stain Results	Organism	Antibiotic
Gram's (+) cocci	S. pneumoniae, S. aureus S. agalactiae (Group B)	Vancomycin and third-generation cephalosporin
Gram's (-) cocci	N. meningitidis	Penicillin G
Gram's (-) coccobacilli	H. influenzae	Third-generation cephalosporin
Gram's (+) bacilli	Listeria monocytogenes	Ampicillin, Pen G + Gentamycin

Gram's (-) bacilli	E. coli, Klebsiella Serratia, Pseudomonas	Ceftazidime +/- aminoglycoside

Recommended Dosages of Antibiotics

Antibiotic	Dosage
Ampicillin	2g IV q 4 h
Cefotaxime	2g IV q 4-6 h
Ceftazidime	2g IV q 8 h
Ceftriaxone	2g IV q 12 h
Gentamycin	Load 1.5 mg/kg IV, then 1-2mg/kg q8h
Nafcillin/Oxacillin	1.5-2g IV q4h
Penicillin G	4 million units IV q4h
Rifampin	600 mg po q 12-24 h
Trimethoprim-sulfamethoxazole	10 mg/kg IV q 12 h
Vancomycin	1.5-2 g IV q12h

A. In areas characterized by high resistance to penicillin, vancomycin plus a third-generation cephalosporin should be the first-line therapy. H. influenzae is usually adequately covered by a third-generation cephalosporin. The drug of choice for N. meningitidis is penicillin or ampicillin.

B. In patients who are at risk for Listeria meningitis, ampicillin must be added to the regimen. S. agalactiae (Group B) is covered by ampicillin, and adding an aminoglycoside provides synergy. Pseudomonas and other Gram-negative bacilli should be treated with a broad spectrum third-generation cephalosporin (ceftazidime) plus an aminoglycoside. S. aureus may be covered by nafcillin or oxacillin; vancomycin may be needed if the patient is at risk for methicillin-resistant S. aureus.

C. **Corticosteroids.** Audiologic and neurological sequelae in infants older than two months of age are markedly reduced by early administration of dexamethasone in patients with H. influenzae (Hib) meningitis. Dexamethasone should be given at a dose of 0.15 mg/kg every six hours IV for 2-4 days to children with suspected Hib or pneumococcal meningitis. The dose should be given just prior to or with the initiation of antibiotics.

References, see page 268.

Sepsis

Sepsis is the most common cause of death in medical and surgical ICUs. Mortality ranges from 20-60%. The systemic inflammatory response syndrome (SIRS) is an inflammatory response that may be a manifestation of both sepsis and the inflammatory response that results from insults, such as trauma and burns. The term "sepsis" is reserved for patients who have SIRS attributable to documented infection.

Pathophysiology

A. Although gram-negative bacteremia is commonly found in patients with sepsis, gram-positive infection may affect 30-40% of patients. Fungal, viral, and parasitic infections are occasionally encountered as well. Approximately 60% of patients with sepsis have negative blood cultures.

Defining sepsis and related disorders

Term	Definition
Systemic inflammatory response syndrome (SIRS)	The systemic inflammatory response to a variety of severe clinical insults manifested by ≥2 of the following conditions: Temperature >38°C or <36°C, heart rate >90 beats/min, respiratory rate >20 breaths/min or Pa CO2 <32 torr, white blood cell count >12,000 cells/mm3 , <4000 cells/mm 3 , or >10% band cells
Sepsis	The presence of SIRS caused by an infectious process; it is considered severe if hypotension or systemic manifestations of hypoperfusion (lactic acidosis, oliguria, or change in mental status) are present.
Septic shock	Sepsis-induced hypotension despite adequate fluid resuscitation, along with the presence of perfusion abnormalities that may induce lactic acidosis, oliguria, or an acute alteration in mental status.
Multiple organ dysfunction syndrome (MODS)	The presence of altered organ function in an acutely ill patient such that homeostasis cannot be maintained without intervention

B. Sources of bacteremia leading to sepsis include the urinary, respiratory and GI tracts, and skin and soft tissues (including catheter sites). The source of bacteremia is unknown in 30% of patients.

C. Escherichia coli is the most frequently encountered gram-negative organism, followed by Klebsiella, Enterobacter, Serratia, Pseudomonas, Proteus, Providencia, and Bacteroides species. Up to 16% of sepsis cases are polymicrobic.

D. Gram-positive organisms, including Staphylococcus aureus and Staphylococcus epidermidis, are associated with catheter or line-related infections. Fungemias may occur in immunocompromised patients or as superinfections in critically ill patients.

Clinical evaluation

A. Although fever is the most common sign of sepsis, normal body temperatures and hypothermia are common in the elderly. Tachypnea and/or hyperventilation with respiratory alkalosis may occur before the onset of fever or leukocytosis it is often the earliest sign of sepsis.

B. Other common clinical signs of systemic inflammation or impaired organ perfusion include altered mentation, oliguria, and tachycardia. Manifestations of sepsis-related altered mental status range from mild disorientation and lethargy to confusion, agitation, and frank obtundation.

C. In the early stages of sepsis, tachycardia is associated with increased cardiac output; peripheral vasodilation; and a warm, well-perfused appearance. As shock develops, vascular resistance continues to fall, hypotension ensues and myocardial depression progresses and results in decreased cardiac output. During the later stages of septic shock, vasoconstriction and cold extremities develop.

D. Laboratory findings. In the early stages of sepsis, arterial blood gas measurements usually reveal respiratory alkalosis. As shock ensues, metabolic acidosis--or mixed metabolic acidosis with respiratory alkalosis--becomes apparent. Hypoxemia is common.

Manifestations of Sepsis	
Clinical features	**Laboratory findings**
Temperature instability	Respiratory alkaloses
Tachypnea	Hypoxemia
Hyperventilation	Increased serum lactate levels
Altered mental status	Leukocytosis and increased
Oliguria	neutrophil concentration
Tachycardia	Eosinopenia
Peripheral vasodilation	Thrombocytopenia
	Anemia
	Proteinuria
	Mildly elevated serum bilirubin
	levels

1. Leukocytosis accompanied by an increased percentage of neutrophils is frequently an early finding in sepsis. Eosinopenia is also commonly encountered. Thrombocytopenia occurs early and can be severe.

2. Disseminated intravascular coagulation is seen in patients with profound sepsis. It is characterized by thrombocytopenia, elevated prothrombin and partial thromboplastin times, decreased fibrinogen levels, and elevated levels of fibrin degradation products.

3. Anemia may be caused by dilution from resuscitation with intravenous solutions, bleeding, chronic disease, and acute inflammation.

4. Renal manifestations of sepsis range from minimal proteinuria to acute tubular necrosis and renal failure. Renal insufficiency may occasionally be attributable to an acute glomerulonephritis or interstitial nephritis. Shock may result in oliguria, azotemia, and acute tubular necrosis or cortical necrosis.

5. Liver function abnormalities range from mildly elevated serum bilirubin levels in the early stages to severe hepatocellular damage with markedly elevated transaminase levels in the later stages.

E. Hemodynamics

1. The hallmark of early septic shock is a dramatic drop in systemic vascular resistance, which may precede a decrease in blood pressure.

2. Cardiac output rises in response to the fall in systemic blood pressure. This is referred to as the "hyperdynamic state" in sepsis. Shock results if the increase in cardiac output is insufficient to maintain blood pressure. Diminished cardiac output may also occur as systemic blood pressure falls.

Treatment of sepsis

A. **Resuscitation.** During the initial resuscitation of a hypotensive patient with sepsis, large volumes of IV fluid should be given to support systemic blood pressure and cardiac output. Initial resuscitation may require 4 to 6 L of crystalloid. Fluid infusion volumes should be titrated to obtain a pulmonary capillary wedge pressure of 10 to 20 mm Hg. Other indices of organ perfusion include oxygen delivery, serum lactate levels, arterial blood pressure, and urinary output.

B. **Vasopressor and inotropic therapy** is necessary if hypotension persists despite aggressive fluid resuscitation.
   1. **Dopamine** is a first-line agent for sepsis-associated hypotension. It has combined dopaminergic, alpha-adrenergic and beta-adrenergic activities. Begin with 5 µg/kg/min and titrate the dosage to the desired blood pressure response, usually a systolic blood pressure of greater than 90 mm Hg.
   2. **Epinephrine or norepinephrine infusions** may be used if hypotension persists despite high dosages of dopamine (20 µg/kg/min), or if dopamine causes excessive tachycardia. These agents have alpha-adrenergic and beta-adrenergic effects and cause peripheral vasoconstriction and increased cardiac contractility.
   3. **Dobutamine** can be added to increase cardiac output and oxygen delivery through its beta-adrenergic inotropic effects.

Vasoactive and Inotropic Drugs	
Agent	**Dosage**
Dopamine	**Inotropic Dose:** 5-10 mcg/kg/min **Vasoconstricting Dose:** 10-20 mcg/kg/min
Dobutamine	**Inotropic:** 5-10 mcg/kg/min **Vasodilator:** 15-20 mcg/kg/min
Norepinephrine	**Vasoconstricting dose:** 2-8 mcg/min
Phenylephrine	**Vasoconstricting dose:** 20-200 mcg/min
Epinephrine	**Vasoconstricting dose:** 1-8 mcg/min

C. **Diagnosis and management infection**
   1. **Initial treatment of life-threatening sepsis** usually consists of a third-generation cephalosporin (ceftazidime, cefotaxime, ceftizoxime), ticarcillin/clavulanic acid, or imipenem. An aminoglycoside (gentamicin, tobramycin, or amikacin) should also be included. Antipseudomonal coverage is important for hospital- or institutional-acquired infections. Appropriate choices include an antipseudomonal penicillin or cephalosporin or an aminoglycoside.
   2. **Methicillin-resistant staphylococci.** If line sepsis or an infected implanted device is a possibility, vancomycin should be added to the regimen to cover

for methicillin-resistant Staph aureus and methicillin-resistant Staph epidermidis.

3. **Intra-abdominal or pelvic infections** are likely to involve anaerobes therefore, treatment should include either ticarcillin/clavulanic acid ampicillin/sulbactam, piperacillin/tazobactam, imipenem, cefoxitin o cefotetan. An aminoglycoside should be included. Alternatively metronidazole with an aminoglycoside and ampicillin may be initiated.

4. **Biliary tract infections.** When the source of bacteremia is thought to be the biliary tract, cefoperazone, piperacillin plus metronidazole piperacillin/tazobactam, or ampicillin/sulbactam with an aminoglycoside should be used.

Dosages of antibiotics used in sepsis

Agent	Dosage
Cefotaxime (Claforan)	2 gm q4-6h
Ceftizoxime (Cefizox)	2 gm IV q8h
Cefoxitin (Mefoxin)	2 gm q6h
Cefotetan (Cefotan)	2 gm IV q12h
Ceftazidime (Fortaz)	2 g IV q8h
Ticarcillin/clavulanate (Timentin)	3.1 gm IV q4-6h (200-300 mg/kg/d)
Ampicillin/sulbactam (Unasyn)	3.0 gm IV q6h
Piperacillin/tazobactam (Zosyn)	3.375-4.5 gm IV q6h
Piperacillin, ticarcillin, mezlocillin	3 gm IV q4-6h
Meropenem (Merrem)	1 gm IV q8h
Imipenem/ Cilastatin (Primaxin)	0.5-1.0 gm IV q6h
Gentamicin or tobramycin	2 mg/kg IV loading dose, then 1.7 mg/kg IV q8h
Amikacin (Amikin)	7.5 mg/kg IV loading dose; then 5 mg/kg IV q8h
Vancomycin	1 gm IV q12h
Metronidazole (Flagyl)	500 mg IV q6-8h

5. **Multiple-antibiotic-resistant enterococci**
   a. An increasing number of enterococcal strains are resistant to ampicillin and gentamicin. The incidence of vancomycin-resistant enterococci (VRE) is rapidly increasing.
   b. Quinupristin/dalfopristin (Synercid) is a parenteral agent active against

strains of vancomycin-resistant enterococci, except E. faecium and E. faecalis.
  c. Linezolid (Zyvox) is an oral or parenteral agent active against vancomycin-resistant enterococci, including E. faecium and E. faecalis.

References, see page 268.

Diverticulitis

By age 50, one-third of adults have diverticulosis coli; two-thirds have diverticulosis by age 80. Diverticulitis or diverticular hemorrhage occurs in 10-20% of patients with diverticulosis. Causes of diverticulosis include aging, elevation of colonic intraluminal pressure, and decreased dietary fiber. Eighty-five percent are found in the sigmoid colon.

I. Clinical presentation of diverticulitis
  A. Diverticulitis is characterized by the abrupt onset of unremitting left-lower quadrant abdominal pain, fever, and an alteration in bowel pattern. Diverticulitis of the transverse colon may simulate ulcer pain; diverticulitis of the cecum and redundant sigmoid may resemble appendicitis.
  B. **Physical exam.** Left-lower quadrant tenderness is characteristic. Abdominal examination is often deceptively unremarkable in the elderly and in persons taking corticosteroids.

Differential Diagnosis of Diverticulitis	
Elderly	**Middle Aged and Young**
Ischemic colitis Carcinoma Volvulus Colonic Obstruction Penetrating ulcer Nephrolithiasis/urosepsis	Appendicitis Salpingitis Inflammatory bowel disease Penetrating ulcer Urosepsis

II. Diagnostic evaluation
  A. **Plain X-rays** may show ileus, obstruction, mass effect, ischemia, or perforation.
  B. **CT scan** is the test of choice to evaluate acute diverticulitis. The CT scan can be used for detecting complications and ruling out other diseases.
  C. **Contrast enema.** Water soluble contrast is safe and useful in mild-to-moderate cases of diverticulitis when the diagnosis is in doubt.
  D. **Endoscopy.** Acute diverticulitis is a relative contraindication to endoscopy; perforation should be excluded first. Endoscopy is indicated when the diagnosis is in doubt to exclude the possibility of ischemic bowel, Crohn's disease, or carcinoma.
  E. **Complete blood count** may show leukocytosis.

III. Treatment
A. Outpatient treatment
1. **Clear liquid diet**
2. **Oral antibiotics**
   a. Ciprofloxacin (Cipro) 500 mg PO bid **AND**
   b. Metronidazole (Flagyl) 500 mg PO qid.

B. Inpatient treatment
1. Severe cases require hospitalization for gastrointestinal tract rest (NPO), intravenous fluid hydration, and antibiotics. Nasogastric suction is initiated if the patient is vomiting or if there is abdominal distention.
2. Antibiotic coverage should include enteric gram-negative and anaerobic organisms
   a. Ampicillin 1-2 gm IV q4-6h **AND**
   b. Gentamicin or tobramycin 100-120 mg IV (1.5-2 mg/kg), then 80 mg IV q8h (5 mg/kg/d) **AND**
   c. Metronidazole (Flagyl) 500 mg IV q6-8h (15-30 mg/kg/d) **OR**
   d. Cefoxitin (Mefoxin) 2 gm IV q6h **OR**
   e. Piperacillin-tazobactam (Zosyn) 3.375-4.5 gm IV q6h.

C. Failure to improve or deterioration are indications for reevaluation and consideration of surgery. Analgesics should be avoided because they may mask acute deterioration, and they may obscure the need for urgent operation.
D. Oral antibiotics should be continued for 1-2 weeks after resolution of the acute attack. Ciprofloxacin, 500 mg PO bid.
E. After the acute attack has resolved, clear liquids should be initiated, followed by a low residue diet for 1-2 weeks, followed by a high-fiber diet with psyllium.

IV. Surgical therapy
A. An emergency sigmoid colectomy with proximal colostomy is indicated for attacks of diverticulitis associated with sepsis, peritonitis, obstruction, or perforation.
B. Elective sigmoid resection is indicated for second or subsequent attacks of diverticulitis, or for attacks with complications managed nonoperatively (eg, percutaneous CT-guided drainage of an abscess), or carcinoma.
C. Operative procedures
1. **Single-stage procedure.** This procedure is usually performed as an elective procedure after resolution of the acute attack of diverticulitis. The segment containing inflamed diverticulum (usually sigmoid colon) is resected with primary anastomosis. A bowel prep is required.
2. **Two-stage procedure.** This procedure is indicated for acute diverticulitis with obstruction or perforation with an unprepared bowel. The first stage consists of resection of the involved segment of colon with end colostomy and either a mucous fistula or a Hartmann rectal pouch. The second stage consists of a colostomy take-down and reanastomosis after 2-3 months.

References, see page 268.

Urinary Tract Infection

An estimated 40 percent of women report having had a urinary tract infections (UTI) at some point in their lives. UTIs are the leading cause of gram-negative bacteremia.

I. Acute uncomplicated cystitis in young women

A. Sexually active young women have the highest risk for UTIs. Their propensity to develop UTIs is caused by a short urethra, delays in micturition, sexual activity, and the use of diaphragms and spermicides.

B. Symptoms of cystitis include dysuria, urgency, and frequency without fever or back pain. Lower tract infections are most common in women in their childbearing years. Fever is absent.

C. A microscopic bacterial count of 100 CFU/mL of urine has a high positive predictive value for cystitis in symptomatic women. Ninety percent of uncomplicated cystitis episodes are caused by *Escherichia coli*; 10 to 20 percent are caused by coagulase-negative *Staphylococcus saprophyticus* and 5 percent are caused by other Enterobacteriaceae organisms or enterococci. Up to one-third of uropathogens are resistant to ampicillin, but the majority are susceptible to trimethoprim-sulfamethoxazole (85 to 95 percent) and fluoroquinolones (95 percent).

D. Young women with acute uncomplicated cystitis should receive urinalysis (examination of spun urine) and a dipstick test for leukocyte esterase.

E. A positive leukocyte esterase test has a sensitivity of 75 to 90 percent in detecting pyuria associated with a UTI. The dipstick test for nitrite indicates bacteriuria. Enterococci, *S. saprophyticus* and Acinetobacter species produce false-negative results on nitrite testing.

F. Three-day antibiotic regimens offer the optimal combination of convenience, low cost and efficacy comparable to seven-day or longer regimens.

G. Trimethoprim-sulfamethoxazole (Bactrim, Septra), 1 DS tab bid for 3 days, remains the antibiotic of choice in the treatment of uncomplicated UTIs in young women.

H. A fluoroquinolone is recommended for patients who cannot tolerate sulfonamides or trimethoprim, who have a high frequency of antibiotic resistance because of recent antibiotic treatment, or who reside in an area with significant resistance to trimethoprim-sulfamethoxazole. Treatment should consist of a three-day regimen of one of the following:

  1. Ciprofloxacin (Cipro), 250 mg bid.

  2. Ofloxacin (Floxin), 200 mg bid.

I. A seven-day course should be considered in pregnant women, diabetic women and women who have had symptoms for more than one week and thus are at higher risk for pyelonephritis.

II. Recurrent cystitis in young women

A. Up to 20 percent of young women with acute cystitis develop recurrent UTIs. The causative organism should be identified by urine culture. Multiple infections caused by the same organism require longer courses of antibiotics and possibly further diagnostic tests. Women who have more than three UTI recurrences within one year can be managed using one of three preventive strategies:

  1. Acute self-treatment with a three-day course of standard therapy.

  2. Postcoital prophylaxis with one-half of a trimethoprim-sulfamethoxazole double-strength tablet (40/200 mg) if the UTIs have been clearly related to intercourse.

  3. Continuous daily prophylaxis for six months: Trimethoprim-sulfamethoxazole, one-half tablet/day (40/200 mg); norfloxacin (Noroxin), 200 mg/day; cephalexin (Keflex), 250 mg/day.

III. Pyelonephritis

A. Acute uncomplicated pyelonephritis presents with a mild cystitis-like illness and accompanying flank pain; fever, chills, nausea, vomiting, leukocytosis and abdominal pain; or a serious gram-negative bacteremia. The microbiologic features of acute uncomplicated pyelonephritis are the same as cystitis, except that *S. saprophyticus* is a rare cause.

B. The diagnosis should be confirmed by urinalysis with examination for pyuria and/or white blood cell casts and by urine culture. Urine cultures demonstrate more than 100,000 CFU/mL of urine. Blood cultures are positive in 20%.

C. Oral therapy should be considered in women with mild to moderate symptoms. Since *E. coli* resistance to ampicillin, amoxicillin and first-generation cephalosporins exceeds 30 percent, these agents should not be used for the treatment of pyelonephritis. Resistance to trimethoprim-sulfamethoxazole exceeds 15 percent; therefore, empiric therapy with ciprofloxacin (Cipro), 250 mg twice daily is recommended.

D. Patients who are too ill to take oral antibiotics should initially be treated parenterally with a third-generation cephalosporin, a broad-spectrum penicillin, a quinolone or an aminoglycoside. Once these patients have improved clinically, they can be switched to oral therapy.

E. The total duration of therapy is usually 14 days. Patients with persistent symptoms after three days of appropriate antimicrobial therapy should be evaluated by renal ultrasonography or computed tomography for evidence of urinary obstruction. In the small percentage of patients who relapse after a two-week course, a repeated six-week course is usually curative.

IV. Urinary tract infection in men

A. Urinary tract infections most commonly occur in older men with prostatic disease, outlet obstruction or urinary tract instrumentation. In men, a urine culture growing more than 1,000 CFU of a pathogen/mL of urine is the best sign of a urinary tract infection, with a sensitivity and specificity of 97 percent. Men with urinary tract infections should receive seven days of antibiotic therapy (trimethoprim-sulfamethoxazole or a fluoroquinolone).

B. Urologic evaluation should be performed routinely in adolescents and men with pyelonephritis or recurrent infections. When bacterial prostatitis is the source of a urinary tract infection, eradication usually requires antibiotic therapy for six to 12 weeks.

References, see page 268.

Syphilis

Syphilis, an infection caused by *Treponema pallidum*, is usually sexually transmitted and is characterized by episodes of active disease interrupted by periods of latency.

I. Clinical evaluation

A. Primary syphilis

1. The incubation period for syphilis is 10-90 days; 21 days is average. The lesion begins as a painless, solitary nodule that becomes an indurated ulceration (chancre) with a ham-colored, eroded surface, and a serous discharge found on or near the genitalia. Atypical lesions are frequent and

may take the form of small multiple lesions.
2. The chancre is usually accompanied by painless, enlarged regional lymph nodes. Untreated lesions heal in 1-5 weeks.
3. The diagnosis is made by the clinical appearance and a positive darkfield examination; the serologic test (VDRL, RPR) is often negative in the first 4-6 weeks after infection.

B. Secondary syphilis

1. Twenty-five percent of untreated patients progress to secondary syphilis 2-6 months after exposure. Secondary syphilis lasts for 4-6 weeks.
2. Bilateral, symmetrical, macular, papular, or papulosquamous skin lesions become widespread. The lesions are non-pruritic and frequently involve the palms, soles, face, trunk and extremities. Condyloma lata consists of rash and moist lesions. Secondary syphilis is highly infectious. Mucous membranes are often involved, appearing as white patches in the mouth, nose, vagina, and rectum.
3. Generalized nontender lymphadenopathy and patchy alopecia sometimes occur. A small percentage of patients have iritis, hepatitis, meningitis, fever, and headache.
4. The serologic test (VDRL, RPR) is positive in >99% of cases; the test may be falsely negative because of the prozone phenomenon caused by high antigen titers. Retesting of a diluted blood sample may be positive. No culture test is available.

C. Latent syphilis consists of the interval between secondary syphilis and late syphilis. Patients have no signs or symptoms, only positive serological tests.

D. Late syphilis is characterized by destruction of tissue, organs, and organ systems.

1. **Late benign syphilis.** Gummas occur in skin or bone.
2. **Cardiovascular syphilis.** Medial necrosis of the aorta may lead to aortic insufficiency or aortic aneurysms.
3. **Neurosyphilis**
   a. Spinal fluid shows elevated WBCs, increased total protein, and positive serology.
   b. Pupillary changes are common; the Argyll Robertson pupil accommodates but does not react to light.
   c. Neurosyphilis may cause general paresis or tabes dorsalis--degeneration of the sensory neurons in the posterior columns of the spinal cord.

II. Serology

A. Nontreponemal tests

1. Complement fixation tests (VDRL or RPR) are used for screening; they become positive 4-6 weeks after infection. The tests start in low titer and, over several weeks, may reach 1:32 or higher. After adequate treatment of primary syphilis, the titer becomes nonreactive within 9-18 months.
2. False-positive tests occur in hepatitis, mononucleosis, viral pneumonia, malaria, varicella, autoimmune diseases, diseases associated with increased globulins, narcotic addicts, leprosy, and old age.

B. Treponemal tests

1. Treponemal tests include the FTA-ABS test, TPI test, and microhemagglutination assay for T. pallidum (MHA-TP). A treponemal test should be used to confirm a positive VDRL or RPR.
2. Treponemal tests are specific to treponema antibodies and will remain positive after treatment. All patients with syphilis should be tested for HIV.

III. Treatment of primary or secondary syphilis

A. Primary or secondary syphilis. Benzathine penicillin G, 2.4 million units IM in a single dose.

B. Patients who have syphilis and who also have symptoms or signs suggesting neurologic disease (meningitis) or ophthalmic disease (uveitis) should be evaluated for neurosyphilis and syphilitic eye disease (CSF analysis and ocular slit-lamp examination).

C. Penicillin allergic patients. Doxycycline 100 mg PO 2 times a day for 2 weeks.

D. Follow-up and retreatment

   1. Early syphilis--repeat VDRL at 3, 6, and 12 months to ensure that titers are declining.
   2. Syphilis >1 year--also repeat VDRL at 24 months.
   3. Neurosyphilis-- also repeat VDRL for 3 years.
   4. **Indications for retreatment**
      a. Clinical signs or symptoms persist or recur.
      b. Four-fold increase in the titer of a nontreponemal test (VDRL).
      c. Failure of an initially high titer nontreponemal test (VDRL) to show a 4-fold decrease within a year.
   5. Sex partners should be evaluated and treated.

IV. Treatment of latent syphilis

A. Patients who have latent syphilis who have acquired syphilis within the preceding year are classified as having early latent syphilis. Latent syphilis of unknown duration should be managed as late latent syphilis.

B. Treatment of early latent syphilis. Benzathine penicillin G, 2.4 million units IM in a single dose.

C. Treatment of late latent syphilis or latent syphilis of unknown duration. Benzathine penicillin G 2.4 million units IM each week x 3 weeks.

D. All patients should be evaluated clinically for evidence of late syphilis (aortitis, neurosyphilis, gumma, iritis).

E. Indications for CSF examination before treatment

   1. Neurologic or ophthalmic signs or symptoms
   2. Other evidence of active syphilis (aortitis, gumma, iritis)
   3. Treatment failure
   4. HIV infection
   5. Serum nontreponemal titer >1:32, unless duration of infection is known to be <1 year
   6. Nonpenicillin therapy planned, unless duration of infection is known to be <1 year.

F. CSF examination includes cell count, protein, and CSF-VDRL. If a CSF examination is performed and the results are abnormal, the patient should be treated for neurosyphilis.

V. Treatment of late syphilis

A. Benzathine penicillin G 2.4 million units IM weekly x 3 weeks. Penicillin allergic patients are treated with doxycycline, 100 mg PO bid x 4 weeks.

B. Patients with late syphilis should undergo CSF examination before therapy.

VI. Treatment of neurosyphilis

A. Central nervous system disease can occur during any stage of syphilis. Evidence of neurologic involvement (eg, ophthalmic or auditory symptoms, cranial nerve palsies) warrants a CSF examination. Patients with CSF abnormalities should have follow-up CSF examinations to assess response to treatment.

B. Treatment of neurosyphilis. Penicillin G 2-4 million units IV q4h for 10-14 days. Alternatively, penicillin G procaine 2.4 million units IM daily plus probenecid 500 mg PO qid, both for 10-14 days, can be used.

C. Follow-up. If CSF pleocytosis was present initially, CSF examination should be repeated every 6 months until the cell count is normal.

References, see page 268.

Gastrointestinal Disorders

Peptic Ulcer Disease

Peptic ulcer disease is diagnosed in 500,000 patients each year in the United States. Patients with peptic ulcer disease should be treated as having an infectious illness caused by the bacterium *Helicobacter pylori*. Peptic ulcer disease due to *H pylori* infection can be cured with a combination of antimicrobial and antisecretory drugs.

I. **Pathophysiology**
   A. Helicobacter pylori (HP), a spiral-shaped, flagellated organism, is the most frequent cause of peptic ulcer disease (PUD). Nonsteroidal anti-inflammatory drugs (NSAIDs) and pathologically high acid-secreting states (Zollinger-Ellison syndrome) are less common causes. More than 90% of ulcers are associated with H. pylori. Eradication of the organism cures and prevents relapses of gastroduodenal ulcers.
   B. **Complications of peptic ulcer disease** include bleeding, duodenal or gastric perforation, and gastric outlet obstruction (due to inflammation or strictures).

I. **Clinical evaluation**
   A. **Symptoms of PUD** include recurrent upper abdominal pain and discomfort. The pain of duodenal ulceration is often relieved by food and antacids and worsened when the stomach is empty (eg, at nighttime). In gastric ulceration, the pain may be exacerbated by eating.
   B. **Nausea aud vomiting** are common in PUD. Hematemesis ("coffee ground" emesis) or melena (black tarry stools) are indicative of bleeding.
   C. **Physical examination.** Tenderness to deep palpation is often present in the epigastrium, and the stool is often guaiac-positive.

Classic presentation of uncomplicated peptic ulcer disease

Epigastric pain (burning, vague abdominal discomfort, nausea)
    Often nocturnal
    Occurs with hunger or hours after meals
    Usually temporarily relieved by meals or antacids
Persistence or recurrence over months to years
History of self-medication and intermittent relief

   D. **NSAID-related gastrointestinal complications**. NSAID use and *H pylori* infection are independent risk factors for peptic ulcer disease. The risk is 5 to 20 times higher in persons who use NSAIDs than in the general population. Misoprostol (Cytotec) has been shown to prevent both NSAID ulcers and related complications. The minimum effective dosage is 200 micrograms twice daily; total daily doses of 600 micrograms or 800 micrograms are significantly more effective.

Laboratory and diagnostic testing
   A. Alarm signs and symptoms that suggest gastric cancer are indications for early endoscopy or upper gastrointestinal radiology studies.

Indications for early endoscopy	
Anorexia Dysphagia Gastrointestinal bleeding (gross or occult) New-onset symptoms in persons ≥45 yr of age	Presence of a mass Unexplained anemia Unexplained weight loss Vomiting (severe)

B. Noninvasive testing for H pylori

1. In the absence of alarm symptoms for gastric cancer, most patients with dyspepsia should undergo evaluation for *H pylori* infection with serologic testing for *H pylori* antigens.

2. **Serologic tests** to detect *H pylori* antibodies are the preferred testing method. Serologic testing is highly sensitive, but it cannot be used for follow-up after therapy because antibody titers fall slowly and may remain elevated for a year or longer. Rapid office-based serologic kits have a sensitivity of 90% and a specificity of 85%.

3. **Urea breath tests** measure the carbon dioxide produced when *H pylori* urease metabolizes urea labeled with radioactive carbon (13C or 14C). The 13C test does not involve a radioactive isotope and, unlike the 14C test, can be used in children and pregnant women. With the 13C test, exhaled breath samples are usually sent to a central testing facility. The 14C test, which exposes the patient to a small dose of radiation, can be analyzed in a hospital's nuclear medicine laboratory. Urea breath tests have a sensitivity and specificity of 90-99%. The urea breath test is the best method of confirmation of care.

4. **Stool testing** for H pylori antigens has an accuracy for pretreatment testing of *H pylori* that is similar to that of other available tests.

5. **Biopsy-based testing** performed at endoscopy can provide valuable information via histologic testing, rapid urease tests, and culture. Sensitivity of the tests for *H pylori* ranges from 80% to 100%, and specificity exceeds 95%.

IV. Treatment of peptic ulcer disease

A. Combination therapy

1. Dual therapy is not recommended because cure rates for all regimens are less than 85%. Recommended triple therapies consist of a bismuth preparation or proton pump inhibitor or H2 receptor antagonist plus two antibiotics.

Triple therapies for peptic ulcer disease

BMT therapy:
Bismuth subsalicylate (Pepto-Bismol), 2 tablets with meals and at bedtime for 14 days
and
Metronidazole (Flagyl), 250 mg with meals and at bedtime (total daily dose, 1,000 mg) for 14 days
and
Tetracycline, 500 mg with meals and at bedtime (total daily dose, 2 g) for 14 days
or
A prepackaged triple-therapy agent (**Helidac**), to be taken qid for 14 days, consists of 525 mg bismuth subsalicylate, 250 mg metronidazole, and 500 mg tetracycline; an H_2-blocker or proton pump inhibitor should be added (Omeprazole [Prilosec], 20 mg qd or lansoprazole [Prevacid], 15 mg qd).

Ranitidine bismuth citrate (Tritec), 1 tablet (400 mg) bid for 14 days
and
Tetracycline, 500 mg bid for 14 days
and
Clarithromycin (Biaxin) **or** metronidazole (Flagyl), 500 mg bid for 14 days

Omeprazole (Prilosec), 20 mg bid, **or** lansoprazole (Prevacid), 30 mg bid
and
Clarithromycin (Biaxin), 250 or 500 mg bid for 14 days
and
Metronidazole (Flagyl), 500 mg bid, **or** amoxicillin, 1 g bid for 14 days
or
A prepackaged triple-therapy agent (**Prevpac**), to be taken bid for 14 days, consists of 30 mg lansoprazole, 1 g amoxicillin, and 500 mg clarithromycin.

2. The *H pylori* eradication rate is 96% for patients who take more than 60% of their medication.

B. Confirmation of cure of *H pylori* infection
1. Is it always necessary to confirm cure of *H pylori* infection. About 75% of patients presumed to have uncomplicated peptic ulcer disease due to *H pylori* infection are cured after one course of therapy.
2. The urea breath test is the best method for assessing the effectiveness of therapy. The stool antigen test appears to be only slightly less accurate, and its use should be considered when breath testing is not available.
3. Confirmation of cure must be delayed until at least 4 to 6 weeks after completion of antimicrobial therapy. Treatment with proton pump inhibitors must be discontinued at least 1 week before urea breath testing to confirm cure. H2-receptor antagonists have no effect on the urea breath test and need not be discontinued before confirmation testing.

C. Treatment of NSAID-related ulcers
1. When the ulcer is caused by NSAID use, healing of the ulcer is greatly facilitated by discontinuing the NSAID. Acid antisecretory therapy with an H2-blocker or proton pump inhibitor speeds ulcer healing. Proton pump inhibitors are more effective in inhibiting gastric acid production and are often used to heal ulcers in patients who require continuing NSAID treatment.
2. If serologic or endoscopic testing for H pylori is positive, antibiotic treatment is necessary.
3. **Acute H_2-blocker therapy**
   a. **Ranitidine (Zantac)**, 150 mg bid or 300 mg qhs.

          b. Famotidine (Pepcid), 20 mg bid or 40 mg qhs.
          c. Nizatidine (Axid Pulvules), 150 mg bid or 300 mg qhs.
          d. Cimetidine (Tagamet), 400 mg bid or 800 mg qhs.
      4. Proton pump inhibitors
          a. Omeprazole (Prilosec), 20 mg qd.
          b. Lansoprazole (Prevacid), 15 mg before breakfast qd.
V. Surgical treatment of peptic ulcer disease
    A. Indications for surgery. Exsanguinating hemorrhage, >5 units transfusion in 24 hours, rebleeding during same hospitalization, intractability, perforation, gastric outlet obstruction, endoscopic signs predictive of rebleeding.
    B. Unstable patients should receive a truncal vagotomy, oversewing of bleeding ulcer bed, and pyloroplasty.

References, see page 268.

Gastroesophageal Reflux Disease

About 18% of the adult population in the United States have heartburn at least once a week. Gastroesophageal reflux describes the movement of gastric acid into the esophagus. The major antireflux barrier is the lower esophageal sphincter (LES) located at the esophagogastric junction. Patients with disordered esophageal motility from connective-tissue diseases or primary motility disorders and those with hyposalivation from chronic xerostomia, cigarette smoking, or anticholinergic medications are predisposed to increased severity of GERD.

I. Clinical evaluation
    A. Heartburn, defined as a retrosternal burning sensation radiating to the pharynx and acid regurgitation are classic symptoms of GERD. They usually occur postprandially, especially after large meals.
    B. Symptoms may be exacerbated by recumbency, straining, and bending over and are usually improved by antacids. These symptoms are specific enough that their presence establishes the diagnosis of GERD without confirmatory tests.

II. Complications
    A. Esophagitis with ulceration may result in gastrointestinal hemorrhage, which is reported in about 2% of patients with reflux esophagitis.
    B. Esophageal strictures form in about 10% of patients with GERD. These patients are managed with periodic dilations and acid suppression with proton pump inhibitors.
    C. Barrett's esophagus. Metaplastic changes in the esophageal mucosa that result from GERD are referred to as Barrett's esophagus. The presence of columnar appearing epithelium more than 3 cm above the proximal gastric folds is criterion for diagnosis. The reported incidence of adenocarcinoma in Barrett's esophagus, which is considered a premalignant condition, is 1 in 52 patient years.
    D. Extraesophageal manifestations of GERD may include noncardiac chest pain, chronic hoarseness and cough, and asthma

III. Diagnosis
    A. Esophageal endoscopy is the most popular test for initial evaluation of GERD symptoms. Barium swallow modified by a barium-coated test meal is the most sensitive test for evaluation of dysphagia. The observation of reflux of free barium into the esophagus establishes the diagnosis of GERD.

B. Ambulatory esophageal pH monitoring is the best test to establish the presence of abnormal acid esophageal reflux, although it provides no information about the esophageal structure or mucosa.

. **Treatment**

Lifestyle modifications recommended for all patients with GERD

Stop smoking cigarettes
Lose excess weight
Eat small meals
Reduce consumption of caffeine, chocolate, fatty foods, alcohol, onions, peppermint, and spearmint
Elevate head of bed 6 to 9 in.
Avoid tight-fitting garments

A. Antacids. Antacids work by neutralizing gastric acid and are indicated for treatment of occasional heartburn. Antacids have a very short duration of action, necessitating frequent dosing.

B. Histamine antagonists
   1. Histamine$_2$ (H$_2$) receptor antagonists are moderately effective for treating GERD. These drugs are safe, with rare side effects. However, cimetidine may cause mental status changes, antiandrogenic activity (gynecomastia), and inhibition of the cytochrome P-450 system, which may alter levels of drugs metabolized by this pathway (eg, theophylline, warfarin, phenytoin).
   2. The indicated oral doses for the treatment of reflux esophagitis are cimetidine (Tagamet), 800 mg twice daily; ranitidine (Zantac), 150 mg two to four times daily; famotidine (Pepcid), 20 mg to 40 mg twice daily; and nizatidine (Axid), 150 mg twice daily. The efficacy of all the H$_2$ receptor antagonists is equivalent.

C. Proton pump inhibitors
   1. The proton pump inhibitors (PPIs), omeprazole (Prilosec) and lansoprazole (Prevacid), are the most effective acid-suppressing medications available. These drugs inhibit the proton pump.
   2. The usual dosage for treatment of reflux esophagitis is 20 to 40 mg of omeprazole (Prilosec) daily or 30 mg of lansoprazole (Prevacid) daily. At these doses, reflux symptoms are abolished in most patients. PPIs are safe and well tolerated. Side effects of headache, abdominal pain and diarrhea are rare.

D. Patients with classic symptoms who are less than 40 years old and who have had symptoms for less than 10 years do not require diagnostic studies. Indications for upper gastrointestinal endoscopy include onset of new symptoms in older patients with long-standing GERD, the presence of alarm symptoms, atypical or equivocal symptoms, and failure of full-dose H$_2$ receptor antagonist therapy.

Alarm symptoms in patients with suspected GERD
Hematemesis
Melena
Dysphagia
Unexplained weight loss
Frequent vomiting

V. Antireflux surgery is now commonly performed laparoscopically. They involve reduction of the hiatal hernia and wrapping of the proximal stomach around the distal esophagus (Nissen fundoplication). Antireflux surgery is reserved for patients who do not respond to medical therapy and for patients who prefer surgical treatment to long-term medication use. After antireflux surgery, about 90% of patients are symptom-free at 1 year, and 60% to 80% remain asymptomatic at long-term follow-up.

References, see page 268.

Viral Hepatitis

Acute viral hepatitis consists of hepatocellular necrosis and inflammation caused by hepatitis A virus (HAV), hepatitis B virus (HBV), hepatitis C virus (HCV), hepatitis D virus (HDV), or hepatitis E virus (HEV). Chronic viral hepatitis is seen with HBV, HCV, and HDV infection. Hepatitis A and hepatitis E virus do not cause a chronic carrier state or chronic liver disease.

I. **Clinical manifestations of viral hepatitis**
    A. **Acute viral hepatitis**
        1. **Symptoms of acute hepatitis** include anorexia, fatigue, myalgias and nausea, developing 1-2 weeks prior to the onset of jaundice. Weight loss and distaste for food and cigarettes may occur, followed by headache, arthralgias, vomiting, and right upper quadrant tenderness.
        2. Symptoms of hepatitis A, B and C are indistinguishable, except that patients with hepatitis A are more frequently febrile. Five to 10% of patients will develop a serum-sickness syndrome following infection with HBV, characterized by fever, rash, and arthralgias.
        3. **Physical examination.** Jaundice occurs in less than one-half of hepatitis patients. Jaundice can be observed when the bilirubin is greater than 2 mg/dL and is most easily observed under the tongue or in the sclera. Hepatomegaly and/or splenomegaly may also occur.
    B. **Chronic hepatitis**
        1. Chronic hepatitis most frequently presents as fatigue in patients with HBV, HCV, or HDV infection; jaundice is rarely present. The major difference between chronic hepatitis caused by HBV, compared to HCV, is a higher rate of cirrhosis that develops with HCV.
        2. In both hepatitis B and hepatitis C, evidence of chronic liver disease may include amenorrhea, muscle wasting, gynecomastia, and spider angiomata. As the disease progresses, asterixis, ascites, hepatic encephalopathy, peripheral edema, easy bruisability, testicular atrophy, bleeding, and esophageal varices may develop.

3. Chronic hepatitis requires a liver biopsy to confirm the diagnosis and to assess severity so as to determine whether treatment is needed. A major complication of chronic hepatitis is hepatocellular carcinoma.

Diagnosis of acute hepatitis

A. Laboratory findings in acute hepatitis

1. Aspartate aminotransferase (AST) and alanine aminotransferase (ALT) enzymes increase during the prodromal phase of hepatitis and may reach 20 times normal. The peak usually occurs when the patients are jaundiced, then rapidly falls during recovery.
2. In icteric patients, the bilirubin continues to increase as the aminotransferases decline and may reach 20 mg/dL. There are equal proportions of direct and indirect bilirubin.
3. The international normalized ratio is usually normal in acute hepatitis, but it can become prolonged in patients with severe hepatitis. The INR is a marker of prognosis.
4. If acute viral hepatitis is suspected, serologic tests should include IgM anti-HAV, IgM anti-HBc, HBsAg, and anti-HCV. In patients with fulminant hepatic failure or known previous infection with HBV, an anti-HDV should also be ordered.

Hepatitis Panels and Tests

Panel	Marker Detected
Acute hepatitis panel	IgM anti-HAV, IgM anti-HBc, HBsAg, anti-HCV
To monitor HBV	HBsAg, HBeAg, anti-HBe, HBsAg, HBeAg, total anti-HBc
HBV immunity panel	Anti-HBs, total anti-HBc
Individual Tests	**Marker Detected**
Immunity to HBV	Anti-HBs (post-vaccination)
Immunity to HAV	Anti-HAV
To screen for HBV infection	HBsAg for pregnant women
To monitor HCV infection	Anti-HCV

Clinical evaluation of acute hepatitis

1. Initially, patients should be evaluated for other etiologies of liver disease that can cause elevated liver enzymes.
2. **Common causes of elevated aminotransferase levels**
   a. **Infection.** Pneumococcal bacteremia, sepsis, Epstein-Barr virus, cytomegalovirus, herpes simplex virus, Varicella-zoster virus, syphilis, tuberculosis, mycobacterium avium complex.
   b. **Drugs and toxins.** Acetaminophen, benzenes, carbon tetrachloride, halothane, isoniazid, ketoconazole, 6-mercaptopurine, phenytoin, propylthiouracil, rifampin.
   c. **Vascular anoxia.** Budd-Chiari syndrome, congestive heart failure, veno-occlusive disease.

   d. **Metabolic.** Alpha-1-anti-trypsin deficiency, hemochromatosis, Wilson
      disease.
   e. **Others.** Alcoholic liver disease, choledocholithiasis, nonalcoho
      steatohepatitis, malignancy, shock.
   f. **Autoimmune hepatitis** occurs primarily in young women with system
      manifestations of autoimmune phenomena. These patients have positiv
      tests for antinuclear antibody and anti-Sm antibody.
   g. **Wilson's disease** is an autosomal recessive condition that results in tox
      copper accumulation in the liver as well as other organs. Diagnosis can b
      made by identifying Kayser-Fleischer rings in the eyes, an elevated urina
      copper, or low serum ceruloplasmin.

Blood Studies for Evaluating Elevations of Serum Liver Enzymes	
Disease to be Ruled Out	**Suggested Blood Test**
Alpha1-antitrypsin deficiency	Alpha-1-antitrypsin
Autoimmune chronic hepatitis	ANA, anti-Sm antibody
Hemochromatosis	Serum iron, TIBC, ferritin
Hepatitis B	HBsAg, HBeAg, anti-HBc
Hepatitis C	Anti-HCV
Primary biliary cirrhosis	Anti-mitochondrial antibody
Wilson's disease	Ceruloplasmin

III. Hepatitis A virus (HAV)
   A. Hepatitis A is usually an acute, self-limited infection, which does not result in
      chronic carrier state. Low-grade fever (<101° F) is common at the onset, wi
      malaise, anorexia, dark urine, and pale stools. Fulminant hepatic failure resultin
      in encephalopathy or death is rare.
   B. Transmission is by the fecal-oral route, and hepatitis A should be suspected
      infection occurs following ingestion of contaminated food or shellfish,
      institutionalized persons, children in day care centers, or if travel to an enderr
      area.
   C. The diagnosis is confirmed by the presence of IgM anti-HAV. The IgM anti-HA
      titer decreases over several months. The IgG anti-HAV rises and persis
      indefinitely and affords immunity to subsequent HAV exposure.
   D. **Treatment of acute hepatitis A infection** consists of antipyretics. Ninety-nir
      percent of acute hepatitis A will resolve without sequelae.

IV. Hepatitis B virus (HBV)
   A. The hepatitis B virus is composed of a double-stranded DNA molecule, co
      antigens and surface antigens. Incubation is 45-160 days. Transmission
      parenteral or sexual, with serum, semen and saliva shown to be contagious.
   B. Hepatitis B is difficult to distinguish from hepatitis A, but it usually has a mo
      protracted course. The diagnosis of acute hepatitis B is made by the demonstr
      tion of HBsAg in the serum and IgM antibody to hepatitis B core antigen (an
      HBc IgM), which appears at the same time as symptoms. Anti-HBc IgM gradua

declines during recovery.

C. In children born to women positive for HBsAg, the transmission rate is 10-40%. In homosexual males, the prevalence rate is 70%. Transmission among adolescents is primarily through sexual intercourse. Asymptomatic acute illness accounts for 40-50% of all infections.

D. Laboratory diagnosis of hepatitis B

1. Antibody to HBsAg (anti-HBs) develops after active infection and serves as an indicator of immunity. Anti-HBs alone is also detectable in the serum of individuals who have been vaccinated against HBV or who have been given hepatitis B immune globulin (HBIG).
2. IgM anti-HBc indicates recent HBV infection within the preceding 4-6 months.
3. Presence of HBeAg indicates active viral replication and high infectivity. Antibody to HBeAg (anti-HBe) develops in most people infected with HBV.
4. The persistence of HBsAg for six months after the diagnosis of acute HBV indicates progression to chronic hepatitis B.

E. Prognosis

1. Over 90% of adult patients with acute hepatitis B recover uneventfully. The mortality rate from acute hepatitis B is 1-2%.
2. **Chronic hepatitis** will develop in 6-10%, manifest by persistent HBsAg positivity.
3. **Fulminant hepatic failure** occurs in <1%, and it is characterized by prolongation of the INR, hyperbilirubinemia, and encephalopathy.

F. Management of acute hepatitis B

1. **Indications for hospitalization** include inability to maintain intake of nutrition and fluid, encephalopathy, bleeding, or INR >2.0.
2. **Bed rest** is not mandatory in uncomplicated cases. Diet should be free of fried or fatty foods.

G. Management of chronic hepatitis B

1. **Interferon Alfa**
   a. Interferon therapy is indicated for patients with at least a two-fold increase in ALT level for at least six months, presence of HBsAg and hepatitis B DNA titer. A liver biopsy should be done to stage the extent of liver involvement.
   b. Interferon is administrated as 5-10 million units SC three times a week for 16 weeks. Beneficial outcome of treatment with interferon is defined as disappearance of HBV DNA and HBeAg, normalization of ALT level, and improvement in histologic features. Successful treatment is obtained in 25 to 40 percent of cases.
2. **New antivirals.** Ribavirin (Virazole) has shown some limited success in the treatment of chronic hepatitis B.
3. **Liver transplantation** is a poor option in patients who develop cirrhosis from hepatitis B. Hepatitis B reinfection in the grafted liver usually results in allograft failure in one to two years.

V. Hepatitis C

A. Anti-HCV antibody is positive in 70-90% of patients with hepatitis C, although there is a prolonged interval between onset of illness and seroconversion. The test does not distinguish acute from chronic infection.

B. Clinical features of acute hepatitis C are indistinguishable from those of other viral hepatitides. Clinically recognized acute hepatitis C infection occurs less commonly than with HAV or HBV, and the majority of patients are asymptomatic.

C. Multiple transfusions, injection drug use, or high-risk sexual activity increase the index of suspicion for HCV. Perinatal transmission can occur in the 3rd trimester; in HCV-infected mothers, the offspring are infected 50% of the time.

    D. Heterosexual or household contacts have a 1-14% prevalence of anti-HCV. Between homosexuals, the attack rate is 2.9% per year.

    E. Prognosis. Fifty percent of patients with acute hepatitis C will progress to chronic liver disease, and 20% of these will develop cirrhosis. Patients with chronic hepatitis C are at risk for hepatocellular carcinoma.

    F. Treatment of hepatitis C
- **1. Acute hepatitis C** is usually is not severe, requiring only symptomatic therapy.
- **2.** All hepatitis C patients and their close contacts should receive the hepatitis B vaccine. Consuming significant amounts of alcohol may lead to rapid progression of disease.
- **3. Chronic HCV hepatitis**
   - **a. Interferon Alfa**
      - **(1)** Chronic HCV hepatitis is treated with interferon alfa. A liver biopsy is required before interferon therapy. The standard dosage is 3 million units SQ three times per week for six months.
      - **(2)** Response is measured by observing normalization of serum ALT levels. Loss of detectable HCV RNA may also be used as a criterion. Fifty percent of patients respond, with 50 percent of those responders relapsing within one year.
   - **b. Ribavirin** in combination with interferon is helpful, especially following liver transplantation.
   - **c. Liver transplantation** for treatment of hepatitis C is now common, although 19% of patients develop cirrhosis following transplantation.

VI. Hepatitis D

    A. Hepatitis D develops in patients who are coinfected with both HBV and HDV. Drug addicts and hemophiliacs are frequently affected, and infection can result in acute or chronic hepatitis.

    B. The clinical manifestations of HDV infection are indistinguishable from HBV alone; however, coinfected patients are at higher risk for fulminant hepatic failure. Cirrhosis may develop in up to 70%.

    C. An anti-HDV test should be ordered in patients with fulminant hepatitis or in patients known to be HBsAg positive who suffer a clinical deterioration.

    D. Treatment of hepatitis D. Interferon alfa may be administered as 10 million units three times per week for at least 12 months. Results have not been encouraging, and any durable response may require treatment for life.

VII. Hepatitis E

    A. No tests are available for diagnosis of hepatitis E. The clinical course is self-limited and similar to that of HAV. This infection should be suspected in individuals recently returning from India, Southeast Asia, Middle East, North Africa, and Mexico.

    B. The incubation period is 30-40 days, and treatment consists of supportive care.

VIII. Hepatitis G is a parenterally transmitted virus. It shares about 25 percent of its viral genome with the hepatitis C virus and may also cause chronic infection. Persistent infection with hepatitis G virus is common but does not seem to lead to chronic disease.

IX. Prevention of hepatitis

    A. Prevention of hepatitis A
- **1.** Employees of child care facilities and travelers to third world countries should be vaccinated against hepatitis A, and they should avoid uncooked shellfish, fruits, vegetables or contaminated water.
- **2.** Vaccination is given 2 weeks prior to exposure, with a booster dose anytime between 6 and 12 months. Children and adults exposed to hepatitis A at

home or in child care facilities should receive immune globulin (0.02 mg/kg).
- **B. Prophylactic therapy for hepatitis B**
  1. **Passive immunization** with hepatitis B immune globulin (HBIG) is recommended for:
     a. Accidental needlestick or mucosal exposure to HBsAg.
     b. Accidental transfusion of HBSAG-positive blood products.
     c. Spouses and/or sexual contacts of acute cases.
     d. Infants born to HBsAg-positive mothers.
  2. **Recommendations for active immunization**
     a. **Pre-exposure.** Infants, children, adolescents, health care workers, hemodialysis patients, homosexual males, illicit drug abusers, recipients of multiple blood products, sexual and household contacts of HBV carriers, prison inmates, heterosexually active persons with multiple partners, travelers to HBV-endemic areas.
     b. **Post-exposure (in conjunction with HBIG).** Infants born to HBsAg positive mothers; sexual contacts of acute hepatitis B cases; needlestick exposure to HBV; vaccine recipients with inadequate anti-HBs and needlestick exposure.
  3. There are two hepatitis B vaccines available, Recombivax HB and Engerix-B. Vaccination at zero, one and two months appears to result in protective antibody against HBV occurs in 90-95% of vaccinated individuals.
  4. **Infants born to HBsAg-positive women** should receive HBIG (0.5 mL) and hepatitis B vaccine.
  5. **Postexposure prophylaxis following sexual exposure** to HBV consists of HBIG and simultaneous hepatitis B vaccination with completion of the vaccine series at 1 and 6 months.
- **C. Hepatitis C.** There is no immune globulin preparation or vaccine available.

References, see page 268.

Acute Pancreatitis

The incidence of acute pancreatitis ranges from 54 to 238 episodes per 1 million per year. Patients with mild pancreatitis respond well to conservative therapy, but those with severe pancreatitis may have a progressively downhill course to respiratory failure, sepsis and death.

- **I. Etiology**
  - **A.** Numerous conditions are associated with acute pancreatitis. The most common causes are excessive ethanol intake and cholelithiasis, accounting for 65-80 percent of cases. Alcohol-induced pancreatitis occurs after the patient has consumed large quantities of alcohol. Following alcoholic and gallstone-related pancreatitis, the next largest category is idiopathic pancreatitis. It is estimated that in 10 percent of patients no cause can be found.
  - **B.** Elevation of serum triglycerides (>1,000 mg per dL) has been causally linked with acute pancreatitis. Autodigestion of the pancreas, believed to be primarily due to activation of trypsin, causes the pathologic changes found in acute pancreatitis.

Selected Causes of Acute Pancreatitis	
Alcoholism	Infections
Cholelithiasis	Microlithiasis
Drugs	Pancreas divisum
Hypertriglyceridemia	Trauma
Idiopathic causes	

Medications Associated with Acute Pancreatitis	
Asparaginase (Elspar)	Mercaptopurine (Purinethol)
Azathioprine (Imuran)	Pentamidine (Nebupent)
Didanosine (Videx)	Sulfonamides
Estrogens	Tetracyclines
Ethacrynic acid (Edecrin)	Thiazide diuretics
Furosemide (Lasix)	Valproic acid (Depakene)

II. Clinical presentation

A. Symptoms. Midepigastric pain, nausea and vomiting are the typical symptoms associated with acute pancreatitis. The abdominal pain frequently radiates to the back. The pain is sudden in onset, progressively increases in intensity and becomes constant.

B. Physical examination
1. Patients with acute pancreatitis appear ill. The severity of pain often causes the patient to move continuously in search of a more comfortable position. Findings that suggest severe pancreatitis include hypotension, tachypnea with decreased basilar breath sounds, and flank (Grey Turner's sign) or periumbilical (Cullen's sign) ecchymoses indicative of hemorrhagic pancreatitis. If fever is present, infection should be ruled out.
2. Abdominal distention and tenderness in the epigastrium are common. Voluntary or involuntary guarding, rebound tenderness, and hypoactive or absent bowel sounds indicate peritoneal irritation.

III. Laboratory tests

A. Leukocytosis with a left shift and an elevated hematocrit (hemoconcentration) and hyperglycemia are common. Prerenal azotemia may result from dehydration. Hypoalbuminemia, hypertriglyceridemia and hypocalcemia may be present. Hyperbilirubinemia with mild elevations of transaminases and alkaline phosphatase are common.

B. Amylase. An elevated amylase level often confirms the clinical diagnosis of pancreatis. Although most patients present with hyperamylasemia.

Selected Conditions Other Than Pancreatitis Associated with Amylase Elevation	
Pancreatic type origin Carcinoma of the pancreas Common bile duct obstruction Post-ERCP Mesenteric infarction Pancreatic trauma Perforated viscus Renal failure Salivary type origin	Acute alcoholism Diabetic ketoacidosis Lung cancer Ovarian neoplasm Renal failure Ruptured ectopic pregnancy Salivary gland infection Macroamylase Macroamylasemia

  C. Lipase measurements are more specific for pancreatitis than amylase levels but less sensitive. Hyperlipasemia may also occur in patients with renal failure, perforated ulcer disease, bowel infarction and bowel obstruction.

  D. Abdominal radiographs may reveal non-specific findings such as "sentinel loops" (dilated loops of small bowel in the vicinity of the pancreas), ileus and, occasionally, pancreatic calcifications.

  E. Ultrasonography. demonstrates the entire pancreas in only 20 percent of patients with acute pancreatitis. Its greatest utility is in evaluation of patients with possible gallstone disease.

  F. Computed tomography(CT) is the imaging modality of choice in acute pancreatitis. In 14-29% of patients, CT findings will be normal, usually indicating mild disease. Pancreatic necrosis, a marker for the severity of pancreatitis and potential infection, may be discerned by CT. Pseudocysts and abscesses are well-delineated with CT scanning.

IV. Prognosis. Ranson's criteria is used to determine prognosis in acute pancreatitis. Patients with two or fewer risk factors have a mortality rate of less than 1 percent; those with three or four risk factors, a mortality rate of 16 percent; five or six risk factors, a mortality rate of 40 percent; and seven or eight risk factors, a mortality rate approaching 100 percent.

Ranson's Criteria for Acute Pancreatitis	
At admission	**During initial 48 hours**
1. Age >55 years 2. WBC >16,000 per mm³ 3. Blood glucose >200 mg per dL 4. Serum LDH >350 IU per L 5. AST (SGOT) >250 U per L	1. Hematocrit drop >10 percentage points 2. BUN rise >5 mg per dL 3. Arterial pO_2 <60 mm Hg 4. Base deficit >4 mEq per L 5. Serum calcium <8.0 mg per dL 6. Estimated fluid sequestration > 6 L

V. Treatment

  A. Most cases of acute pancreatitis will improve within three to seven days with conservative therapy. Management consists of prevention and early detection of the complications of severe pancreatitis. Vigorous intravenous hydration is necessary because patients may sequester liters of fluid, leading to intravascular depletion, prerenal azotemia and shock. A decrease in urine output to less than 30 mL per hour is an indication of inadequate fluid replacement.

  B. Patients should take nothing by mouth to minimize pancreatic secretions. Total parenteral nutrition should be instituted for those patients fasting for more than five days in order to prevent malnutrition. A nasogastric tube is warranted in patients with nausea and vomiting or ileus.

C. **Pain control.** The use of morphine is discouraged because it may cause Oddi's sphincter spasm, which may exacerbate the pancreatitis. Meperidine (Demerol) (25-100 mg IM q4-6h) is favored. Other injectable agents such as ketorolac (Toradol) are also used.

D. **Antibiotics.** Routine use of antibiotics is not recommended in most cases of acute pancreatitis. In cases of infectious pancreatitis treatment with cefoxitin, cefotetan, ampicillin/sulbactam, or imipenem is appropriate.
   1. Cefoxitin (Mefoxin) 1-2 gm IV q6h.
   2. Cefotetan (Cefotan) 1-2 gm IV q12h.
   3. Ampicillin/sulbactam (Unasyn) 1.5-3.0 gm IV q6h.

E. Pseudocyst is suggested by continuing abdominal pain, vomiting, nausea, epigastric tenderness, abdominal mass, and hyperamylasemia. CT is diagnostic. CT scanning should be performed to detect pseudocyst and/or abscess in patients with continued clinical deterioration or failure to improve. Pseudocysts smaller than 5 cm in diameter will resorb without intervention. Pseudocysts greater than 5 cm usually require surgical intervention after the wall has matured.

F. Alcoholics may require alcohol withdrawal prophylaxis with chlordiazepoxide 25-100 mg IV/IM q6h x 3 days, thiamine 100 mg IM/IV qd x 3d; folic acid 1 mg IM/IV qd x 3d; multivitamin qd.

References, see page 268.

Lower Gastrointestinal Bleeding

The spontaneous remission rate for lower gastrointestinal bleeding, even with massive bleeding, is 80%. No source of bleeding can be identified in 12%, and bleeding is recurrent in 25%. Bleeding has usually ceased by the time the patient presents to the emergency room.

I. **Clinical evaluation**
   A. The severity of blood loss and hemodynamic status should be assessed immediately. Initial management consists of resuscitation with crystalloid solutions (lactated Ringers solution) and blood products if necessary.
   B. The duration and quantity of bleeding should be assessed; however, the duration of bleeding is often underestimated.
   C. Risk factors that may have contributed to the bleeding include nonsteroidal anti-inflammatory drugs, anticoagulants, colonic diverticulosis, renal failure, coagulopathy, colonic polyps and hemorrhoids.
   D. Patients may have a history of hemorrhoids, diverticulosis, inflammatory bowel disease, peptic ulcer, gastritis, cirrhosis, or esophageal varices.
   E. **Hematochezia.** Bright red or maroon blood per rectum suggests a lower GI source; however, 11-20% of patients with an upper GI bleed will have hematochezia as a result of rapid blood loss.
   F. **Melena.** Sticky, black, foul-smelling stools suggest a source proximal to the ligament of Treitz, but melena can also result from bleeding in the small intestine or proximal colon.
   G. **Malignancy** may be indicated by a change in stool caliber, anorexia, weight loss and malaise.

H. **Associated findings**
1. **Abdominal pain** may result from ischemic bowel, inflammatory bowel disease, or a ruptured aortic aneurysm.
2. **Painless, massive bleeding** suggests vascular bleeding from diverticula, angiodysplasia or hemorrhoids.
3. **Bloody diarrhea** suggests inflammatory bowel disease or an infectious origin.
4. **Bleeding with rectal pain** is seen with anal fissures, hemorrhoids, and rectal ulcers.
5. **Chronic constipation** suggests hemorrhoidal bleeding. New onset constipation or thin stools suggests a left-sided colonic malignancy.
6. **Blood on the toilet paper or dripping** into the toilet water after a bowel movement suggests a perianal source.
7. **Blood coating the outside of stool** suggests a lesion in the anal canal.
8. **Blood streaking or mixed in with the stool** may result from a polyp or malignancy in the descending colon.
9. **Maroon colored stools** often indicate small bowel and proximal colon bleeding.

II. **Physical examination**
   A. **Postural hypotension** indicates a 20% blood volume loss; whereas, overt signs of shock (pallor, hypotension, tachycardia) indicate a 30-40% blood loss.
   B. **The skin** may be cool and pale with delayed capillary refill if bleeding has been significant.
   C. **Stigmata of liver disease,** including jaundice, caput medusae, gynecomastia, and palmar erythema, should be sought because these patients frequently have GI bleeding.

III. **Differential diagnosis of lower gastrointestinal bleeding**
   A. **Angiodysplasia and diverticular disease** of the right colon account for the vast majority of episodes of acute lower gastrointestinal bleeding. Most acute LGI bleeding originates from the colon; however, 15-20% of episodes arise from the small intestine and the upper gastrointestinal tract.
   B. **Elderly patients.** Diverticulosis and angiodysplasia are the most common causes of lower GI bleeding.
   C. **Younger patients.** Hemorrhoids, anal fissures, and inflammatory bowel disease are more common causes.

IV. **Diagnosis and management of lower gastrointestinal bleeding**
   A. Rapid clinical evaluation and resuscitation should precede diagnostic or therapeutic studies. Intravenous fluids (1-2 liters) should be infused over 10-20 minutes to restore intravascular volume, and blood should be transfused if there is rapid ongoing blood loss or if hypotension or tachycardia is present. Coagulopathy is corrected with fresh frozen plasma or platelets.
   B. When small amounts of bright red blood are passed per rectum, the lower gastrointestinal tract can be assumed to be the source.
   C. In patients with large-volume maroon stools, nasogastric tube aspiration should be performed to exclude massive upper gastrointestinal hemorrhage.
   D. If the nasogastric aspirate contains no blood, then anoscopy and sigmoidoscopy should be performed to determine whether a colonic mucosal abnormality (ischemic or infectious colitis) or hemorrhoids might be the cause of bleeding.
   E. If these measures fail to yield a diagnosis, rapid administration of polyethylene glycol-electrolyte solution (CoLyte or GoLYTELY) should be initiated orally or by means of a nasogastric tube; 4 L of the lavage solution is given over a 2- to 3-hour period. This allows for diagnostic and therapeutic colonoscopy and adequately prepares the bowel should emergency operation become necessary.

V. Definitive management of lower gastrointestinal bleeding

A. Colonoscopy

1. Colonoscopy is the procedure of choice for diagnosing colonic causes of gastrointestinal bleeding. It should be performed after adequate preparation of the bowel. If the bowel cannot be adequately prepared because of persistent, acute bleeding, a bleeding scan or angiography is preferable.
2. Endoscopy may be therapeutic for angiodysplastic lesions, polyps, and tumors, which can be coagulated.
3. If colonoscopy fails to reveal a source for the bleeding, the patient should be observed because, in about 80% of cases, bleeding ceases spontaneously.

B. Bleeding scan.
The technetium-labeled ("tagged") red blood cell bleeding scan can detect bleeding sites when bleeding is intermittent. If the result is positive, the next step is colonoscopy or angiography.

C. Angiography

1. Selective mesenteric angiography detects arterial bleeding that occurs at a rate of 0.5 mL/min or faster. Diverticular bleeding causes pooling of contrast medium within a diverticulum.
2. Bleeding angiodysplastic lesions appear as abnormal vasculature. When active bleeding is seen with diverticular disease or angiodysplasia, selective arterial infusion of vasopressin is effective in 90%.

D. Surgery

1. If bleeding continues and no source has been found, surgical intervention is warranted.
2. Surgical resection may be indicated for patients with recurrent diverticular bleeding, or for patients who have had persistent bleeding from colonic angiodysplasia and have required blood transfusions. Treatment of lower gastrointestinal bleeding involves resection of the involved segment.

VI. Angiodysplasia

A. Angiodysplastic lesions are small vascular tufts that are formed by capillaries, veins, and venules, appearing as red dots or spider-like lesions 2 to 10 mm in diameter.

B. Angiodysplastic lesions develop secondary to chronic colonic distention, and they have a prevalence of 25% in elderly patients.

C. The most common site of bleeding is the right colon. Most patients with angiodysplasia have recurrent minor bleeding; however, massive bleeding is not uncommon.

VII. Diverticular disease

A. Diverticular disease is the most common cause of acute lower gastrointestinal bleeding. Sixty to 80% of bleeding diverticula are located in the right colon. Ninety percent of all diverticula are found in the left colon.

B. Diverticular bleeding tends to be massive, but it stops spontaneously in 80% of patients, and the rate of rebleeding is only 25%.

VIII. Colon polyps and colon cancers

A. These disorders rarely cause significant acute LGI hemorrhage. Left-sided and rectal neoplasms are more likely to cause gross bleeding than right sided lesions. Right sided lesions are more likely to cause anemia and occult bleeding.

B. Diagnosis and treatment consists of colonoscopic excision or surgical resection.

IX. Inflammatory bowel disease

A. Ulcerative colitis can occasionally cause severe GI bleeding associated with abdominal pain and diarrhea.

B. Colonoscopy and biopsy is diagnostic, and therapy consists of medical treatment of the underlying disease; resection is required occasionally.

X. Ischemic colitis
A. This disorder is seen in elderly patients with known vascular disease; abdominal pain may be postprandial and associated with bloody diarrhea or rectal bleeding. Severe blood loss is unusual but can occur.
B. Abdominal films may reveal "thumbprinting", caused by submucosal edema. Colonoscopy reveals a well-demarcated area of hyperemia, edema, and mucosal ulcerations. The splenic flexure and descending colon are the most common sites.
C. Most episodes resolve spontaneously; however, vascular bypass or resection may occasionally be required.

XI. Hemorrhoids
A. Hemorrhoids rarely cause massive acute blood loss. In patients with portal hypertension, rectal varices should be sought.
B. **Diagnosis** is by anoscopy and sigmoidoscopy. Treatment consists of a high fiber diet, stool softeners, and/or hemorrhoidectomy.

References, see page 268.

Acute Diarrhea

Acute diarrhea is defined as diarrheal disease of rapid onset, often with nausea, vomiting, fever, and abdominal pain. Most episodes of acute gastroenteritis will resolve within 3 to 7 days.

I. Clinical evaluation of acute diarrhea
A. The nature of onset, duration, frequency, and timing of the diarrheal episodes should be assessed. The appearance of the stool, buoyancy, presence of blood or mucus, vomiting, or pain should be determined.
B. Contact with a potential source of infectious diarrhea should be sought.
C. **Drugs that may cause diarrhea** include laxatives, magnesium-containing compounds, sulfa-drugs, and antibiotics.

II. Physical examination
A. **Assessment of volume status.** Dehydration is suggested by dry mucous membranes, orthostatic hypotension, tachycardia, mental status changes, and acute weight loss.
B. **Abdominal tenderness**, mild distention and hyperactive bowel sounds are common in acute infectious diarrhea. The presence of rebound tenderness or rigidity suggests toxic megacolon or perforation.
C. **Evidence of systemic atherosclerosis** suggests ischemia. Lower extremity edema suggests malabsorption or protein loss.

III. Acute infectious diarrhea
A. **Infectious diarrhea** is classified as noninflammatory or inflammatory, depending on whether the infectious organism has invaded the intestinal mucosa.
B. **Noninflammatory** infectious diarrhea is caused by organisms that produce a toxin (enterotoxigenic E coli strains, Vibrio cholerae). Noninflammatory, infectious diarrhea is usually self-limiting and lasts less than 3 days.
C. **Blood or mucus** in the stool suggests inflammatory disease, usually caused by bacterial invasion of the mucosa (enteroinvasive E coli, Shigella, Salmonella, Campylobacter). Patients usually have a septic appearance and fever; some have abdominal rigidity and severe abdominal pain.
D. **Vomiting out of proportion to diarrhea** is usually related to a neuroenterotoxin-

mediated food poisoning from Staphylococcus aureus or Bacillus cereus, or rotavirus (in an infant), or Norwalk virus (in older children or adults). The incubation period for neuroenterotoxin food poisoning is less than 4 hours, while that of a viral agent is more than 8 hours.

E. **Traveler's diarrhea** is a common acute diarrhea. Three or four unformed stools are passed/per 24 hours, usually starting on the third day of travel and lasting 2-3 days. Anorexia, nausea, vomiting, abdominal cramps, abdominal bloating, and flatulence may also be present.

F. **Antibiotic-related diarrhea**
   1. Antibiotic-related diarrhea ranges from mild illness to life-threatening pseudomembranous colitis. Overgrowth of Clostridium difficile causes pseudomembranous colitis. Amoxicillin, cephalosporins and clindamycin have been implicated most often, but any antibiotic can be the cause.
   2. Patients with pseudomembranous colitis have high fever, cramping, leukocytosis, and severe, watery diarrhea. Latex agglutination testing for C difficile toxin can provide results in 30 minutes.
   3. **Enterotoxigenic E coli**
      a. The enterotoxigenic E coli include the E coli serotype 0157:H7. Grossly bloody diarrhea is most often caused by E. coli 0157:H7, causing 8% of grossly bloody stools.
      b. Enterotoxigenic E coli can cause hemolytic uremic syndrome, thrombotic thrombocytopenic purpura, intestinal perforation, sepsis, and rectal prolapse.

IV. **Diagnostic approach to acute infectious diarrhea**
   A. An attempt should be made to obtain a pathologic diagnosis in patients who give a history of recent ingestion of seafood (Vibrio parahaemolyticus), travel or camping, antibiotic use, homosexual activity, or who complain of fever and abdominal pain.
   B. Blood or mucus in the stools indicates the presence of Shigella, Salmonella, Campylobacter jejuni, enteroinvasive E. coli, C. difficile, or Yersinia enterocolitica.
   C. Most cases of mild diarrheal disease do not require laboratory studies to determine the etiology. In moderate to severe diarrhea with fever or pus, a stool culture for bacterial pathogens (Salmonella, Shigella, Campylobacter) is submitted. If antibiotics were used recently, stool should be sent for Clostridium difficile toxin.

V. **Laboratory evaluation of acute diarrhea**
   A. **Fecal leukocytes** is a screening test which should be obtained if moderate to severe diarrhea is present. Numerous leukocytes indicate Shigella, Salmonella, or Campylobacter jejuni.
   B. **Stool cultures for bacterial pathogens** should be obtained if high fever, severe or persistent (>14 d) diarrhea, bloody stools, or leukocytes is present.
   C. **Examination for ova and parasites** is indicated for persistent diarrhea (>14 d), travel to a high-risk region, gay males, infants in day care, or dysentery.
   D. **Blood cultures** should be obtained prior to starting antibiotics if severe diarrhea and high fever is present.
   E. **E coli 0157:H7 cultures.** Enterotoxigenic E coli should be suspected if there are bloody stools with minimal fever, when diarrhea follows hamburger consumption or when hemolytic uremic syndrome is diagnosed.
   F. **Clostridium difficile cytotoxin** should be obtained if diarrhea follows use of an antimicrobial agent.
   G. **Rotavirus antigen test (Rotazyme)** is indicated for hospitalized children <2 years old with gastroenteritis. The finding of rotavirus eliminates the need for

antibiotics.
VI. Treatment of acute diarrhea
A. Fluid and electrolyte resuscitation
1. **Oral rehydration.** For cases of mild to moderate diarrhea in children, Pedialyte or Ricelyte should be administered. For adults with diarrhea, flavored soft drinks with saltine crackers are usually adequate.
2. **Intravenous hydration** should be used if oral rehydration is not possible.
B. Diet. Fatty foods should be avoided. Well-tolerated foods include complex carbohydrates (rice, wheat, potatoes, bread, and cereals), lean meats, yogurt, fruits, and vegetables. Diarrhea often is associated with a reduction in intestinal lactase. A lactose-free milk preparation may be substituted if lactose intolerance becomes apparent.
VII. Empiric antimicrobial treatment of acute diarrhea
A. Febrile dysenteric syndrome
1. If diarrhea is associated with high fever and stools containing mucus and blood, empiric antibacterial therapy should be given for Shigella or Campylobacter jejuni.
2. Norfloxacin (Noroxin) 400 mg bid **OR**
3. Ciprofloxacin (Cipro) 500 mg bid.
B. Travelers' diarrhea. Adults are treated with norfloxacin 400 mg bid, ciprofloxacin 500 mg bid, or ofloxacin 300 mg bid for 3 days.

References, see page 268.

Chronic Diarrhea

Diarrhea is considered chronic if it lasts longer than 2 weeks.

I. Clinical evaluation of chronic diarrhea
A. Initial evaluation should determine the characteristics of the diarrhea, including volume, mucus, blood, flatus, cramps, tenesmus, duration, frequency, effect of fasting, stress, and the effect of specific foods (eg, dairy products, wheat, laxatives, fruits).
B. Secretory diarrhea
1. Secretory diarrhea is characterized by large stool volumes (>1 L/day), no decrease with fasting, and a fecal osmotic gap <40.
2. **Evaluation of secretory diarrhea** consists of a giardia antigen, Entamoeba histolytica antibody, Yersinia culture, fasting serum glucose, thyroid function tests, and a cholestyramine (Cholybar, Questran) trial.
C. Osmotic diarrhea
1. Osmotic diarrhea is characterized by small stool volumes, a decrease with fasting, and a fecal osmotic gap >40. Postprandial diarrhea with bloating or flatus also suggests osmotic diarrhea. Ingestion of an osmotically active laxative may be inadvertent (sugarless gum containing sorbitol) or covert (with eating disorders).
2. **Evaluation of osmotic diarrhea**
   a. Trial of lactose withdrawal.
   b. Trial of an antibiotic (metronidazole) for small-bowel bacterial overgrowth.
   c. Screening for celiac disease (anti-endomysial antibody, antigliadin antibody).
   d. Fecal fat measurement (72 hr) for pancreatic insufficiency.

    e. Trial of fructose avoidance.

    f. Stool test for phenolphthalein and magnesium if laxative abuse is suspected.

    g. Hydrogen breath analysis to identify disaccharidase deficiency or bacterial overgrowth.

D. Exudative diarrhea

    1. Exudative diarrhea is characterized by bloody stools, tenesmus, urgency, cramping pain, and nocturnal occurrence. It is most often caused by inflammatory bowel disease, which may be suggested by anemia, hypoalbuminemia, and an increased sedimentation rate.

    2. Evaluation of exudative diarrhea consists of a complete blood cell count, serum albumin, total protein, erythrocyte sedimentation rate, electrolyte measurement, Entamoeba histolytica antibody titers, stool culture, Clostridium difficile antigen test, ova and parasite testing, and flexible sigmoidoscopy and biopsies.

References, see page 268.

Neurologic Disorders

Ischemic Stroke

Ischemic stroke is the third leading cause of death in the United States and the most common cause of neurologic disability in adults. Approximately 85 percent of strokes are ischemic in nature.

Clinical evaluation of the stroke patient
A. A rapid evaluation should determine the time when symptoms started. Other diseases that may mimic a stroke, including seizure disorder, hypoglycemia, complex migraine, dysrhythmia or syncope, should be excluded.
B. Markers of vascular disease such as diabetes, angina pectoris and intermittent claudication, are suggestive of ischemic stroke. A history of atrial fibrillation or MI suggests a cardiac embolic stroke.

Physical examination
A. Assessment should determine whether the patient's condition is acutely deteriorating or relatively stable. Airway and circulatory stabilization take precedence over diagnostic and therapeutic interventions.
B. **Neurologic exam.** Evaluation should include the level of consciousness, orientation; ability to speak and understand language; cranial nerve function, especially eye movements and pupil reflexes and facial paresis; neglect, gaze preference, arm and leg strength, sensation, and walking ability.
C. A semiconscious or unconscious patient probably has a hemorrhage. A patient with an ischemic stroke may be drowsy but is unlikely to lose consciousness unless the infarcted area is large.

CT Scanning and diagnostic studies
A. All patients with signs of stroke should undergo a noncontrast head CT to screen for bleeding and to rule out expanding lesions such as subdural hematomas, epidural hematomas, or other indications for emergent surgery.
B. A complete blood count (CBC) including platelets, international normalized ratio (INR), activated partial thromboplastin time (aPTT), serum electrolytes, and a rapid blood glucose should be obtained. ECG, and chest x-ray should be ordered. If the patient is a candidate for thrombolytic therapy, typed and cross-match should be obtained. Arterial blood gas and lumbar puncture should be obtained when indicated.

Management of ischemic stroke
A. **Tissue plasminogen activator (tPA, Activase).** Use of t-PA within three hours of ischemic stroke onset may substantially improve long-term functional outcome compared with placebo, even when the 6 percent incidence of intracerebral hemorrhage in t-PA recipients is considered. For every 100 patients given t-PA, 12 more experience complete neurologic recovery than with placebo. The t-PA dose must be given within three hours of stroke onset. When a patient awakens from sleep with a neurologic deficit, onset of stroke must be assumed to be the time that sleep commenced. It is sometimes difficult to be certain of the exact time of stroke onset at initial evaluation; if time of onset is uncertain, t-PA should not be given.
B. The CT scan must document the absence of intracranial bleeding before treatment. Patients with severe ischemic strokes have a higher risk of t-PA-associated brain hemorrhage, but they also have the most to gain.

Criteria for Thrombolysis of Patients with Acute Ischemic Stroke Using Tissue Plasminogen Activator

Inclusion criteria
Age greater than 18 years
Clinical diagnosis of ischemic stroke, with onset of symptoms within three hours of initiation of treatment
Noncontrast CT scan with no evidence of hemorrhage

Exclusion criteria
History
Stroke or head trauma in previous three months
History of intracranial hemorrhage that may increase risk of recurrent hemorrhage
Major surgery or other serious trauma in previous 14 days
Gastrointestinal or genitourinary bleeding in previous 21 days
Arterial puncture in previous seven days
Pregnant or lactating patient
Clinical findings
Rapidly improving stroke symptoms
Seizure at onset of stroke
Symptoms suggestive of subarachnoid hemorrhage, even if CT scan is normal
Persistent systolic pressure greater than 185 mm Hg or diastolic pressure greater than 110 mm Hg, or patient is requiring aggressive therapy to control blood pressure
Clinical presentation consistent with acute myocardial infarction or postmyocardial infarction pericarditis requires cardiologic evaluation before treatment
Imaging results
CT scan with evidence of hemorrhage
CT scan with evidence of hypodensity and/or effacement of cerebral sulci in more than one-third of middle cerebral artery territory
Laboratory findings
Glucose level less than 50 mg per dL (2.8 mmol per L) or greater than 400 mg per dL (22.2 mmol per L)
Platelet count less than 100,000 per mm^3 (100 $\times\times$ 10^9 per L)
Patient is taking warfarin and has abnormal International Normalized Ratio
Patient has received heparin within 48 hours, and partial thromboplastin time is elevated

---

C. **Aspirin** produces a small reduction in the likelihood of death or sever disability. The risk of death or disability is reduced by about one case per 10 patients treated with early aspirin. Aspirin or other antiplatelet agents should b initiated after the CT scan has excluded hemorrhage and 24 hours after t-P in the absence of contraindications.

D. **Heparin.** Heparin has no benefit in the treatment of ischemic stroke.

E. **Cytoprotective agents.** These agents increase the tolerance of neurons ischemia. Large trials testing citicoline, clomethiazole and glycine antagoni should be completed soon.

Initial Management of Acute Stroke

Determine whether stroke is ischemic or hemorrhagic by computed tomography

Consider administration of t-PA if less than three hours from stroke onset
General management:
- Blood pressure (avoid hypotension)
- Assure adequate oxygenation
- Administer intravenous glucose
- Take dysphagia/aspiration precautions
- Consider prophylaxis for venous thrombosis if patient is unable to walk
- Suppress fever, if present
- Assess stroke mechanism (eg, atrial fibrillation, hypertension)
- Consider aspirin therapy if ischemic stroke and no contraindications (not within 24 hours of t-PA)

F. Labored or weak respirations are an indication for intubation and ventilation.
G. **Dosage and administration.** The dose of t-PA for acute ischemic stroke is 0.9 mg/kg with a maximum dose of 90 mg. Ten percent of the dose is given as a bolus dose, and the remainder is given over 60 minutes. No heparin or antiplatelet agents (aspirin) should be administered until 24 hours after initiation of t-PA treatment and a 24-hour safety CT has ruled out intracranial hemorrhage.
H. **Blood pressure management in thrombolytic therapy**
   1. Arterial blood pressure should be kept just below a 185 mm Hg during the first 24 hours to minimize the risk of intracerebral hemorrhage.
   2. Severe hypertension should be controlled with labetalol, administered at an initial dose of 10 mg IV over 1-2 minutes. The dose may be repeated or doubled every 10-20 minutes if needed, or an IV infusion of 2 mg/min may be initiated. If the response is unsatisfactory, then an infusion of sodium nitroprusside starting at a dose of 0.25 mcg/kg/min is recommended.

General care
A. **Blood pressure**
   1. Acute stroke produces an increase in blood pressure in 80% of patients. Minimal or moderate elevations in blood pressure do not require urgent pharmacological treatment, since there generally is a spontaneous decline in blood pressure over time.
   2. Antihypertensive intervention is not required unless the systolic blood pressure is greater than 220 mmHg or diastolic pressure exceed 120 mm Hg. A rapid reduction in the blood pressure is unnecessary and may be harmful. A reduction to systolic blood pressures of 200-230 mmHg and to diastolic pressures of 100-120 mmHg is adequate.
B. **Fever.** In patients with acute stroke, fever is not uncommon. Fever should be suppressed. Mild elevations in body temperature will worsen the neurologic outcome from ischemic insults.
C. **Hyperglycemia.** Hyperglycemia may be deleterious to the ischemic penumbra. Glucose levels should be kept below 150 mg per dL (8.3 mmol per L).

ferences, see page 268.

Transient Ischemic Attack

A transient ischemic attack (TIA) is a temporary focal neurologic deficit caused by th brief interruption of local cerebral blood flow. The prevalence of TIAs 1.6-4.1 percer Stroke occurs in one-third of patients who have a TIA. The duration of a foc neurologic deficit that leads to cerebral infarction has arbitrarily been determined to b 24 hours or greater.

I. Differential diagnosis and symptoms

Common Clinical Findings Associated with Ischemia in Various Arterial Distributions	
Anterior cerebral artery Weakness in contralateral leg Sensory loss in contralateral leg, with or without weakness or numbness in proximal contralateral arm **Middle cerebral artery** Contralateral hemiparesis Deviation of head and eyes toward side of lesion Contralateral hemianesthesia Contralateral hemianopia Aphasia (if dominant hemisphere is affected) Unawareness of stroke (if nondominant hemisphere is affected)	**Lenticulostriate arteries** Pure motor hemiparesis (lacunar syndrome) **Posterior cerebral artery** Visual field disturbance Contralateral sensory loss Amnesia **Vertebrobasilar arteries** Vertigo Nausea and vomiting Ataxia Nystagmus

II. Pathophysiology.

The most frequent mechanism of TIA is embolization by thrombus from an atherosclerotic plaque in a large vessel (stenotic carotid artery TIAs may also occur as manifestations of intracranial atherosclerotic disea (lacunar TIAs) or large-vessel occlusion. In addition, they can be associated wi atrial fibrillation or mitral valve prolapse, carotid or vertebral dissection, a hypercoagulable states (antiphospholipid antibody syndrome).

III. Evaluation of TIA symptoms

A. The primary objective when evaluating a patient with a transient ischemic atta (TIA) is to determine whether the ischemic insult has occurred in the anteri or posterior circulation.

B. **Anterior circulation ischemia** causes motor or sensory deficits of th extremities or face, amaurosis fugax, aphasia, and/or homonymo hemianopia.

C. **Posterior circulation ischemia** causes motor or sensory dysfunction association with diplopia, dysphasia, dysarthria, ataxia, and/or vertigo.

D. Assessment should determine the activity in which the patient was engag and the patient's physical position at the onset of the attack. A description of t specific symptoms of the attack should be obtained, including the speed w which they developed, whether they were bilateral or unilateral, and th duration.

E. History of hypertension, diabetes, cardiac disease, previous TIA or stro cigarette smoking, or use of street drugs should be sought.

F. Differentiating TIAs from other entities

1. **Seizures** almost always involve a change in the level of consciousness

awareness, excessive motor activity and confusion, none of which characterizes a TIA.

2. **Syncope**. Changes in cardiac output produce generalized, rather than focal, cerebral ischemia, characterized by loss of consciousness and a rapid heartbeat (often due to an arrhythmia).

3. **Benign positional vertigo.** Recurrent waves of dizziness, which last 2-10 seconds and are related to movement (standing up or sitting down), are characteristic.

G. Physical examination

1. Heart rate and rhythm and the blood pressure in both arms, peripheral pulses, skin lesions (petechiae of embolic origin), and skin manifestations of connective tissue disease should be assessed.

2. Carotid bruits may suggest carotid stenosis. Ophthalmoscopic examination can detect arterial or venous occlusion and emboli.

3. **Neurologic examination**

   a. The neurologic examination should be normal in TIA patients unless the patient has had a previous stroke or is currently experiencing a TIA or stroke.

   b. Evaluation should include the level of consciousness, orientation, ability to speak and understand language; cranial nerve function, especially eye movements and pupil reflexes and facial paresis. Neglect, gaze preference, arm and leg strength, sensation, and walking ability should be assessed.

Conditions That Can Masquerade as Stroke	
Todd's paralysis (postepileptic paralysis) Hypoglycemia Complicated migraine Conversion disorder or malingering	Brain tumor Drug overdose Bell's palsy

IV. Laboratory studies

Initial Evaluation of a Patient with Transient Ischemic Attack
Complete blood cell count with platelet count
Chemistry profile (including cholesterol and glucose levels)
Prothrombin time and activated partial thromboplastin time
Erythrocyte sedimentation rate
Syphilis serology
Electrocardiography
Cranial computed tomography (particularly with hemispheric transient ischemic attack)
Noninvasive arterial imaging (ultrasonography, magnetic resonance angiography)

A. **Complete blood count** with differential rules out profound anemia, polycythemia, leukocytosis, thrombocytopenia and thrombocytosis. The chemistry profile may demonstrate hypoglycemia that can present with focal neurologic deficits or hyperglycemia that can worsen the outcome after stroke.

B. **Prothrombin time and an activated partial thromboplastin time** are needed to rule out coagulopathies. The erythrocyte sedimentation rate serves as a screening test for autoimmune disorders. Syphilis serology screens for neurosyphilis.

C. **Electrocardiogram** (ECG) is used to detect arrhythmias (eg, atrial fibrillation) as the cause of ischemia. Computed tomographic (CT) scanning of the head is necessary to rule out intracranial bleeding or tumors. CT may reveal the vascular distribution of previous ischemic events.

D. **Carotid duplex studies** are recommended in all patients with TIA symptoms. These tests (eg, Doppler plus B-mode imaging) detect extracranial carotid disease.

E. **Echocardiography** may be helpful in identifying atrial thrombus in patients with atrial fibrillation. Transcranial Doppler ultrasonography can reveal intracranial stenosis of the middle cerebral or posterior cerebral arteries.

F. **Magnetic resonance angiography** is used to detect stenosis in extracranial or intracranial cerebral arteries. Arteriography is reserved for suspected intracranial vasculitis or arterial dissection.

G. **Special testing for hypercoagulable states** (antiphospholipid antibodies) protein C and S, antithrombin III should be reserved for use in patients less than 50 years of age, patients with a history of thrombotic disease and patients in whom no other cause of TIA is found. Holter monitoring is recommended for use in patients who had palpitations.

H. **Lumbar puncture** may be warranted if central nervous system infection is suspected or the presenting symptoms suggest subarachnoid hemorrhage but the CT scan is negative.

V. **Treatment**

A. **Reduction of risk factors**

1. Aggressive treatment of chronic hypertension should maintain the systolic blood pressure below 140 mm Hg and the diastolic blood pressure below 90 mm Hg.

2. Cigarette smoking and consumption of three or more alcohol drinks per day should be discouraged.

3. Atrial fibrillation is one of the strongest independent risk factors for stroke. Warfarin (Coumadin) or aspirin is effective for stroke prevention in patients with atrial fibrillation.

B. **Carotid endarterectomy guidelines**

1. Surgery is recommended in symptomatic patients with 70 percent carotid stenosis.

2. Surgery may be considered in symptomatic patients with carotid stenosis of 50 to 69 percent. The risks and benefits of surgery should be carefully considered in these patients.

3. Surgery should not be considered in patients with carotid stenosis of less than 50 percent.

C. **Stroke prevention, antithrombotic therapy**

1. **Aspirin.** Because aspirin inactivates cyclooxygenase activity for the life of platelets, thromboxane A_2 cannot be produced. Aspirin in a dosage of 50 to 325 mg per day is recommended for all TIA patients for stroke prevention.

2. **Ticlopidine (Ticlid)** inhibits platelet aggregation and is recommended for patients who can not tolerate aspirin. The dosage is 250 mg PO bid. Adverse events include neutropenia, thrombocytopenia, diarrhea, rash, abnormal liver function tests and elevated cholesterol levels. Close

monitoring of complete blood count is required for the first three months.
3. **Clopidogrel (Plavix)**, 75 mg qd, is recommended for patients who can not tolerate aspirin. Clopidogrel has fewer side effects than ticlopidine.

References, see page 268.

Alzheimer's Disease

Alzheimer's disease currently affects about 4 million people in the United States. This neurodegenerative disease causes selective neuronal loss in brain regions involved in memory, language, personality, and cognition. The earliest symptom of Alzheimer's disease is usually the insidious onset and progression of memory loss. Initially, this memory loss can be difficult to differentiate from common age-associated benign forgetfulness. However, patients with age-associated benign forgetfulness are aware of the deficit and their activities of daily living are minimally impaired.

I. **Pathogenesis**
   A. Age is the major risk factor for development of Alzheimer's disease. The incidence of Alzheimer's disease increases with age, doubling every 5 years between ages 60 and 85. Limited education and a history of head trauma may also be factors in development of disease.
   B. The presenilin 1 gene is the most common site of mutations responsible for early-onset Alzheimer's disease. Genetic testing should be restricted to patients with early-onset Alzheimer's disease and a strong family history of dementia.
   C. Onset of dementia symptoms after age 60 occurs in about 90% of patients with Alzheimer's disease. No causative mutations have been found in this group of patients, but a susceptibility gene, apolipoprotein E (*APOE*), has been identified. Although the presence of the *APOE* gene increases the risk of Alzheimer's disease, evaluation of the *APOE* genotype is not useful in the absence of symptoms of Alzheimer's disease because many people without the disease carry this allele.

II. **Diagnosis**

Criteria for diagnosis of Alzheimer's disease

Dementia established by clinical examination and documented by the Mini-Mental State Examination or similar examination

Deficits in two or more areas of cognition (ie, language, memory, perception)

Progressive worsening of memory and other cognitive function; as disease progresses, patient experiences impairment in activities of daily living and altered behavioral patterns

No disturbance of consciousness

Onset between ages 40 and 90, but most often after age 65

Absence of other systemic disorder or brain disease that may account for deficits in memory and cognition

---

   A. Computed tomographic scanning and magnetic resonance imaging often show generalized and hippocampal atrophy in patients with Alzheimer's disease. These tests are not sensitive enough to establish a diagnosis. Imaging is useful in excluding a diagnosis of stroke, tumor, or hydrocephalus.

   B. Delirium should be excluded and coexisting conditions that worsen dementia by reviewing medications, screening for depression, and ruling out nutritional deficiencies, diabetes mellitus, uremia, alterations in electrolytes and thyroid disease.

III. Treatment of Alzheimer's disease

   A. Cholinesterase inhibitors. In Alzheimer's disease, the levels of enzymes responsible for the synthesis of acetylcholine are reduced by 58% to 90% in selected areas of the brain.

   B. In patients with mild-to-moderate Alzheimer's disease, cholinesterase inhibitors result in a small but statistically significant improvement in cognitive ability.

   C. Donepezil (Aricept) requires only once-daily dosing, and routine monitoring by laboratory testing is not required. Tacrine (Cognex) requires four-times-daily dosing and frequent monitoring of serum transaminase levels.

   D. Rivastigmine (Exelon) is another acetylcholinesterase inhibitor. It is administered twice daily and has a similar efficacy and side-effect profile to donepezil.

Drug Treatments for Dementia		
Medication	**Typical dosage**	**Comments**
Donepezil (Aricept)	5 to 10 mg once daily	Equal efficacy and fewer side effects than tacrine; elevated hepatic transaminase levels are rare; diarrhea and abdominal pain occur occasionally.
Rivastigmine (Exelon)	3-6 mg bid	
Ibuprofen (Motrin)	400 mg two to three times daily	Gastrointestinal or renal toxicity.
Conjugated estrogens (Premarin)	0.625 mg daily	Prescribe for women; add cyclic progestin for patients with an intact uterus.
Vitamin E	800 to 2,000 IU daily	Mild antioxidant effects.

   E. Estrogen replacement therapy has a significant protective effect and may delay the expression of Alzheimer's disease.

   F. Nonsteroidal anti-inflammatory drugs (NSAIDs) such as aspirin and ibuprofen have been associated with a lower incidence of dementia. Because of the risks of gastrointestinal and renal toxicity, these agents cannot be routinely recommended as a preventive measure.

   G. Vitamin E supplementation may significantly slow the progression of moderate Alzheimer's disease. Vitamin E supplementation may be considered in persons with dementia or those who are at risk for the disease. Dosages of up to 2,000 IU daily are used.

   H. Ginkgo biloba extract has been reported to delay symptom progression in dementia, but little is known about the long-term effects of the extract, and it can not be recommended.

IV. Management of behavior problems in Alzheimer's disease

   A. Delusions are treated with an antipsychotic agent such as haloperidol (Haldol)

or risperidone (Risperdal).
B. Agitation should be treated with a short-acting antianxiety agent such as lorazepam (Ativan) or buspirone (BuSpar).
C. Depression is managed with a selective serotonin reuptake inhibitor, beginning at one-half the usual dosage. If sedation is also desirable, trazodone (Desyrel) is useful.

References, see page 268.

Seizure Disorders and Epilepsy

Epilepsy is a disorder that consists of recurrent seizures. Epilepsy occurs in 1 to 2 percent of the general population. The incidence of epilepsy is highest in infancy. It decreases during childhood and is lowest in adolescence. The incidence markedly increases in elderly patients.

I. Classification
  A. Seizure disorders are classified according to their clinical features. At their onset, seizures may be partial (affecting only one area of the brain) or generalized (ie, affecting the whole brain). Partial seizures may be simple or complex.
  B. If the patient remains fully conscious, the seizure is classified as simple. However, if the focal discharge involves brain regions that control awareness or if the seizure is sufficiently widespread to cause the patient to lose consciousness, the seizure is classified as complex.
  C. Complex partial seizures usually begin with arrested motion and a blank stare. Automatisms, such as simple hand movements, oral-buccal behaviors, including lip-smacking or swallowing, and involuntary vocalizations may occur initially or during the seizure.

II. Clinical evaluation
  A. The history should assess the duration of seizures and the nature of behaviors that occur during a seizure. At the termination of a seizure, the patient may be confused, fatigued or disoriented. Simple and complex partial seizures can generalize to produce tonic-clonic seizures.
  B. Absence seizures, which begin during childhood, are typically brief, usually lasting 10 seconds or less. The patient does not have an aura, and there are no lingering or postictal effects after the seizure. Arrested motion and a blank stare are the hallmarks of this type of seizure. Patients with absence seizures display a characteristic electroencephalographic pattern of generalized spike-and-wave discharges occurring at a rate of three per second.
  C. Convulsions represent the most common type of generalized seizures. Most generalized convulsions begin with a tonic phase in which sustained contraction of all muscles occurs, with extended legs and flexed or extended arms. This phase lasts for several seconds and is followed by a clonic phase characterized by rhythmic contractions of the limbs. After the violent muscle contractions subside, the patient enters a postictal phase in which breathing resumes and unresponsiveness is followed by gradual recovery of consciousness.

III. Diagnostic evaluation
  A. Laboratory evaluation should include blood glucose levels, BUN, electrolytes and liver enzymes. A complete blood count may suggest a systemic condition, such as infection, a platelet abnormality or anemia.

B. Epilepsy in children is typically idiopathic. In patients over age 30, a cause is found in only 15 to 23 percent of adults. Strokes are a common cause of seizures in patients over age 65.

C. Lumbar puncture. If a patient is febrile or has altered cognitive function, such as behavioral changes, cerebrospinal fluid studies should be performed. Children with typical febrile seizures may not require lumbar puncture. Lumbar puncture should be performed only after the presence of an intracranial mass or increased intracranial pressure has been excluded; computed tomographic (CT) scanning may be used to make this determination.

D. Electroencephalography. Focal or generalized seizure patterns interrupting background patterns confirm a diagnosis of epilepsy. The diagnostic yield of an EEG can be improved if the patient is sleep-deprived.

E. Magnetic resonance imaging (MRI) is the preferred study for epilepsy. MRI can help establish a precise diagnosis in patients with intractable complex partial seizures arising from temporal lobe structures; many of these patients have mesial temporal atrophy or sclerosis.

IV. Differential diagnosis

A. Sensory or motor dysfunction may be caused by transient ischemia. Embolic cerebrovascular disease, extracranial carotid or basilar artery disease or migraine may precipitate transient ischemic events. Hypoglycemia in diabetes can cause seizures.

B. Drug and alcohol abuse as well as withdrawal from these substances can also result in alterations of consciousness and seizures. Some drugs lower the seizure threshold and can facilitate seizure development.

Drugs that Can Precipitate Seizures

Alcohol use and withdrawal
Amphetamine use and withdrawal
Barbiturate use and withdrawal
Benzodiazepine use and withdrawal
Cocaine use and withdrawal
Meperidine (Demerol) use and withdrawal
Phenothiazine use and withdrawal
Theophylline use

V. Treatment

A. Therapy should be started with a single drug. If possible, seizure control should be achieved by increasing the dosage of the initial drug rather than by adding a second agent. If seizure control cannot be achieved with the first drug, a second agent may be added. Dosage adjustments should be based on clinical response rather than serum drug levels.

B. Monitoring drug levels is usually not necessary in patients with good seizure control who are taking a well-tolerated drug. However, monitoring can be useful when determining adherence to therapy, assessing unexplained changes in seizure control or evaluating toxic effects.

Antiepileptic Drugs

| | Recommended daily dosage | | |
	Adults	Children (per kg of body weight)	Dosing intervals
Carbamazepine (Tegretol)	600 to 1,600 mg	20 to 40 mg	Three or four times per day
Ethosuximide (Zarontin)	750 to 1,5000 mg	4 to 5 mg	Twice per day
Gabapentin (Neurontin)	900 mg up to 6,000 mg		Three or four times per day
Lamotrigine (Lamictal)	200 to 800 mg		Twice per day
Phenobarbital (Solfoton)	1 to 4 mg per kg	2 to 5 mg	Once or twice per day
Phenytoin (Dilantin)	200 to 500 mg	5 mg up to a maximum of 300 mg	Once or twice per day
Primidone (Mysoline)	500 to 1,000 mg	10 to 20 mg	Three or four times per day
Tiagabine (Gabitril Filmtabs)	32 to 56 mg		Three or four times per day
Topiramate (Topamax)	400 to 800 mg		Twice per day
Valproic acid (Depakene, Depakote)	15 to 60 mg per kg	15 to 60 mg	Three or four times per day

C. The drugs of choice for treatment of partial seizures are carbamazepine and phenytoin. Each of these agents is highly effective for this indication. Valproic acid is also effective in the treatment of partial seizures.

D. Gabapentin, lamotrigine, tiagabine and topiramate are also effective in controlling partial seizures. Each of these latter four drugs is usually used in a combination.

Drugs of Choice for Seizure Disorders

Type of seizure disorder	Drug
Child hood epilepsy	
Absence spells	Ethosuximide (Zarontin), valproic acid (Depakote)
Absence spells with generalized seizures	Valproic acid
Juvenile myoclonic epilepsy	Valproic acid
Temporal lobe epilepsy	Phenytoin (Dilantin), carbamazepine (Tegretol)
Partial complex seizures	Phenytoin, carbamazepine
Simple partial seizures	Carbamazepine, phenytoin
Generalized tonic-clonic seizures	Phenytoin, carbamazepine, valproic acid

Side Effects of Common Antiepileptic Drugs

Drug	Type of side effect			
	Central nervous system	Gastrointestinal	Hematologic	Dermatologic
Carbamazepine (Tegretol)	Diplopia Sedation Neuropathy	Liver dysfunction	Leukopenia Aplastic anemia Folate deficiency anemia	Rashes, bullae Hypertrichosis
Phenytoin (Dilantin)	Sedation Gait disturbances Nystagmus, ataxia Confusion Neuropathy	Liver dysfunction	Decreased lymphocyte count Aplastic anemia Folate deficiency anemia	Rashes, bullae Hypertrichosis
Barbiturates	Sedation Hyperactivity in children Neuropathy	Liver dysfunction	Aplastic anemia Folate deficiency anemia	Rashes, bullae
Valproic acid (Depacon, Depakene, Depakote)	Neuropathy Coma	Hepatic failure	Aplastic anemia Thrombocytopenia Folate deficiency anemia	Rashes, bullae Alopecia

Ethosuximide (Zarontin)	Neuropathy		Aplastic anemia Folate deficiency anemia	Rashes Lupus erythematosus

References, see page 268.

Migraine Headache

Migraine affects 15% to 17% of women and 6% of men. Headaches can generally be grouped into three major categories: migraine, tension-type, and organic.

Clinical evaluation

A. **Migraine** headaches are usually unilateral, and the acute attack typically lasts from 4 to 24 hours. Migraine headaches can occur with an aura or without an aura. The aura may consist of focal neurologic symptoms starting 5 to 30 minutes before onset of an acute headache attack.

B. The most common aura symptoms associated with migraine include scotomata (blind spots), teichopsia (fortification spectra, or the sensation of a luminous appearance before the eyes), photopsia (flashing lights), and paresthesias, as well as visual and auditory hallucinations, diplopia, ataxia, vertigo, syncope, and hyperosmia.

C. **Tension-type headache** is characterized by steady, aching pain of mild to moderate intensity, often as a band-like pain around the head. Gastrointestinal and neurologic signs and symptoms usually do not occur.

D. **Physical examination** should assess the fundus of the eye, neck rigidity, and identify infectious processes of the nose and throat. The temporal artery may appear dilated and pulsating. Neurologic symptoms should be evaluated with computed tomographic scanning.

Pathophysiology of migraine

A. Migraine headache is probably generated by a nucleus in the brainstem. The central generator is the contralateral dorsal raphe nucleus of the midbrain. After the dorsal raphe central generator turns on, there is an activation of the trigeminovascular system. This system connects the generator to the meningeal blood vessels, which dilate and become inflamed, a process referred to as neurogenic inflammation.

B. Two key serotonin (5-HT) receptors, 5-HT_{1B} and 5-HT_{1D}, reverse the migraine processes. The 5-HT_{1D} receptors are vasoconstrictive and are located in the lumen of the meningeal vessels.

Features of Migraine Headache and Headache Caused by Serious Underlying Disease

Migraine headache	Headache caused by serious underlying disease
History	
• Chronic headache pattern similar from attack to attack • Gastrointestinal symptoms • Aura, especially visual • Prodrome	• Onset before puberty or after age 50 (tumor) • "Worst headache ever" (subarachnoid hemorrhage) • Headache occurring after exertion, sex, or bowel movement (subarachnoid hemorrhage) • Headache on rising in the morning (increased intracranial pressure, tumor) • Personality changes, seizures, alteration of consciousness (tumor) • Pain localized to temporal arteries or sudden loss of vision (giant cell arteritis) • Very localized headache (tumor, subarachnoid hemorrhage, giant cell arteritis)
Physical examination	
• No signs of toxicity • Normal vital signs • Normal neurologic examination	• Signs of toxicity (infection, hemorrhage) • Fever (sinusitis, meningitis, or other infection) • Meningismus (meningitis) • Tenderness of temporal arteries (giant cell arteritis) • Focal neurologic deficits (tumor, meningitis, hemorrhage) • Papilledema (tumor)
Laboratory tests and neuroimaging	
• Normal results	• Erythrocyte sedimentation rate >50 mm/hr (giant cell arteritis) • Abnormalities on lumbar puncture (meningitis, hemorrhage) • Abnormalities on CT or MRI (tumor, hemorrhage, aneurysm)

III. **Treatment of migraine**
  A. **5-HT$_{1D}$ receptor agonists ("Triptans")**
    1. **Sumatriptan (Imitrex)**
       a. Sumatriptan (Imitrex) is available in three forms: subcutaneous injection, nasal spray, and oral tablet. Injectable sumatriptan comes as a 6 mg dose for use with an autoinjector. Subcutaneous sumatriptan is the most effective triptan. It works extremely quickly with 50% headache response at 30 minutes, a one-hour headache response of 77%, and more than 80% at two hours. Recurrence of migraine within 24 hours after headache response with injectable sumatriptan is 34-38%. Recurrence

with the spray and tablet is 35-40%.

b. Nasal spray sumatriptan. 20 mg is the optimal dose, with a two-hour headache response of 64%. Almost 40% have headache response at 30 minutes. The spray comes in a single-use device. When sniffed, it causes a terrible taste in the back of the throat; therefore, patients should spray it once in one nostril and not sniff in.

c. The sumatriptan oral tablet has a bioavailability of 14%. The optimal starting dose is 50 mg, with a 61% headache response at two hours.

d. Maximum sumatriptan dosages are two 6-mg subcutaneous doses, two 20-mg nasal sprays, or four 50-mg tablets per 24 hours. However, if a patient needs to switch, she can use one injection or one spray plus two tablets in the same day, or one injection plus one spray in 24 hours.

e. All triptans can cause subjective "triptan sensations," which include heat feelings and flushing, numbness, paresthesias, tiredness and tightening, and heaviness of neck, jaw, and chest. Triptans can narrow coronary arteries. These drugs are contraindicated in coronary artery disease, vascular disease, uncontrolled hypertension, basilar or hemiplegic migraine or within 24 hours of another triptan or ergot.

f. Sumatriptan is the most used triptan. The injection has the fastest onset for a triptan, and the highest overall efficacy.

2. **Zolmitriptan (Zomig)**

a. Zolmitriptan has an oral bioavailability of 40%. Zolmitriptan is contraindicated with MAO-A inhibitors. The optimal dose is 2.5 mg. The maximum dose is 10 mg per 24 hours. Two-hour headache response is 62-65%. Recurrence rate averages about 30%. Adverse events are triptan sensations, similar to sumatriptan tablets.

b. Zolmitriptan is superior to oral sumatriptan (50 mg) for headache response at two hours, 67.1% vs. 63.8%, respectively. Zolmitriptan has a longer duration of action than sumatriptan.

3. **Naratriptan (Amerge)** has good oral bioavailability (63-74%) and a longer T 1/2 (6 hours) than sumatriptan. It works more slowly, and in a lower percentage of patients, than the other three triptans. Two-hour headache response for the optimal dose of 2.5 mg is 48%. The maximum dose is 5 mg per 24 hours. Naratriptan should not be used in patients with rapid onset migraine or who wake up with migraine. Naratriptan should only be selected for those patients who are sensitive to side effects.

4. **Rizatriptan (Maxalt)**

a. Rizatriptan (Maxalt) is a high-efficacy, quick-onset triptan, like sumatriptan and zolmitriptan. Oral bioavailability is more than 40%.

b. Rizatriptan has two doses, 5 and 10 mg, and two forms, traditional tablet and mint-flavored, orally dissolvable tablet or melt. Two-hour headache response for the optimal dose (10 mg) is 67-77%. Recurrence rate is 30-47%.

c. The melt is not absorbed through the buccal mucosa, but rather dissolves on the tongue, is swallowed, and then is absorbed in the gastrointestinal tract. Its efficacy is the same as the traditional tablet, with a two-hour headache response of 66-74%. Adverse events for rizatriptan are similar to those seen with sumatriptan and zolmitriptan tablets.

d. Propranolol raises the circulating rizatriptan level, so patients on propranolol should be given the 5-mg rizatriptan dose. Others should take the 10-mg dose. The maximum rizatriptan dose is 30 mg per 24 hours, but 15 mg per 24 hours for patients on propranolol.

5. **Triptan selection**
   a. Patients with migraine should receive a triptan as the first-line medication. If they have significant nausea, with or without vomiting, an oral drug is not recommended. Rather, a parenteral or nasal spray should be used.
   b. Sumatriptan provides the greatest versatility and should be prescribed to most patients in multiple forms to allow a patient various modes of treatment. The 6-mg subcutaneous injection offers the greatest speed and the highest efficacy of any triptan.
   c. Zolmitriptan has superior headache response to oral sumatriptan at two hours, and less chance of recurrence or use of rescue medicine over the next 24 hours.
   d. Rizatriptan may work sooner than oral sumatriptan. The rizatriptan melt could be taken discretely without water and can be used while driving or at a movie.
   e. Naratriptan has fewer side effects, slower onset, and the lowest recurrence rate of the triptans.

Drugs for Treatment of Migraine and Tension Headache

Drug	Dosage
NSAIDs	
Ibuprofen (Motrin)	400-800 mg, repeat as needed in 4 hr
Naproxen sodium (Anaprox DS)	550-825 mg, repeat as needed in 4 hr
5-HT$_1$ Receptor Agonists ("Triptans")	
Sumatriptan (Imitrex)	6 mg SC; can be repeated in 1 hour; max 2 injections/day 50 mg PO; can be repeated in 2 hours; max 100 mg 20 mg intranasally; can be repeated after 2 hours; max 40 mg/day Max in combination: two injections or sprays; or one of either plus two tablets
Naratriptan (Amerge)	2.5-mg tablet, can be repeated 4 hours later; max 5 mg/day
Rizatriptan (Maxalt)	5- or 10-mg tablet or wafer (MLT); can be repeated in 2 hours; max 100 mg/day, 5 mg/day in patients on propranolol
Zolmitriptan (Zomig)	2.5 mg PO; can be repeated in 2 hours; max 10 mg/day
Ergot Alkaloids	
Dihydroergotamine DHE 45	1 mg IM; can be repeated twice at 1-hour intervals (max 3 mg/attack)
Migranal Nasal Spray	1 spray (0.5 mg)/nostril, repeated 15 minutes later (2 mg/dose; max 3 mg/24 hours)

Drug	Dosage
Ergotamine 1 mg/caffeine 100 mg (Ercaf, Gotamine, Wigraine)	2 tablets PO, then 1 q30min, x 4 PRN (max 6 tabs/attack)
Ergotamine (Ergomar)	2-mg sublingual tablet, can be repeated q30min x 2 PRN (max 3 tabs/attack)
Butalbital combinations	
Aspirin 325 mg, caffeine 40 mg, butalbital 50 mg (Fiorinal)	2 tablets, followed by 1 tablet q4-6h as needed
Acetaminophen 325 mg, butalbital 50 mg (Phrenilin)	2 tablets, followed by 1 tablet as q4-6h needed
Isometheptene combination	
Isometheptene 65 mg, acetaminophen 325 mg, dichloral-phenazone 100 mg (Midrin)	2 tablets, followed by 1 tablet as needed q4-6h prn
Opioid Analgesics	
Butorphanol (Stadol NS)	One spray in one nostril; can be repeated in the other nostril in 60-90 minutes; the same two-dose sequence can be repeated in 3 to 5 hours

B. Prophylaxis against migraine
   1. Patients with frequent or severe migraine headaches or those refractory to symptomatic treatment may benefit from prophylaxis. Menstrual or other predictable migraine attacks may sometimes be prevented by a brief course of an NSAID, taken for several days before and during the first few days of menstruation.
   2. **Beta-adrenergic blocking agents** are used most commonly for continuous prophylaxis. Propranolol, timolol, metoprolol (Lopressor), nadolol (Corgard) and atenolol (Tenormin) have been effective.
   3. **Tricyclic antidepressants** can prevent migraine and may be given concurrently with other prophylactic agents. Amitriptyline (Elavil) in a dosage ranging from 10 to 50 qhs is commonly used.
   4. **Valproate (Depakote)**, an anticonvulsant, has been effective in decreasing migraine frequency. Its effectiveness is equal to that of propranolol. Adverse effects include nausea, weight gain and fatigue. Valproate taken during pregnancy can cause congenital abnormalities.

Drugs for Prevention of Migraine

Drug	Dosage
Propranolol (Inderal)	80 to 240 mg/day, divided bid, tid or qid
Timolol (Blocadren)	10 to 15 mg bid
Divalproex sodium (Depakote)	250 mg bid

Drug	Dosage
Amitriptyline (Elavil)	25-50 mg qhs

References, see page 268.

Vertigo

The clinical evaluation of vertigo begins with the patient's description of symptoms and the circumstances in which they occur. Many drugs can cause dizziness. Common nonvestibular causes (eg, hyperventilation, orthostatic hypotension, panic disorder) are often diagnosed.

I. **History and physical examination**
   A. Patients may use the term "dizziness" to describe one or more different sensations. These sensations include vertigo (spinning), light-headedness, unsteadiness and motion intolerance. The onset of symptoms, whether the sensation is constant or episodic, how often episodes occur and the duration of episodes should be assessed. Activities or movements that provoke or worsen a patient's dizziness should be sought as well as activities that minimize symptoms. Rotational vertigo when rolling over in bed is highly suggestive of BPPV.
   B. Vertigo is a sensation of movement of the self or of one's surroundings. Patients may describe vertigo as a sensation of floating, giddiness or disorientation. The duration of vertiginous symptoms and whether head movement provokes symptoms (positional vertigo) or if attacks occur without provocation (spontaneous vertigo) should be assessed.
   C. Hearing loss, tinnitus and aural fullness should be sought. Vision, strength and sensation, coordination, speech and swallowing should be evaluated. Double vision or hemiplegia strongly suggest a central nervous system lesion rather than a peripheral vestibular disorder. History for cardiac disease, migraine, cerebrovascular disease, thyroid disease and diabetes should be sought.

Drugs Associated with Dizziness

Class of drug	Type of dizziness	Mechanism
Alcohol	Positional vertigo	Specific-gravity difference in endolymph vs cupula
Intoxication	CNS depression	Disequilibrium Cerebellar dysfunction
Tranquilizers	Intoxication	CNS depression
Anticonvulsants	Intoxication Disequilibrium	CNS depression Cerebellar dysfunction
Antihypertensives	Near faint	Postural hypotension

...ass of drug	Type of dizziness	Mechanism
...minoglycosides	Vertigo Disequilibrium Oscillopsia	Asymmetric hair-cell loss Vestibulospinal reflex loss Vestibulo-ocular reflex loss

D. Physical examination should evaluate orthostatic blood pressure changes followed by a complete head and neck examination as well as otologic and neurologic examinations. A pneumatic otoscope should be used to confirm normal tympanic membrane mobility. Balance, gait, cerebellar and cranial nerve function, and nystagmus should be evaluated.

E. Nystagmus consists of involuntary eye movements caused by asymmetry of signals from the right and left vestibular systems. Nystagmus of peripheral vestibular origin is usually horizontal with a slight or dramatic rotary component. Nystagmus of central origin is usually predominantly vertical.

F. The Dix-Hallpike test is particularly helpful to elicit nystagmus associated with BPPV. This maneuver stimulates the posterior semicircular canal, which is the semicircular canal most commonly involved in BPPV.

G. An audiogram should be performed if a specific cause of dizziness cannot be found after a thorough history and physical examination. Additional testing may include electronystagmography, auditory evoked brainstem response testing, radiologic imaging of the brain, brainstem and temporal bone and selected blood tests. Auditory evoked brainstem response testing measures the integrity of the auditory system and is useful to screen for acoustic tumors. Magnetic resonance imaging (MRI) should be reserved for patients with unilateral otologic symptoms or neurologic symptoms or those in whom dizziness persists despite appropriate treatment.

Benign paroxysmal positional vertigo

A. The most common cause of peripheral vestibular vertigo is BPPV. This condition is characterized by sudden, brief and sometimes violent vertigo after a change in head position. The sensation of vertigo usually lasts for only a few seconds. This form of vertigo is often noticed when a patient lies down, arises or turns over in bed. BPPV does not cause hearing loss, ear fullness or tinnitus. BPPV can occur at any age but is most commonly seen in elderly persons. Although usually unilateral, bilateral BPPV occurs in up to 15 percent of patients. Nystagmus is characteristic of BPPV.

B. BPPV is caused by displacement of otoconia from the utricle or saccule into the posterior semicircular canal. Therefore, when a patient moves the head into a provocative position, the otoconia provoke movement of the endolymphatic fluid inside the semicircular canal, creating a sensation of vertigo.

C. Treatment of BPPV. In-office physical therapy, known as repositioning maneuvers, redirects displaced otoconia into the utricle. This form of treatment is effective in 85 to 90 percent of patients. Another type of exercise that is performed at home also attempts to redirect displaced otoconia and is effective in 60 to 70 percent of patients.

D. During these exercises, the patient initially sits upright on the edge of a bed or couch. Then the patient rapidly lies down on his side with the affected ear down. Vertigo usually occurs. After the vertigo subsides (or after one minute if no vertigo occurs), the patient rapidly turns in a smooth arc to the opposite side. After vertigo associated with this movement subsides (or after one minute if no vertigo occurs), the patient slowly sits upright. The entire maneuver is repeated five times twice per day until the patient no longer experiences vertigo for two

successive days. Surgical treatment is reserved for the 2 to 5 percent of case
that fail to respond to nonsurgical treatment.

III. Vestibular neuronitis

A. Vestibular neuronitis is characterized by acute onset of intense verti
associated with nausea and vomiting that is unaccompanied by any neurolog
or audiologic symptoms. The symptoms usually reach their peak within
hours and then gradually subside. During the first 24 to 48 hours of a verti
nous episode, severe truncal unsteadiness and imbalance are present.

B. Vestibular neuronitis is presumed to have a viral etiology because it is oft
associated with a recent history of a flu-like illness. Management of the init
stage of vestibular neuronitis includes bed rest and the use of antiemetics (e
promethazine [Phenergan]) and vestibular suppressants (eg, diazepa
[Valium]). After the patient is able to stand, the brain begins compensating
the acute loss of unilateral vestibular function. The compensation process m
be enhanced by performance of vestibular exercises twice per day for eight
10 weeks.

IV. Meniere's disease

A. Meniere's disease is characterized by fluctuating hearing loss, tinnitus, episo
vertigo and, occasionally, a sensation of fullness or pressure in the ear. Verti
rapidly follows and is typically severe, with episodes occurring abruptly a
without warning. The duration of vertigo is usually several minutes to hou
Unsteadiness and dizziness may persist for days after the episode of verti

B. Diseases with similar symptoms include syphilis, acoustic neuroma a
migraine. Isolated episodes of hearing loss or vertigo may precede
characteristic combination of symptoms by months or years.

C. Meniere's disease results from excessive accumulation of endolymphatic fl
(endolymphatic hydrops). As inner-ear fluid pressure increases, symptoms
Meniere's disease develop.

D. Diuretics (eg, triamterene-hydrochlorothiazide [Dyazide, Maxzide]) and a lo
salt diet are the mainstays of treatment. This combined regimen reduc
endolymphatic fluid pressure. Other preventive measures include use
vasodilators and avoidance of caffeine and nicotine. Acute vertiginous episod
may be treated with oral or intravenous diazepam. Promethazine
glycopyrrolate (Robinul) is effective in the treatment of nausea.

E. Surgical treatments are an option when appropriate prophylactic measures
to prevent recurrent episodes of vertigo. Surgical procedures used in
treatment of Meniere's disease range from draining excess endolymphatic fl
from the inner ear (endolymphatic shunt) to severing the vestibular nerve (w
hearing preservation). In selected cases, a chemical labyrinthectomy may
performed. Chemical labyrinthectomy involves the injection of a vestibuloto
gentamicin (Garamycin) solution into the middle ear.

Antivertiginous and Antiemetic Drugs		
Classes and agents	Dosage	Comments
Antihistamines		
Dimenhydrate (Benadryl)	50 mg PO q4-6h or 100-mg supp. q8h	Available without prescription, mild sedation, minimal side effects
Meclizine (Antivert)	25-50 mg PO q4-6h	Mild sedation, minimal side effects
Promethazine (Phenergan)	25-50 mg PO, IM, or suppository q4-6h	Good for nausea, vertigo, more sedation, extrapyramidal effects
Monoaminergic agents		
Amphetamine	5 or 10 mg PO q4-6h	Stimulant, can counteract sedation of antihistamines, anxiety
Ephedrine	25 mg PO q4-6h	Available without prescription
Benzodiazepine		
Diazepam (Valium)	5 or 10 mg PO q6-8h	Sedation, little effect on nausea
Phenothiazine		
Prochlorperazine (Compazine)	5-25 mg PO, IM, or suppository q4-6h	Good antiemetic; extrapyramidal side effects, particularly in young patients

References, see page 268.

Chronic Fatigue Syndrome

Chronic fatigue is relatively common, but criteria-based chronic fatigue syndrome (CFS) is rare. Fatigue is defined as severe mental and physical exhaustion that differs from somnolence or lack of motivation and is not attributable to exertion or diagnosable disease. Chronic fatigue is defined as persistent or relapsing fatigue lasting 6 or more consecutive months. CFS is characterized by severe disabling fatigue lasting more than 6 months and symptoms that feature impairments in concentration and short-term memory, sleep disturbances, and musculoskeletal pain. About 24% of patients complain of fatigue.

I.   **Common causes of chronic fatigue**
   A. The differential diagnosis of fatigue includes many infections, malignancies, endocrinopathies, and connective tissue disease. The psychiatric illnesses include depression, anxiety, bipolar disease, and somatoform and psychotic disorders. Depression is one of the most common underlying diagnoses when fatigue is a primary complaint.
   B. **Anxiety.** Both depression and anxiety tend to be accompanied by sleep disturbance symptoms. Anemia characteristically will cause a more generalized physical fatigue without sleep disturbances. Asthma and other lung diseases are common causes of fatigue.

Common causes of fatigue		
Diagnosis	Frequency in primary care	Fatigued patients (%)
Depression	Very common	18
Environment (lifestyle)	Very common	17
Anxiety, anemia, asthma	Very common	14
Diabetes	Very common	11
Infections	Common	10
Thyroid, tumors	Common	7
Rheumatologic	Common	5
Endocarditis, cardio-vascular	Common	8
Drugs	Common	5

   C. **Diabetes** should be considered in the obese patient with fatigue. Hypothyroidism and hyperthyroidism are easily treatable causes of fatigue. Tumors and other malignancies may cause tiredness. Many infections cause fatigue, including viruses, tuberculosis, Lyme disease, and HIV infection.
   D. **Rheumatologic disorders,** including rheumatoid arthritis, systemic lupus erythematosus and fibromyalgia, are common causes of fatigue.
   E. **Endocarditis** is a very rare cause of fatigue associated with valvular and other cardiovascular diseases.
   F. **Drugs** that may cause fatigue including analgesics, psychotropics, antihypertensives, and antihistamines. Over-the-counter medications and substance abuse (caffeine, alcohol, and illicit drugs) may cause fatigue.
II. **Clinical evaluation**
   A. Evaluation of chronic fatigue should exclude diseases associated with fatigue. The time of onset of symptoms and the nature of the fatigue should be determined. Chronic fatigue syndrome is characterized by fatigue that is typically present throughout the day (even upon awakening), worsens with exercise, and is not improved with rest.
   B. Fever, chills, night sweats, weight loss or anorexia may be seen in chronic fatigue syndrome; however, infectious disease or malignancy should also be considered. Confusion and cognitive difficulties are reported by nearly all chronic fatigue syndrome patients.
   C. Headaches, myalgias, arthralgias, and painful adenopathy are common complaints in chronic fatigue syndrome, although the presence of arthritis may also suggest connective tissue diseases. Anhedonia is suggestive of depression.
   D. Recent travel, insect bites, tick exposure, skin rashes, and use of prescription and over-the-counter drugs should be sought.

E. Physical examination. Specific physical findings such as nonexudative pharyngitis, lymphadenopathy, skin rashes, muscle tenderness and orthostatic hypotension are often seen in chronic fatigue syndrome patients. The Romberg test and tandem gait test may be abnormal in up to 20% of chronic fatigue syndrome patients.

Criteria for chronic fatigue syndrome

Clinically evaluated, unexplained, persistent or relapsing chronic fatigue of new or definite onset; not the result of ongoing exertion; not substantially alleviated by rest; and causes substantial reduction in previous levels of occupational, educational, social, or personal activities; and

Occurs concomitantly with four or more of the following symptoms, all of which must have persisted or recurred during 6 or more consecutive months of illness and must not have predated the fatigue:
Short-term memory or concentration impairment
Sore throat
Tender cervical or axillary lymph nodes
Muscle pain or multijoint pain without joint swelling or redness
Headaches of a new type, pattern, or severity
Unrefreshing sleep
Postexertional malaise lasting more than 24 hours

Laboratory evaluation of chronic fatigue

For all patients
Complete blood cell count with differential
Erythrocyte sedimentation rate
Urinalysis
Other tests based on findings
Thyroid stimulating hormone
Blood Chemistry levels:
Alanine aminotransferase
Aspartate aminotransferase
Blood urea nitrogen
Electrolytes
Glucose
Heterophil antibody test (Monospot)
Serologic studies for Lyme or HIV antibody titers

III. Management of the fatigued patient

A. Regular exercise will improve functional capacity, mood, and sleep. Regular sleep habits should be advised. In those complaining of depressive symptoms or sleep disturbance, an antidepressant or sleep hypnotic is indicated. A sedating antidepressant, such as amitriptyline (Elavil) 25 mg qhs, may be helpful for complaints of insomnia or restlessness. If the primary complaints are hypersomnia and psychomotor retardation, a selective serotonin reuptake inhibitor is indicated.

B. For physical symptoms such as headaches, myalgias, or arthralgias, nonsteroidal anti-inflammatory agents may be helpful. Therapies for which no effectiveness has been demonstrated in CFS include vitamins, acyclovir, gamma globulin, folic acid, cyanocobalamin, and magnesium.

C. **Antidepressants**
1. Selective serotonin reuptake inhibitors (SSRIs) are the drugs of choice. Fluoxetine (Prozac), paroxetine (Paxil), sertraline (Zoloft), and fluvoxamine (LuVox) are effective in reducing fatigue, myalgia, sleep disturbance, and depression.
2. For the patient who has significant difficulty with insomnia or with pain, paroxetine at bedtime is recommended because it is mildly sedating. Fluoxetine is useful in patients who complain of lack of energy because it has activating properties. Fluoxetine often improves cognitive functioning, especially concentrating ability.
3. Initial dosage should be low because many CFS patients are sensitive to side effects.
   a. Fluoxetine (Prozac) 20 mg PO qAM; 20-40 mg/d [20 mg].
   b. Paroxetine (Paxil) 10 mg qAM; increase as needed to max of 40 mg/d. [10, 20, 30, 40 mg].
   c. Fluvoxamine (LuVox) 50-100 mg qhs; max 300 mg/d [50, 100 mg]
   d. Sertraline (Zoloft) 50-100 mg PO qAM [50, 100 mg].

D. **Omega-3 and omega-6 fatty acids**, in the form of fish oil supplements, may bring some improvement.

IV. **Prognosis**. CFS is a chronic illness, but 40-60% of patients improve within1-3 years after diagnosis. The mean duration of illness prior to diagnosis is 52.6 months.

References, see page 268.

Dermatologic and Allergic Disorders

Herpes Simplex Virus Infections

Herpes simplex virus (HSV) affects more than one-third of the world's population. HSV exists as types 1 and 2, which have affinities for different body sites. Ninety percent of infections caused by HSV-2 are genital, and 90 percent of those caused by HSV-1 are oral.

I. Diagnosis

A. The diagnosis of genital HSV infection may be made clinically, but laboratory confirmation is recommended in patients presenting with primary or suspected recurrent infection. The gold standard of diagnosis is viral isolation by tissue culture, although this process can take as long as four to five days, and the sensitivity rate is only 70 to 80 percent. Viral culture is still the diagnostic test of choice for HSV skin infections.

B. Polymerase chain reaction enzyme-linked immunosorbent assay (PCR-ELISA) is extremely sensitive (96 percent) and specific (99 percent) but expensive. For this reason, it is not used for the diagnosis of skin lesions but is the test of choice for diagnosing HSV encephalitis.

II. Antiviral medications

A. Acyclovir is an acyclic guanosine analog. Oral bioavailability is only 15 to 30 percent. The dosage must be adjusted in patients with renal failure. Acyclovir is a safe and extremely well-tolerated drug. Toxicity is rare, but in patients who are dehydrated or who have poor renal function, the drug can crystallize in the renal tubules, leading to a reversible creatinine elevation or, rarely, acute tubular necrosis. Adverse effects, usually mild, include nausea, vomiting, rash and headache.

B. Valacyclovir is the l-valine ester prodrug of acyclovir. It has an oral bioavailability three to five times greater than that of acyclovir, and it is safe and well tolerated.

C. Famciclovir is the oral form of penciclovir, a purine analog similar to acyclovir. Oral bioavailability is 77 percent. Mechanism and efficacy are similar to those of acyclovir.

III. Genital herpes

A. Genital HSV infection is usually transmitted through sexual contact. About 21.9 percent of all persons in the United States 12 years of age or older have serologic evidence of HSV-2 infection. Risk factors include multiple sexual partners, increasing age, female gender, low socioeconomic status and human immunodeficiency virus (HIV) infection.

B. Clinical presentation

1. Primary genital herpes has an incubation period of two to 12 days, with a mean of four days, followed by a prodrome of itching, burning or erythema. Multiple transient, painful vesicles then appear on the penis, perineum, vulva, vagina or cervix, and tender inguinal lymphadenopathy may follow. The initial ulceration crusts and heals by 14 to 21 days. Systemic symptoms include fever, headache, malaise, abdominal pain and myalgia. Recurrences are usually less severe and shorter in duration than the initial outbreak.

2. Approximately 90 percent of those infected are unaware that they have herpes infection and may unknowingly shed virus and transmit infection.

C. Treatment of primary infection
1. **Acyclovir (Zovirax)** is effective in reducing symptoms. The oral acyclovir dosage for treatment of primary genital herpes is 400 mg PO tid or 200 mg five times daily for 10 days. Intravenous administration may be required in immunocompromised patients and those with severe disseminated infection. Topical acyclovir is much less effective than oral or intravenous acyclovir.
2. **Valacyclovir (Valtrex)**, 400 mg PO tid, is indicated for the treatment of primary genital herpes but costs more than acyclovir.
3. **Famciclovir (Famvir)**, 250 mg PO tid for 7-10 days, is as effective as acyclovir in the treatment of initial genital herpes infection, although it may be twice as expensive.

D. Treatment of recurrent infection
1. Recurrences of herpes are often mild and infrequent. Drug therapy to prevent recurrences is reserved for patients who have more than six outbreaks per year.
2. Acyclovir (Zovirax) has been used to suppress recurrences of genital herpes, decreasing the frequency by as much as 80 percent.
3. Famciclovir and valacyclovir are as effective as acyclovir in suppressing recurrent genital herpes. Valacyclovir has the advantage of once-daily dosing. Famciclovir must be given twice daily to be effective.

Dosages and Characteristics of Chronic Suppressive Treatment Regimens for Recurrent Genital Herpes Infection		
Drug	**Dosage**	**Decrease in recurrence rate (percentage)**
Acyclovir (Zovirax)	400 mg twice daily [200, 400, 800 mg]	78 to 79
Famciclovir (Famvir)	250 mg twice daily [125, 250, 500 mg]	79
Valacyclovir (Valtrex)	1 g once daily [500 mg]	78 to 79

4. **Episodic therapy** is intended to diminish symptoms and infectivity during recurrences. Acyclovir, taken within minutes to hours after the prodrome of recurrence begins, exerts a minimal benefit in recurrent genital herpes infections. Famciclovir and valacyclovir are slightly more effective for the treatment of recurrent infections.

Dosages and Cost of Antiviral Agents for Treatment of Episodic Genital Herpes	
Drug	**Dosage**
Acyclovir (Zovirax)	200 mg 5 times daily for 5 days 800 mg twice daily for 5 days
Famciclovir (Famvir)	125 mg twice daily for 5 days
Valacyclovir (Valtrex)	500 mg twice daily for 5 days

IV. Orolabial herpes
  A. Orolabial herpes (gingivostomatitis) is the most prevalent form of mucocutaneous herpes infection; 35 to 60 percent of persons in the United States show serologic evidence of having been infected by HSV-1. Overall, the highest rate of infection occurs during the preschool years. Female gender, history of sexually transmitted diseases and multiple sexual partners are risk factors.
  B. Clinical presentation
    1. Primary herpetic gingivostomatitis usually affects children under the age of five. It typically takes the form of painful vesicles and ulcerative erosions on the tongue, palate, gingiva, buccal mucosa and lips. Edema, halitosis and drooling may be present, and tender submandibular or cervical lymphadenopathy is common.
    2. Systemic symptoms include fever (38.4 to 40°°C [101 to 104°°F]), malaise and myalgia. The duration of the illness is two to three weeks, and oral shedding of virus may continue for as long as 23 days.
    3. Recurrences typically occur two or three times a year. The duration is shorter and the discomfort less severe than in primary infections. UV radiation may trigger recurrence of orolabial HSV-1.
  C. Treatment of primary infection
    1. Topical acyclovir has not proved to accelerate healing. Topical penciclovir (Denavir), applied every two hours for four days, reduces clinical healing time by one day.
    2. Oral acyclovir, in a dosage of 200 mg five times daily for five days, accelerates loss of crusts by one day in adults and can reduce the mean duration of pain by 36 percent. Acyclovir decreases the duration of oral lesions in primary infection from 10 days to four days. Standard analgesic therapy with acetaminophen or ibuprofen should also be advised.
  D. Treatment of recurrent infection
    1. Oral acyclovir (400 mg bid) is effective in reducing by 50 to 78 percent the frequency of herpes labialis. Oral acyclovir lessens the severity of lesions when they occur. Short-term prophylactic therapy (400 mg bid) with acyclovir may be desirable in some patients who anticipate intense exposure to UV light (eg, skiers, or in those who work outdoors) or before special occasions, such as a wedding.
    2. **Famciclovir (Famvir),** in a dosage of 250 mg tid for five days, accelerates healing time from 5.8 days to 3.0 days.
V. Patient counseling
  A. Patients should be warned about HSV autoinoculation from one body site to another. Infected areas should be patted dry rather than wiped dry. Sunscreen and lip balm are recommended to reduce recurrent disease.
  B. Patients should abstain from sexual activity while lesions are present. Use of latex condoms is encouraged because of asymptomatic viral shedding.
  C. The risk of neonatal transmission must be explained to the patient.
  D. Recommended testing includes evaluation for gonorrhea, chlamydia, syphilis, genital warts, and human immunodeficiency virus (HIV).

References, see page 268.

Herpes Zoster and Postherpetic Neuralgia

Herpes zoster (shingles) results from reactivation of the varicella-zoster virus. Herpes zoster is a sporadic disease with an estimated lifetime incidence of 10 to 20 percent. The incidence of herpes zoster increases sharply with advancing age, roughly doubling in each decade past the age of 50 years. Herpes zoster is uncommon in persons less than 15 years old.

I. Pathophysiology

A. Varicella-zoster virus is a highly contagious DNA virus. Varicella represents the primary infection in the nonimmune person. During the primary infection, the virus gains entry into the sensory dorsal root ganglia, where the virus remains latent for decades. Reactivation of the virus occurs following a decrease in virus-specific cell-mediated immunity. The reactivated virus causes a dermatomal distribution of pain and skin lesions.

B. Although herpes zoster is not as contagious as the primary varicella infection, persons with reactivated infection can transmit varicella-zoster virus to nonimmune contacts. About 20 percent of patients with herpes zoster develop postherpetic neuralgia. The most established risk factor is age; this complication occurs nearly 15 times more often in patients more than 50 years of age.

II. Clinical evaluation

A. Herpes zoster typically presents with a prodrome consisting of hyperesthesia, paresthesias, burning dysesthesias or pruritus along the affected dermatome(s). The prodrome generally lasts one to two days but may precede the appearance of skin lesions by up to three weeks.

B. The skin lesions begin as a maculopapular rash that follows a dermatomal distribution in a "belt-like pattern." The maculopapular rash evolves into vesicles with an erythematous base. The vesicles are painful, and their development is often associated with the occurrence of flu-like symptoms. Although any vertebral dermatome may be involved, T5 and T6 are most commonly affected. The most frequently involved cranial nerve dermatome is the ophthalmic division of the trigeminal nerve. The vesicles crust over within seven to 10 days.

C. **Postherpetic neuralgia** is defined as pain that persists for longer than one to three months after resolution of the rash. Affected patients usually report constant burning, lancinating pain. Symptoms tend to abate over time. Less than one quarter of patients still experience pain at six months after the herpes zoster eruption, and fewer than one in 20 has pain at one year.

III. Treatment of herpes zoster

A. **Antiviral agents** have been shown to decrease the duration of herpes zoster rash and the severity of pain associated with the rash. Benefits have been demonstrated in patients who received antiviral agents within 72 hours after the onset of rash.

B. **Acyclovir (Zovirax)** therapy appears to produce a moderate reduction in the development of postherpetic neuralgia. Other antiviral agents, specifically valacyclovir (Valtrex) and famciclovir (Famvir), appear to be at least as effective as acyclovir.

C. **Valacyclovir (Valtrex)**, a prodrug of acyclovir, is administered three times daily. Compared with acyclovir, valacyclovir may be slightly better at decreasing the severity of pain associated with herpes zoster, as well as the duration of postherpetic neuralgia.

D. **Famciclovir (Famvir).** The advantages of famciclovir are its dosing schedule (three times daily), its longer intracellular half-life compared with acyclovir and

its better bioavailability compared with acyclovir and valacyclovir.
- **E.** All three antiviral agents are generally well tolerated. The most common adverse effects are nausea, headache, vomiting, dizziness and abdominal pain.

Treatment Options for Herpes Zoster	
Medication	**Dosage**
Acyclovir (Zovirax)	800 mg orally five times daily for 7 to 10 days; 10 mg per kg IV every 8 hours for 7 to 10 days
Famciclovir (Famvir)	500 mg orally three times daily for 7 days
Valacyclovir (Valtrex)	1,000 mg orally three times daily for 7 days
Prednisone (Deltasone)	30 mg orally twice daily on days 1 through 7; then 15 mg twice daily on days 8 through 14; then 7.5 mg twice daily on days 15 through 21

- **F.** Prednisone used in conjunction with acyclovir has been shown to reduce the pain associated with herpes zoster. Some studies with prednisone therapy have shown decreased postherpetic neuralgia pain at three and 12 months. Other studies have demonstrated no benefit.
- **G. Analgesics.** Patients with mild-to-moderate pain may respond to over-the-counter analgesics. Patients with more severe pain may require the addition of a narcotic medication. Lotions containing calamine (eg, Caladryl) may be used on open lesions to reduce pain and pruritus. Once the lesions have crusted over, capsaicin cream (Zostrix) may be applied. The lidocaine (Xylocaine) patch (q4-12h) and nerve blocks have also been reported to be effective in reducing pain.
- **H. Ocular involvement.** Ocular herpes zoster is treated with orally administered antiviral agents and corticosteroids.

V. Treatment of postherpetic neuralgia
- **A.** Although postherpetic neuralgia is generally a self-limited condition, it can last indefinitely.

Treatment of Postherpetic Neuralgia	
Medication	**Dosage**
Topical agents	
Capsaicin cream (Zostrix)	Apply to affected area three to five times daily.
Lidocaine (Xylocaine) patch	Apply to affected area every 4 to 12 hours as needed.

Tricyclic antidepressants	
Amitriptyline (Elavil)	0 to 25 mg orally at bedtime; increase dosage by 25 mg every 2 to 4 weeks until response is adequate, or to maximum dosage of 150 mg per day.
Nortriptyline (Pamelor)	0 to 25 mg orally at bedtime; increase dosage by 25 mg every 2 to 4 weeks until response is adequate, or to maximum dosage of 125 mg per day.
Imipramine (Tofranil)	25 mg orally at bedtime; increase dosage by 25 mg every 2 to 4 weeks until response is adequate, or to maximum dosage of 150 mg per day.
Desipramine (Norpramin)	25 mg orally at bedtime; increase dosage by 25 mg every 2 to 4 weeks until response is adequate, or to maximum dosage of 150 mg per day.
Anticonvulsants	
Phenytoin (Dilantin)	100 to 300 mg orally at bedtime; increase dosage until response is adequate or blood drug level is 10 to 20 µg per mL (40 to 80 µmol per L).
Carbamazepine (Tegretol)	100 mg orally at bedtime; increase dosage by 100 mg every 3 days until dosage is 200 mg three times daily, response is adequate or blood drug level is 6 to12 µg per mL (25.4 to 50.8 µmol per L).
Gabapentin (Neurontin)	100 to 300 mg orally at bedtime; increase dosage by 100 to 300 mg every 3 days until dosage is 300 to 900 mg three times daily or response is adequate.

B. **Analgesics**
1. **Capsaicin (Zostrix-HP)**, an extract from hot chili peppers, is more efficacious for post-herpetic neuralgia than placebo. Capsaicin cream must be applied to the affected area three to five times daily.
2. **Lidocaine patches** reduce pain intensity, with minimal systemic absorption. The effect lasts only four to 12 hours with each application.
3. **Acetaminophen** (eg, Tylenol) and nonsteroidal anti-inflammatory drugs are useful for potentiating the pain-relieving effects of other agents.
C. **Tricyclic antidepressants** that are commonly used in the treatment of postherpetic neuralgia include amitriptyline (Elavil), nortriptyline (Pamelor), imipramine (Tofranil) and desipramine (Norpramin).
D. **Anticonvulsants.** Phenytoin (Dilantin), carbamazepine (Tegretol) and gabapentin (Neurontin) are often used to control neuropathic pain.
E. **Other modalities** used to treat post-herpetic neuralgia include transcutaneous electric nerve stimulation (TENS), biofeedback and nerve blocks.

References, see page 268.

Acne Vulgaris

Acne vulgaris is a polymorphous skin disorder of the sebaceous follicles that begins around the time of puberty and peaks during the teenage years. Prevalence exceeds 85% in teenagers and then declines to about 8% in 25-to 34-year olds and to 3% in 35- to 44-year-olds. More adolescent boys than girls are afflicted.

I. **Pathophysiology of acne**
   A. Acne is a disease of the pilosebaceous follicle, most commonly on the face, neck, and upper trunk. Acne vulgaris arises from increased sebum production. Androgenic hormones produced during the pubertal period enlarge sebaceous glands, causing increased sebum production.
   B. Proliferation of Propionibacterium acnes is felt to play a pivotal role in the pathogenesis of inflammatory acne lesions.

II. **Clinical evaluation.** Acne vulgaris occurs primarily on the face and (to a varying degree) the neck, upper back, chest, and shoulders. Classification is based on the number and predominant type of lesions and on the affected sites. The three distinct types are obstructive acne, inflammatory acne, and acne scars.

III. **Treatment of acne**
   A. Topical agents are generally preferred for comedonal lesions and for superficial inflammatory acne without scarring. Cream is the vehicle of choice in patients with dry or sensitive skin. Topical gels and solutions contain alcohol and are preferred by those with excessively oily skin.
   B. Topical comedolytic agents reduce the formation of the microcomedo by reversing abnormal keratinization process duct. These agents are the cornerstone of obstructive acne treatment and an important adjunct in all patients with inflammatory acne.
      1. **Topical tretinoin (Retin-A)**, a vitamin A derivative, promotes the drainage of preexisting comedones and reduces the formation of new ones. The full cosmetic benefit may not be apparent for 6-12 weeks. Tretinoin should be applied lightly every night at bedtime. Skin irritation (dryness, erythema, and peeling) is common. Patients should avoid excessive sun exposure or should use a protective sunscreen.
      2. Tretinoin (Retin-A) is available in creams (0.025%, 0.05%, 0.1%), gels (0.01%, 0.025%), liquid (0.05%), and a microsphere (Retin-A Micro 0.1%). The liquid is the most irritating. Patients with fair or sensitive skin should begin by using the 0.025% cream every other day and gradually increase to daily use at a higher concentration as tolerated. The microsphere reduces the potential for irritation.
      3. **Adapalene (Differin** 0.1% gel), a naphthoic acid derivative with retinoid activity, is comparable to tretinoin, it appears to be less irritating, and it has anti-inflammatory activity. Adapalene is applied as a thin film daily at bedtime. A therapeutic effect is typically seen within 8-12 weeks. Skin irritation occurs in 10-40% of patients. Users should minimize exposure to sunlight.
      4. **Tazarotene (Tazorac**, 0.05% and 0.1% gel), a synthetic acetylenic retinoid with comedolytic properties, is FDA-approved for topical treatment of mild-to-moderate facial acne. It is applied every evening. Tazarotene is associated with skin irritation. Tazarotene does not offer any significant advantages over tretinoin or adapalene.
   C. **Topical antibiotics** inhibit the growth and activity of P acnes. Choices include clindamycin (Cleocin-T 1% solution, lotion, or gel), erythromycin (A/T/S 2% gel

or solution, Erygel 2% gel, Akne-Mycin 2% ointment, T-Stat 2% solution and pads), sulfacetamide (Klaron 10% lotion), and a 3% erythromycin and 5% benzoyl peroxide gel (Benzamycin). Topical antibiotics are applied twice daily. Skin dryness and irritation are the most common side effects. Antibiotic resistance is possible. Resistance is less likely with the erythromycin and benzoyl peroxide combination, making it an option for patients who have developed resistance to other agents.

D. **Benzoyl peroxide** is an antibacterial, agent that may also have mild comedolytic properties. It is available over-the-counter and in prescription formulations (2.5%, 5%, and 10% lotions, creams, and gels). Benzoyl peroxide is typically applied as a thin film, once or twice daily. Mild redness and scaling are common during the first few weeks.

E. **Azelaic acid (Azelex** 20% cream), a dicarboxylic acid with combined antimicrobial and comedolytic properties, is FDA-approved for mild-to-moderate inflammatory acne. It is massaged in twice daily. Mild skin irritation occurs in 5-10% of patients. Because azelaic acid does not cause photosensitivity, it is an alternative comedolytic agent for patients who are reluctant to refrain from activities that involve significant exposure to the sun. Hypopigmentation is a rare adverse reaction.

F. **Systemic agents**
   1. Oral antibiotics are the foundation of moderate-to-severe inflammatory acne treatment because they reduce ductal concentrations of P acnes. Improvement can generally be seen within 2-3 weeks.
   2. **Tetracycline** is favored because of its better tolerability and lower incidence of P acnes resistance. It is initiated at a dose of 1-2 g/d in 2-4 divided doses. Tetracycline should be taken on an empty stomach. Many individuals whose acne is controlled can be weaned off oral antibiotics after 6 months of therapy, and then topical antimicrobial therapy can be continued for maintenance.
   3. Long-term use is considered safe; the most common side effects are gastrointestinal upset and vulvovaginal candidiasis. Gram-negative folliculitis may occur, typically manifested by the sudden appearance of superficial pustular or cystic acne lesions around the nares and flaring out over the cheeks.
   4. **Minocycline (Minocin)** and trimethoprim/sulfamethoxazole (TMP/SMX [Bactrim, Septra]) have a place in treating some refractory cases. Minocycline can be particularly valuable for patients with treatment-resistant inflammatory acne. Minocycline, like all tetracyclines, is contraindicated in pregnant women and in children younger than 9 years of age because of potential adverse effects on developing bones and teeth.
   5. TMP/SMX is prescribed at a dose of 1 regular-strength tablet, qd or bid. Hematologic and dermatologic side effects have restricted its use to patients with severe acne refractory to other antibiotics and to those who develop gram-negative folliculitis secondary to long-term antibiotic therapy.

G. **Hormone therapy** improves acne by suppressing sebum production. A triphasic oral contraceptive pill containing ethinyl estradiol, 35 μg, and norgestimate (Ortho Tri-Cyclen) has been shown to reduce inflammatory acne lesions by 40%.

H. **Oral isotretinoin** (13-cis-retinoic acid [Accutane]) is the only available agent with the potential both to cure acne. Most patients are started at 0.5-1 mg/kg qd or bid, typically for 15-20 weeks. Isotretinoin may be considered for unresponsive moderate-to-severe inflammatory acne. Virtually all patients will see an 80%-90% reduction in acne lesions within 2-4 months of isotretinoin initiation.

Adverse reactions to isotretinoin include cheilitis, nose bleeds, dry skin and mucous membranes, and photosensitivity. Less common are arthralgias myalgias, headache, nyctalopia, and, in rare cases, pseudotumor cerebri. Isotretinoin can induce abnormalities in liver, hematologic, and lipid functions such as hypertriglyceridemia and hypercholesterolemia. Isotretinoin is a teratogen associated with major fetal malformations. Contraception must be ensured both during use and for at least 1 month after discontinuation.

I. **Comedone extraction** is an office procedure used to disimpact obstructive acne lesions. The obstructing plug can usually be expressed after enlarging the pore with a 25-gauge needle.

J. Intralesional corticosteroid injection can rapidly (within 48-72 hours) resolve large or recalcitrant inflammatory acne lesions and reduce the risk for scarring. A 30-gauge needle is used to inject 0.05-0.3 mL of a solution containing triamcinolone acetonide through the pore of the lesion. The corticosteroid solution is usually diluted with normal saline or lidocaine to a concentration of 0.63-2.5.

References, see page 268.

Contact Dermatitis

Contact dermatitis is an extremely common occurrence in the pediatric age group. There are two major forms of contact dermatitis: irritant and allergic. Irritant contact dermatitis is the most common and occurs when a person is exposed to an agent that has a direct toxic effect on the skin. Common causes of irritant contact dermatitis include overbathing, drooling, prolonged contact with moisture and feces in the diaper, and bubble baths.

Clinical evaluation

A. Contact dermatitis usually first appears in infants 2-6 months of age. Infants and children have rashes on the shoulders, chest, abdomen, and back. Infants usually also have a rash on the face, scalp and around the ears. Children older than 18 months old tend to have rashes on the neck and antecubital and popliteal fossae. Contact dermatitis usually resolves by puberty, but it sometimes recurs at times of stress.

B. Acute lesions are itchy, red, edematous papules and small vesicles which may progress to weeping and crusting lesions. Chronic rubbing and scratching may cause lichenification and hyperpigmentation. The classic triad of atopy consists of asthma, allergic rhinitis, and dermatitis.

Precipitating Factors and Activities in Contact Dermatitis	
Moisture-related	Excessive bathing, excessive hand washing, excessive lip licking, excessive sweating, extended showers or baths, repeated contact with water, swimming, occlusive clothing and footwear

Contact-related	Overuse of soap, bubble-bath, cosmetics, deodorants, detergents, solvents, tight clothing, rough fabrics, wool or mohair
Temperature-related	Exposure to excessive warmth, humidity, over-dressing, hot showers or baths
Emotional	Anger, anxiety, depression, stress
Infective	Bacteria, fungi, viruses
Inhalational	Animal dander, cigarette smoke, dust, perfume

C. Patch testing is useful for evaluation of persistent, localized reactions of th hands, feet, and perioral area. It also may be useful in patients who have atop dermatitis and experience a flare or persistence of disease despite appropriat therapy.

II. Treatment of contact dermatitis

A. **Moisture.** Avoidance of excessive bathing, hand washing, and lip licking i recommended. Showers or baths should be limited to no more than 5 minute After bathing, patients should apply a moisturizer (Aquaphor, Eucerin, Lubriderm petrolatum) to noninflamed skin.

B. **Contact with irritants**
  1. Overuse of soap should be discouraged. Use of nonirritating soaps (eg, Dove Ivory, Neutrogena) should be limited to the axilla, groin, hands, and feet.
  2. Infants often have bright red exudative contact dermatitis (slobber dermatitis on the cheeks, resulting from drooling. A corticosteroid will usually brin improvement.

C. **Topical corticosteroids**
  1. Corticosteroid ointments maintain skin hydration and maximize penetratio Corticosteroid creams may sting when applied to acute lesions.
  2. Mid- and low-potency topical corticosteroids are used twice-daily for chroni atopic dermatitis. High-potency steroids may be used for flare-ups, but th potency should be tapered after the dermatitis is controlled.
  3. Use of high-potency agents on the face, genitalia and skin-folds may caus epidermal atrophy ("stretch marks"), rebound erythema, and susceptibility bruising.

Commonly Used Topical Corticosteroids	
Preparation	Size
Low-Potency Agents	
Hydrocortisone ointment, cream, 1, 2.5% (Hytone)	30 g
Mild-Potency Agents	
Alclometasone dipropionate cream, ointment, 0.05% (Aclovate)	60 g

Preparation	Size
Triamcinolone acetonide cream, 0.1% (Aristocort)	60 g
Fluocinolone acetonide cream, 0.01% (Synalar)	60 g
Medium-Potency Agents	
Triamcinolone acetonide ointment (Aristocort A), 0.1%	60 g
Betamethasone dipropionate cream (Diprosone), 0.05%	45 g
Triamcinolone acetonide cream, ointment, 0.1% (Kenalog)	60 g
Mometasone cream 0.1% (Elocon)	45 g
Fluocinolone acetonide ointment, 0.025% (Synalar)	60 g
Hydrocortisone butyrate 0.1% cream, ointment (Locoid)	45 g
Betamethasone valerate cream, 0.1% (Valisone)	45 g
Hydrocortisone valerate cream, ointment, 0.2% (Westcort)	60 g
High-Potency Agents	
Amcinonide ointment, 0.1% (Cyclocort)	60 g
Betamethasone dipropionate ointment (Diprosone) 0.05%	45 g
Fluocinonide cream, ointment, 0.05% (Lidex)	60 g

4. **Allergic reactions to topical corticosteroids** may occur. Mometasone (Elocon) is the least likely to cause an allergic reaction.
D. **Antihistamines**, such as diphenhydramine or hydroxyzine (Atarax), are somewhat useful for pruritus and are sedating. Nonsedating antihistamines, such as loratadine (Claritin) and fexofenadine (Allegra), are helpful.
E. **Systemic steroids.** Systemic corticosteroids are reserved for severe, widespread reactions to poison ivy, or for severe involvement of the hands, face, or genitals. Prednisone, 1-2 mg/kg, is given PO and tapered over 10-18 days.

*eferences, see page 268.

inea Infections

►out 10-20 percent of persons acquire a dermatophyte infection during their lifetime. ►rmatophyte infections are classified according to the affected body site, such as ►ea capitis (scalp), tinea barbae (beard area), tinea corporis (skin other than bearded ►a, scalp, groin, hands or feet), tinea cruris (groin, perineum and perineal areas), ►ea pedis (feet), tinea manuum (hands) and tinea unguium (nails).

144 Tinea Infections

I. Diagnosis
A. **Microscopy.** Material is scraped from an active area of the lesion, placed in a drop of potassium hydroxide solution, and examined under a microscope. Microscopy is positive if hyphae are identified in fungal infections and pseudohyphae or yeast forms are seen in Candida or Pityrosporum infection.

B. **Cultures** are not routinely performed in suspected tinea infections. However, cultures may be obtained when long-term oral drug therapy is being considered, the patient has a recalcitrant infection, or the diagnosis is in doubt.

II. Tinea capitis
A. Tinea capitis primarily affects school-aged children, appearing as one or more round patches of alopecia. Hair shafts broken off at the scalp may appear as black dots. Sometimes tinea capitis appears as non-specific dandruff, or gray patches of hair, or areas of scales, pustules and erythema. A localized, boggy indurated granuloma called a "kerion" may develop.

B. Tinea capitis should be treated with oral therapy. Griseofulvin (Fulvicin PG, Gris PEG, Grisactin Ultra), itraconazole (Sporanox) and terbinafine (Lamisil) are effective options.

III. Tinea barbae.
Tinea barbae affects the beard area of men who work with animals. It is often accompanied by bacterial folliculitis and inflammation secondary to ingrown hairs. Oral therapy with griseofulvin, itraconazole (Sporanox) or terbinafine (Lamisil) is preferred over topical therapy because the involved hair follicles do not respond well to topical therapy.

IV. Tinea corporis
A. Tinea corporis ("ringworm") often affects children and adults who live in hot, humid climates. The classic presentation of this infection is a lesion with central clearing surrounded by an advancing, red, scaly, elevated border.

B. Since tinea corporis can be asymptomatic, it can spread rapidly among children in day-care settings. Unless only one or two lesions are present, tinea corporis should be treated orally. Terbinafine and itraconazole are equally effective in treating tinea corporis. These agents have a better cure rate than griseofulvin. An alternative is fluconazole (Diflucan), which is given orally once a week for up to four consecutive weeks.

V. Tinea cruris
A. Tinea cruris ("jock itch") usually involves the medial aspect of the upper thigh (groin). Unlike yeast infections, tinea cruris generally does not involve the scrotum or the penis. This dermatophyte infection occurs more often in men than in women and rarely affects children. Erythematous, pruritic plaques often develop bilaterally. Topical therapy is sufficient in most patients with tinea cruris. If the infection spreads to the lower thighs or buttocks, oral therapy with itraconazole or terbinafine is recommended.

VI. Tinea pedis
A. Tinea pedis ("athlete's foot") is the most common dermatophyte infection. Tinea pedis infection is usually related to sweating, warmth, and oclusive footwear. The infection often presents as white, macerated areas in the third or fourth toe web or as chronic dry, scaly hyperkeratosis of the soles and heels.

B. Occasionally, tinea pedis may produce acute, highly inflamed, sterile vesicles at distant sites (arms, chest, sides of fingers). Referred to as the "dermatophytid" or "id" reaction, these vesicles probably represent an immunologic response to the fungus; they subside when the primary infection is controlled. The "id" reaction can be the only manifestation of an asymptomatic web space infection.

C. Tinea pedis is often treated with topical therapy. Oral itraconazole and terbinafine are more efficacious in the treatment of hyperkeratotic tinea pedis. Once-weekly dosing with fluconazole is another option, especially in noncompliant patients.

VII. **Tinea manuum** is a fungal infection of the hands. Tinea manuum presents with erythema and mild scaling on the dorsal aspect of the hands or as a chronic, dry, scaly hyperkeratosis of the palms. When the palms are infected, the feet are also commonly infected. Treatment options are the same as for tinea pedis.

VIII. **Tinea unguium**

A. Tinea unguium is a dermatophyte infection of the nails. It is a subset of onychomycosis, which includes dermatophyte, nondermatophyte and yeast infections of the nails. Toenails are involved more frequently than fingernails. Risk factors for this fungal infection include increasing age, diabetes, poor venous and lymphatic drainage, ill-fitting shoes, and sports participation. Involvement of the toenail usually is extremely resistant to treatment and has a tendency to recur. Chemical or surgical avulsion may be helpful in recalcitrant infection.

B. With distal involvement, the affected nail is hyperkeratotic, chalky and dull. The brownish-yellow debris that forms beneath the nail causes the nail to separate from its bed. Coexistent tinea manuum or tinea pedis is common.

C. Tinea unguium requires oral itraconazole or terbinafine. Itraconazole "pulse" therapy (ie, a series of brief medication courses) is recommended for tinea unguium of the fingernails and toenails. Terbinafine pulse therapy may also be effective. Fluconazole is another alternative.

Topical Treatments for Tinea Pedis, Tinea Cruris and Tinea Corporis

Antifungal agent	Prescrip-tion	Cream	Solution or spray	Lotion	Powder	Frequency of application
Imidazoles						
Clotrimazole 1 percent (Lotrimin, Mycelex)		X	X	X		Twice daily
Miconazole 2 percent (Micatin, Monistat-Derm)		X	X	X	X	Twice daily
Econazole 1 percent (Spectazole)	X	X				Once daily
Ketoconazole 2 percent (Nizoral)	X	X	X			Once daily
Oxiconazole 1 percent (Oxistat)	X	X		X		Once daily or twice daily
Allylamines						
Naftifine 1 percent (Naftin)	X	X				Once daily or twice daily
Terbinafine 1 percent (Lamisil)	X	X	X			Once daily or twice daily
Butenafine 1 percent (Mentax)		X				Once daily or twice daily

Recommended Dosages and Durations of Oral Therapy for Tinea Infections					
Antifungal agent	Tinea capitis	Tinea corporis/cruris	Tinea pedis	Tinea unguium Fingernails	Tinea unguium Toenails
Terbinafine (Lamisil)	Adults: 250 mg per day for four to six weeks Children: 3 to 6 mg per kg per day for six weeks	Adults: 250 mg per day for one to four weeks	250 mg per day for two to six weeks	Continuous: 250 mg per day for six weeks Pulse: 500 mg per day for one week on, three weeks off, for a total of two months	Continuous: 250 mg per day for 12 weeks Pulse: 500 mg per day for one week on, three weeks off, for a total of four months
Itraconazole (Sporanox)	Adults: 100 mg per day for six weeks Children: 3 to 5 mg per kg per day for four to six weeks	100 mg per day for two weeks or 200 mg per day for two weeks or 200 mg per day for one to two weeks	100 mg per day for four weeks	Continuous: 200 mg per day for six weeks Pulse: 200 mg twice daily for one week on, three weeks off, for two months	Continuous: 200 mg per day for 12 weeks Pulse: 200 mg twice daily for one week on, three weeks off, for three to four months
Fluconazole (Diflucan)	50 mg per day for three weeks	150 mg weekly for two to four weeks	150 mg weekly for two to six weeks	Not recommended	Not recommended

IX. Treatment selection

A. **Topical antifungal preparations** have limited efficacy because of the lengthy duration of treatment and high relapse rates.

B. **Oral antifungal agents**
1. Oral therapy is often chosen because of its shorter duration and greater compliance. Oral agents must be used for disease that is extensive, that affects hair and nails, or that does not respond to topical agents.
2. **Terbinafine (Sporanox)** has fewer drug interactions because it minimally affects the cytochrome P_{450} enzyme system. Itraconazole, fluconazole and ketoconazole significantly inhibit this system.
3. **Side effects of fluconazole (Diflucan)** include rash, headache, gastrointestinal disorders and elevated liver function levels. Erythema multiforme may rarely occur.
4. **Side effects of terbinafine (Lamisil)** include skin rashes and gastrointestinal upset. It has been associated with Stevens-Johnson syndrome, blood dyscrasias, hepatotoxicity and ocular disturbances, as well as elevated liver enzyme levels in 0.5%. Some patients have noted losing their sense of taste for up to six weeks.
5. **Topical corticosteroids** are beneficial in the initial stages of treatment because they suppress the inflammatory response and provide symptomatic relief. Because of the possibility of fungal proliferation, topical corticosteroids should not be used alone in the treatment of tinea infections.

References, see page 268.

Common Skin Diseases

I. Alopecia Areata

A. Alopecia areata is characterized by asymptomatic, noninflammatory, non-scarring areas of complete hair loss, most commonly involving the scalp, but the disorder may involve any area of hair-bearing skin.

B. Auto-antibodies to hair follicles are the most likely cause. Emotional stress is sometimes a precipitating factor. The younger the patient and the more widespread the disease, and the poorer the prognosis.

C. Regrowth of hair after the first attack takes place in 6 months in 30% of cases, with 50% regrowing within 1 year, and 80% regrowing within 5 years. Ten to 30% of patients will not regrow hair; 5% progress to total hair loss.

D. Lesions are well defined, single or multiple round or oval areas of total hair loss. Typical "exclamation point" hairs (3-10 mm in size with a tapered, less pigmented proximal shaft) are seen at the margins.

E. **Differential diagnosis** includes tinea capitis, trichotillomania, secondary syphilis, and lupus erythematosus.

F. A VDRL or RPR test for syphilis should be obtained. A CBC, SMAC, sedimentary rate, thyroid function tests, and antinuclear antibody should be completed to screen for pernicious anemia, chronic active hepatitis, thyroid disease, lupus erythematosus, and Addison's disease.

G. **Therapy.** Topical steroids, intralesional steroids, and topical minoxidil may be somewhat effective.

II. Scabies

A. Scabies is an extremely pruritic eruption usually accentuated in the groin, axillae, navel, breasts and finger webs, with sparing the head.

B. Scabies is spread by skin to skin contact. The diagnosis is established by finding the mite, ova, or feces in scrapings of the skin, usually of the finger webs or genitalia.

C. Treatment of choice for nonpregnant adults and children is lindane (Kwell), applied for 12 hours, then washed off.

D. Elimite, a 5% permethrin cream, applied liberally head to toe and rinsed off in 12 hours, is more effective but more expensive than lindane (Kwell).

E. Treatment should be given to all members of an infected household simultaneously. Clothing and sheets must be washed on the day of treatment.

III. Acne Rosacea

A. This condition commonly presents in fair-skinned individuals and is characterized by papules, erythema, and telangiectasias.

B. Initial treatment consists of doxycycline or tetracycline. Once there has been some clearing, topical metronidazole gel (Metro-gel) can prevent remission. Sunblock should be used because sunlight can exacerbate the condition.

IV. Seborrheic Dermatitis

A. Seborrheic dermatitis is often called cradle cap, dandruff, or seborrhea. It has a high prevalence in infancy and then is not common until after puberty. Predilection is for the face, retroauricular region, and upper trunk.

B. Clinical findings

   1. Infants present with adherent, waxy, scaly lesions on the scalp vertex, also known as "cradle cap."

   2. In adults, the eruption is bilaterally symmetrical, affecting the scalp with patchy or diffuse, waxy, yellow, greasy scaling on the forehead, retroauricular region, auditory meatus, eyebrows, cheeks, and nasolabial folds.

   3. Trunk areas affected include the presternal, interscapular regions, umbilicus, intertriginous surfaces of the axilla, inframammary regions, groin, and anogenital crease. Pruritus is mild, and bacterial infection is indicated by vesiculation and oozing.

C. Treatment

   1. Scalp. Selenium sulfide or tar shampoos are useful. Topical corticosteroid lotions are used for difficult lesions.

   2. Face, neck, and intertriginous regions. Hydrocortisone 1 or 2 ½%.

   3. Trunk. Fluorinated steroids can be used if severe lesions are present.

V. Drug eruptions

A. Drug eruptions may be type I, type II, type III, or type IV immunologic reactions. Cutaneous drug reactions may start within 7 days of initiation of the drug or within 4-7 days after the offending drug has been stopped.

B. The cutaneous lesions usually become more severe and widespread over the following several days to 1 week and then clear over the next 7-14 days.

C. Lesions most often start first and clear first from the head and upper extremities to the trunk and lower legs. Palms, soles, and mucous membranes may be involved.

D. Most drug reactions appear as a typical maculopapular drug reaction. Tetracycline is associated with a fixed drug eruption. Thiazide diuretics have a tendency for photosensitivity eruptions.

E. Treatment of drug eruptions

   1. Oral antihistamines are very useful. Diphenhydramine (Benadryl), 25-50 mg q4-6h. Soothing, tepid water baths in Aveeno or corn starch or cool compresses are useful.

   2. Severe signs and symptoms. A 2-week course of systemic steroids (prednisone starting at 60 mg/day and then tapering) will usually stop the symptoms.

F. Erythema Multiforme

1. Erythema multiforme presents as dull red macules or papules on the back of hands, palms, wrists, feet, elbows and knees. The periphery is red and the center becomes blue or darker red, hence the characteristic target or iris lesion.
2. The rash is most commonly a drug reaction caused by sulfa medications or phenytoin (Dilantin). It is also seen as a reaction to herpes simplex virus infections, mycoplasma, and Hepatitis B.
3. Erythema multiforme major or Steven's Johnson syndrome is diagnosed when mucous membrane or eye involvement is present.
4. Prednisone 30-60 mg/day is often given with a 2-4 week taper.
5. For HSV-driven erythema multiforme, acyclovir may be helpful. Ophthalmologic consultation is obtained for ocular involvement.

VI. Paronychias

A. Chronic infections around the edge of the nail, paronychias, are caused almost universally to Candida albicans. Moisture predisposes to Candida.

B. Acute perionychia presents as tender, red, swollen areas of the nail fold. Pus may be seen through the nail plate or at the paronychial fold. The most common causative bacteria are staphylococci, beta-hemolytic streptococci, and gram-negative enteric bacteria. Predisposing factors to perionychia include minor trauma and splinters under the nail.

C. **Diagnosis of paronychial lesions.** Chronic lesions are usually caused by Candida and may be diagnosed by KOH prep or by fungal culture. Acute lesions are usually bacterial and may be cultured for bacteria.

D. **Treatment of chronic candida paronychia**

1. Stop all wet work and apply clotrimazole (Lotrimin) 1% solution tid.
2. Resistant cases can be treated with a 3-6 week oral course of fluconazole (Diflucan), 100 mg PO daily, or itraconazole (Sporanox), 200-400 mg PO daily.

E. **Treatment of acute bacterial paronychia** consists of dicloxacillin 500 mg PO qid, cephalexin (Keflex) 500 mg PO qid, cefadroxil (Duricef) 500 mg PO bid, or erythromycin 500 mg PO qid. If redness and swelling do not resolve, and a pocket of pus remains, drainage is indicated.

VII. Pityriasis versicolor

A. Pityriasis versicolor presents as small perifollicular, scaly, hypopigmented or hyperpigmented patches on the upper trunk in young adults. The perifollicular patches expand over time and become confluent.

B. In pityriasis versicolor, fungus does not grow in standard fungal culture media, but KOH examination shows the abundant "spaghetti and meatballs" pattern of short hyphae and round spores. Pityrosporon ovale is part of the normal flora of skin. It is a yeast infection (not a dermatophyte infection).

C. Topical treatment consists of selenium sulfide 2.5% lotion (Exsel, Selsun) applied overnight once a week for 3 weeks. Topical antifungal creams may also be used.

1. Miconazole (Micatin); apply to affected areas bid; 2% cream.
2. Clotrimazole (Lotrimin), apply to affected area bid for up to 4 wk; cream: 1%,1% lotion.
3. Ketoconazole (Nizoral) apply to affected area(s) qd-bid; 2% cream.

D. Systemic treatment consists of fluconazole (Diflucan), 400 mg, or ketoconazole (Nizoral), 400 mg, given as a single dose.

E. Relapses are very common. Prophylactic therapy, once weekly to monthly, with topical or oral agents should be administered if relapses occur.

VIII. Pityriasis rosea
  A. Pityriasis rosea is an acute inflammatory dermatitis characterized by self-limited lesions distributed on the trunk and extremities. A viral cause is hypothesized. It is most common between the ages of 10 and 35.
  B. **Clinical manifestations**
    1. The initial lesion, called the "herald patch," can appear anywhere on the body, and is 2-6 cm in size, and begins a few days to several weeks before the generalized eruption. The hands, face, and feet are usually spared.
    2. The lesions are oval, and the long axes follow the lines of cleavage. Lesions are 2 cm or less, pink, tan, or light brown. The borders of the lesions have a loose rim of scales, peeling peripherally, called the "collarette." Pruritus is usually minimal.
  C. **Differential diagnosis.** Secondary syphilis (a VDRL is indicated for atypical rashes), drug eruptions, viral exanthems, acute papular psoriasis, tinea corporis.
  D. **Treatment.** Topical antipruritic emollients (Caladryl) relieve itching. Ultraviolet therapy may be used. The disease usually resolves in 2-14 weeks and recurrences are unusual.

References, see page 268.

Bacterial Infections of the Skin

I. Furuncles and carbuncles
  A. A furuncle, or boil, is an acute perifollicular staphylococcal abscess of the skin and subcutaneous tissue. Lesions appear as an indurated, dull, red nodule with a central purulent core, usually beginning around a hair follicle or a sebaceous gland. Furuncles occur most commonly on the nape, face, buttocks, thighs, perineum, breast, and axillae.
  B. A carbuncle is a coalescence of interconnected furuncles that drain through a number of points on the skin surface.
  C. The most common cause of furuncles and carbuncles is coagulase-positive S aureus. Cultures should be obtained from suppurative lesions.
  D. **Treatment of furuncles and carbuncles**
    1. Warm compresses and cleansing.
    2. Dicloxacillin (Pathocil) 500 mg PO qid for 2 weeks.
    3. Manipulation and surgical incision of early lesions should be avoided, because these maneuvers may cause local or systemic extension. However, when the lesions begin to suppurate and become fluctuant, drainage may be performed with a No. 11 blade.
    4. Draining lesions should be covered with topical antibiotics and loose dressings.

II. Superficial Folliculitis
  A. Superficial folliculitis is characterized by small dome-shaped pustules at the ostium of hair follicles. It is caused by coagulase-positive S aureus. Multiple or single lesions appear on the scalp, back, and extremities. In children, the scalp is the most common site.
  B. Gram stain and bacterial culture supports the diagnosis.
  C. **Treatment.** Local cleansing and erythromycin 2% solution applied topically bid to affected areas.

III. Impetigo
  A. Impetigo consists of small superficial vesicles, which eventually form pustules

and develop a honey-colored crust. A halo of erythema often surrounds the lesions.

B. Impetigo occurs most commonly on exposed surfaces such as the extremities and face, where minor trauma, insect bites, contact dermatitis, or abrasions may have occurred.

C. Gram stain of an early lesion or the base of a crust often reveals gram-positive cocci.

D. **Treatment of impetigo**
1. A combination of systemic and topical therapy is recommended for moderate to severe cases of impetigo for a 7- to 10-day course:
   a. Dicloxacillin 250-500 mg PO qid.
   b. Cephalexin (Keflex) 250-500 mg PO qid.
   c. Erythromycin 250-500 mg PO qid is used in penicillin allergic patients.
2. Mupirocin (Bactroban) is highly effective against staphylococci and Streptococcus pyogenes. It is applied bid-tid for 2-3 weeks or until 1 week after lesions heal. Bacitracin (neomycin, polymyxin B) ointment tid may also be used.

E. **Complications**
1. Acute glomerulonephritis is a serious complication of impetigo, with an incidence of 2-5%. It is most commonly seen in children under the age of 6 years old. Treatment of impetigo does not alter the risk of acute glomerulonephritis.
2. Rheumatic fever has not been reported after impetigo.

IV. Cellulitis

A. Cellulitis is a diffuse suppurative bacterial inflammation of the subcutaneous tissue. It is characterized by localized erythema, warmth, and tenderness. Cutaneous erythema is poorly demarcated from uninvolved skin. Cellulitis may be accompanied by malaise, fever, and chills.

B. The most common causes are beta-hemolytic streptococci and S aureus. Complications include gangrene, metastatic abscesses, and sepsis.

C. **Treatment**
1. Dicloxacillin or cephalexin provide coverage for streptococci and staphylococci. Penicillin may be added to increase activity against streptococci.
2. **Antibiotic therapy**
   a. Dicloxacillin (Dycill, Pathocil) 40 mg/kg/day in 4 divided doses for 7-12 days; adults: 500 mg qid.
   b. Cephalexin (Keflex) 50 mg/kg/day PO in 4 divided doses for 7-10 days; adults: 500 mg PO qid.
   c. Amoxicillin/clavulanate (Augmentin) 500 mg tid or 875 mg bid for 7-10 days.
   d. Azithromycin (Zithromax) 500 mg on day 1, then 250 mg PO qd for 4 days.
   e. Erythromycin ethylsuccinate 40 mg/kg/day in 3 divided doses for 7-10 days; adults: 250-500 mg qid.

References, see page 268.

Psoriasis

Psoriasis affects about 2 percent of the U.S. population. The disorder is characterized by red, scaling plaques, ranging from only a few lesions to total involvement of the skin. The primary lesion is a well-demarcated erythematous plaque with a silvery scale.

Clinical evaluation

A. Psoriasis lesions are elevated and erythematous, with thick, silver scales. Scraping off the scale leaves a bleeding point (Auspitz sign). Lesion have a predilection for the sacral region, over extensor surfaces (elbows, knees, lumbosacral), and scalp. Other lesions may appear at sites of trauma (Koebner's phenomenon), such as an excoriation.

B. Medications that can trigger the onset of psoriasis include beta-blockers, lithium, nonsteroidal anti-inflammatory agents, and progesterone-containing oral contraceptives.

C. Mucosal psoriasis consist of circinate, ring-shaped, whitish lesions on the tongue, palate, or buccal mucosa. Onycholysis, or separation of the nail plate from the underlying nail bed, is frequently seen, as well as a yellow-brown discoloration underneath the nail, known as an "oil spot."

D. Psoriatic arthritis occurs in 20-34% of patients with psoriasis. It is characterized by asymmetrical distal oligoarthritis involving small joints; a smaller number of patients have a symmetrical arthritis of the larger joints or a spondyloarthropathy. The arthritis may be mutilating and destructive.

Topical therapy

A. Topical therapy, including corticosteroids, calcipotriene (Dovonex), coal tar products, tazarotene (Tazorac) and anthralin (Anthra-Derm), is the mainstay of treatment for localized disease. The use of emollients should be encouraged.

B. **Topical corticosteroids** are the most commonly prescribed treatment for psoriasis. Topical steroids are classified as low-, medium-, high- and super-high potency agents. In general, treatment is initiated with a medium-strength agent, and high-potency agents are reserved for thick chronic plaques. Low-potency agents are used on the face, on areas where the skin tends to be thinner, and on the groin and axillary areas.

C. Potential side effects from corticosteroids include cutaneous atrophy, telangiectasia and striae, acne eruption, glaucoma, hypothalamus-pituitary-adrenal axis suppression and, in children, growth retardation. Although corticosteroids are rapidly effective in the treatment of psoriasis, they are associated with a rapid flare-up of disease after discontinuation. Consequently, topical corticosteroids are frequently used in conjunction with another agent to maintain control. Topical calcipotriene is often used in combination with topical corticosteroids.

Corticosteroid Potency	
Generic name	**Trade name and strength**
Super-high potency	
Betamethasone dipropionate	Diprolene gel/ointment, 0.05% [45 g]

Generic name	Trade name and strength
Diflorasone diacetate	Psorcon ointment, 0.05% [45 g]
Clobetasol propionate	Temovate cream/ointment, 0.05% [45 g]
Halobetasol propionate	Ultravate cream/ointment, 0.05% [45 g]
Potent	
Amcinonide	Cyclocort ointment, 0.1% [60 g]
Betamethasone dipropionate	Diprosone ointment, 0.05% [45 g]
Desoximetasone	Topicort cream/ointment, 0.25%; gel 0.05% [45 g]
Diflorasone diacetate	Florone ointment, 0.05%; Maxiflor ointment, 0.05% [45 g]
Fluocinonide	Lidex cream/ointment, 0.05% [60 g]
Halcinonide	Halog cream, 0.1% [45 g]
Upper mid-strength	
Betamethasone dipropionate	Diprosone cream, 0.05% [45 g]
Betamethasone valerate	Valisone ointment, 0.1% [45 g]
Diflorasone diacetate	Florone, Maxiflor creams, 0.05%
Mometasone furoate	Elocon ointment, 0.1% [45 g]
Triamcinolone acetonide	Aristocort cream, 0.5% [45 g]
Mid-strength	
Desoximetasone	Topicort LP cream, 0.05% [60 g]
Fluocinolone acetonide	Synalar-HP cream, 0.2%; Synalar ointment, 0.025% [60 g]
Flurandrenolide	Cordran ointment, 0.05% [60 g]
Triamcinolone acetonide	Aristocort, Kenalog ointments, 0.1% [60 g]
Lower mid-strength	
Betamethasone dipropionate	Diprosone lotion, 0.05% [60 g]
Betamethasone valerate	Valisone cream/lotion, 0.1% [45 g]

Generic name	Trade name and strength
Fluocinolone acetonide	Synalar cream, 0.025% [45 g]
Flurandrenolide	Cordran cream, 0.05% [45 g]
Hydrocortisone butyrate	Locoid cream, 0.1% [45 g]
Hydrocortisone valerate	Westcort cream, 0.2% [45 g]
Triamcinolone acetonide	Kenalog cream/lotion, 0.1% [60 g]
Mild	
Alclometasone dipropionate	Aclovate cream/ointment, 0.05% [60 g]
Triamcinolone acetonide	Aristocort cream, 0.1% [60 g]
Desonide	DesOwen cream, 0.05% [60 g]
Fluocinolone acetonide	Synalar cream/solution, 0.01% [60 g]
Betamethasone valerate	Valisone lotion, 0.1% [45 g]

D. Calcipotriene (Dovonex) is a vitamin D_3 analog available in cream, ointment and solution formulations. It inhibits epidermal cell proliferation and enhances normal keratinization. This agent has a slow onset of action, and effects may not be noticeable for up to six to eight weeks. Maximal benefits are achieved when calcipotriene is used in combination with potent topical corticosteroids. Treatment could be initiated with twice-daily applications of a topical corticosteroid and calcipotriene until the lesions are flat. When the lesions have become flat, therapy can then be changed to twice daily use of calcipotriene only, with corticosteroid "pulse" therapy twice daily on weekends only. When the lesions have remained flat and the intensity of their color has declined from bright red to pink, the calcipotriene is used alone. Local irritation occurs in approximately 15 percent. Calcipotriene is not recommended for use on the face or with occlusion.

E. Coal tar is a black viscous fluid which suppresses epidermal DNA synthesis. Coal tar is available as an ointment, cream, lotion, shampoo, bath oil and soap. Coal tar is most effective when it is used in combination with other agents, especially ultraviolet B light. Coal tar is effective when it is combined with topical corticosteroids. Because coal tar is messy and malodorous and can stain clothing, nighttime application is recommended. Tar products can cause folliculitis.

F. Anthralin (Dovonex). If good control of psoriasis is not achieved with topical corticosteroids, alone or in combination with calcipotriene or coal tar, anthralin or tazarotene should be added. Anthralin is available in 0.1 percent to 1 percent ointments, creams and solutions. It is generally used on thick, large plaques of psoriasis. The concentration and duration of contact with each treatment is gradually increased, up to a maximum of 30 minutes per application. Anthralin has a tendency to stain any surface, including the skin, clothing and bathtub.

G. Tazarotene (Tazorac). Topical tazarotene is a topical retinoid. Tazarotene helps to normalize the proliferation and differentiation of keratinocytes and decrease inflammation Tazarotene should usually be used in combination with corticosteroids. The primary side effect of topical tazarotene is minor skin irritation and increased photosensitivity. Tazarotene is pregnancy category X and should be avoided in women of childbearing age.

H. **Sunlight and tanning-bed treatment.** Sun exposure in addition to topical therapy may be beneficial when multiple areas are affected with psoriasis. Patients should be encouraged to obtain natural sunlight exposure or tanning-bed light exposure for a few minutes a day, and then to slowly increase the duration of exposure as tolerated. Unaffected areas should be covered with a sunscreen, especially the face.

III. **Intralesional injections, phototherapy and systemic therapy**

A. Psoriatic plaques that fail to respond to topical therapy may be improved by administration of intralesional corticosteroid injections. Triamcinolone (Kenalog) is injected directly into the dermis of persistent plaques at a concentration of 3 to 10 mg per mL. The patient with refractory lesions may benefit from phototherapy (ultraviolet B alone or psoralens plus ultraviolet A).

B. **Systemic therapies** include methotrexate, etretinate (Tegison), cyclosporine, and hydroxyurea, and these therapies have better than an 80% response rate.

References, see page 268.

Allergic Rhinitis and Conjunctivitis

Allergic rhinitis and allergic conjunctivitis are characterized by inflammation of the nasal mucosa, rhinorrhea, nasal congestion, sneezing, and conjunctival injection. The disorder is episodic, seasonal or perennial. Inhaled, ingested or injected allergens encounter IgE that is bound to mast cell membranes, resulting in mast cell degranulation and symptoms.

I. **Diagnosis**

A. Allergic rhinitis presents with nasal congestion, rhinorrhea, sneezing, nasal or ocular pruritus, excessive lacrimation, and postnasal drip with resulting sore throat and cough. Patients often have asthma or atopic dermatitis in their personal or family history.

B. **Physical examination**

1. The conjunctivae may be injected, and profuse tearing may be present. Some patients present with swollen eyelids and boggy sclera. The nasal mucosa may be congested with a profuse clear discharge.

2. Patients may exhibit "allergic shiners" (darkened circles under the eyes caused by venous pooling) and a crease across the bridge of the nose caused by the "allergic salute" (upward rubbing of the nose).

C. **Laboratory testing**

1. **Nasal smear.** Infectious rhinitis demonstrates a predominance of neutrophils, and allergic disease shows a predominance of eosinophils.

2. **Allergy testing** is useful to identify patients with allergic disease that does not display a clear seasonal pattern. In patients with perennial symptoms, testing may help confirm allergic disease and allow identification of allergens that are avoidable.

II. Treatment

Second-Generation Antihistamines	
Drug	**Adult dose**
Cetirizine (Zyrtec) Fexofenadine (Allegra) Loratadine (Claritin)	10 mg once daily 60 mg twice daily 10 mg once daily

Intranasal Corticosteroids		
Drug	**Trade name**	**Dose (sprays/nostril)**
Beclomethasone	Beconase Vancenase Beconase AQ Vancenase AQ	One spray two to qid One spray bid-qid One to two sprays bid One to two sprays bid
Triamcinolone	Nasacort	Two to four sprays qd
Budesonide	Rhinocort	Two to four sprays bid
Flunisolide	Nasalide	Two sprays bid
Fluticasone	Flonase	Two sprays/day or one spray bid
Mometasone	Nasonex	Two sprays qd

A. **Intranasal steroids** are useful in relieving itching, rhinorrhea and congestion, and they are more effective than antihistamines. The most common side effects are headache and local irritation. Occasionally, patients develop intranasal candidiasis.

B. **Azelastine nasal spray (Astelin)** is an intranasal, topical antihistamine, which may cause somnolence; 2 sprays in each nostril bid.

C. **Ophthalmic therapy**

1. **Ocular corticosteroids** are very effective. Dexamethasone (Decadron) 0.1% ophthalmic soln, 1-2 drops q4-8h. Because these drugs may elevate intraocular pressure and worsen infections, they should be administered with caution.

2. **Antihistamine-vasoconstrictor preparations.** Vasocon-A (naphazoline/antazoline) and Naphcon-A (naphazoline/pheniramine) are over-the-counter antihistamine-decongestants; 1-2 drops q2h as needed; up to 4 times a day. Rebound congestion can occur with long-term use.

3. **Cromolyn (Crolom)**, a mast cell stabilizer, is highly effective for the treatment of allergic conjunctivitis; 1-2 drops in each eye q4-6h.

4. **Lodoxamide (Alomide)**, a mast cell stabilizer, is more potent than cromolyn; 1-2 drops qid.

5. **Levocabastine (Livostin)**, a histamine H1 antagonist, provides relief within a few minutes.

6. **Ketorolac (Acular)** is a topical NSAID; 1 drop qid is effective for seasonal allergic conjunctivitis.

III. Immunotherapy. Allergen immunotherapy is effective in patients with allergic rhinitis, and it may be considered if other measures fail.

References, see page 268.

Renal Disorders

Acute Renal Failure

Acute renal failure is defined as a sudden decrease in renal function sufficient to increase the concentration of nitrogenous wastes in the blood. It is characterized by an increasing BUN and creatinine.

Clinical presentation of acute renal failure

A. **Oliguria** is a common indicator of acute renal failure, and it is marked by a decrease in urine output to less than 30 mL/h. Acute renal failure may be oliguric (<500 L/day) or nonoliguric (>30 mL/h). Anuria (<100 mL/day) does not usually occur in renal failure, and its presence suggests obstruction or a vascular cause.

B. Acute renal failure may less commonly be manifest by encephalopathy, volume overload, pericarditis, bleeding, anemia, hyperkalemia, hyperphosphatemia, hypocalcemia, and metabolic acidemia.

Clinical causes of renal failure

A. **Prerenal insult**

   1. Prerenal insult is the most common cause of acute renal failure, accounting for 70% of cases. Prerenal failure is usually caused by reduced renal perfusion secondary to extracellular fluid loss (diarrhea, diuresis, GI hemorrhage) or secondary to extracellular fluid sequestration (pancreatitis, sepsis), inadequate cardiac output, renal vasoconstriction (sepsis, liver disease, drugs), or inadequate fluid intake or replacement.

   2. Most patients with prerenal azotemia have oliguria, a history of large fluid losses (vomiting, diarrhea, burns), and evidence of intravascular volume depletion (thirst, weight loss, orthostatic hypotension, tachycardia, flat neck veins, dry mucous membranes). Patients with congestive heart failure may have total body volume excess (distended neck veins, pulmonary and pedal edema) but still have compromised renal perfusion and prerenal azotemia because of diminished cardiac output.

   3. Causes of prerenal failure are usually reversible if recognized and treated early; otherwise, prolonged renal hypoperfusion can lead to acute tubular necrosis and permanent renal insufficiency.

B. **Intrarenal insult**

   1. **Acute tubular necrosis (ATN)** is the most common intrinsic renal disease leading to ARF.

      a. **Prolonged renal hypoperfusion** is the most common cause of ATN.

      b. **Nephrotoxic agents** (aminoglycosides, heavy metals, radiocontrast media, ethylene glycol) represent exogenous nephrotoxins. ATN may also occur as a result of endogenous nephrotoxins, such as intratubular pigments (hemoglobinuria), intratubular proteins (myeloma), and intratubular crystals (uric acid).

   2. **Acute interstitial nephritis (AIN)** is an allergic reaction secondary to drugs (NSAIDs, β-lactams).

   3. **Arteriolar injury** occurs secondary to hypertension, vasculitis, microangiopathic disorders.

   4. **Glomerulonephritis** secondary to immunologically mediated inflammation may cause intrarenal damage.

C. **Postrenal insult** results from obstruction of urine flow. Postrenal insult is the least common cause of acute renal failure, accounting for 10%.
   1. Postrenal insult may be caused by extra-renal obstructive uropathy secondary to prostate cancer, benign prostatic hypertrophy, or renal calculi occlusion of the bladder outlet.
   2. Postrenal insult may be caused by intrarenal obstruction of the distal tubules by amyloidosis, uric acid crystals, multiple myeloma, or by methotrexate or acyclovir.

III. Clinical evaluation of acute renal failure

A. **Initial evaluation** of renal failure should determine whether the cause is decreased renal perfusion, obstructed urine flow, or disorders of the renal parenchyma. Recent clinical events and drug therapy should be reviewed, including volume status (orthostatic pulse, blood pressure, fluid intake and output, daily weights, hemodynamic parameters), nephrotoxic medications, and pattern of urine output.

B. **Prerenal azotemia** is likely when there is a history of heart failure or extracellular fluid volume loss or depletion.

C. **Postrenal azotemia** is suggested by a history of decreased size or force of the urine stream, anuria, flank pain, hematuria or pyuria, or cancer of the bladder, prostate or pelvis. Anuria usually results from obstructive uropathy; occasional anuria indicates cessation of renal blood flow or rapidly progressive glomerulonephritis.

D. **Intrarenal insult** is suggested by a history of prolonged volume depletion (often post-surgical), pigmenturia, hemolysis, rhabdomyolysis, or nephrotoxins. Intrarenal insult is suggested by recent radiocontrast, aminoglycoside use, or vascular catheterization. Interstitial nephritis may be implicated by a history of medication rash, fever, or arthralgias. Urinary studies may reveal hematuria, sterile pyuria, eosinophiluria, mild proteinuria (<2 g/24 h) and, rarely, white blood cell casts. NSAID-induced acute interstitial nephritis occurs most often with the use of ibuprofen, fenoprofen, and naproxen.

E. **Chronic renal failure** is suggested by the presence of a disease known to cause chronic renal insufficiency (diabetes mellitus). The presence of normochromic normocytic anemia, hypercalcemia, and hyperphosphatemia also suggests chronic renal insufficiency.

IV. Physical examination

A. Cardiac output, volume status, bladder size, and systemic disease manifestations should be assessed.

B. **Prerenal azotemia** is suggested by impaired cardiac output (neck vein distention, pulmonary rales, pedal edema). Volume depletion is suggested by orthostatic blood pressure changes, weight loss, low urine output, or diuretic use.

C. **Flank, suprapubic, or abdominal masses** may indicate an obstructive cause.

D. **Skin rash** suggests drug-induced interstitial nephritis; palpable purpura suggests vasculitis; nonpalpable purpura suggests thrombotic thrombocytopenic purpura or hemolytic-uremic syndrome, all of which are compatible with intrarenal kidney failure.

E. **Bladder catheterization** is useful to rule out suspected bladder outlet obstruction. A residual volume of more than 100 mL suggests bladder outlet obstruction.

F. **Central venous monitoring** is used to measure cardiac output and left ventricular filling pressure if prerenal failure is suspected.

V. Laboratory evaluation

A. **Spot urine sodium concentration**
   1. Spot urine sodium can help distinguish between prerenal azotemia and acute tubular necrosis.

2. Prerenal failure causes increased reabsorption of salt and water and will manifest as a low spot urine sodium concentration <20 mEq/L and a low fractional sodium excretion <1%, and a urine/plasma creatinine >40. Fractional excretion of sodium (%) = ([urine sodium/plasma sodium] ÷ [urine creatinine/plasma creatinine] x 100).

3. If tubular necrosis is the cause, the spot urine concentration will be >40 mEq/L, and fractional excretion of sodium will be >1%.

B. Urinalysis

1. **Normal urine sediment** is a strong indicator of prerenal azotemia or may be an indicator of obstructive uropathy.

2. **Hematuria, pyuria, or crystals** may be associated with postrenal obstructive azotemia.

3. **Abundant cells, casts, or protein** suggests an intrarenal disorder.

4. **Red cells** alone may indicate vascular disorders. RBC casts and abundant protein suggest glomerular disease (glomerulonephritis).

5. **White cell casts and eosinophilic casts** indicate interstitial nephritis.

6. **Renal epithelial cell casts and pigmented granular casts** are associated acute tubular necrosis.

C. Ultrasound is useful for evaluation of suspected postrenal obstruction (nephrolithiasis) after bladder outlet obstruction has been ruled out by catheterization. The presence of small (<10 cm in length), scarred kidneys is diagnostic of chronic renal insufficiency.

VI. Management of acute renal failure

A. Reversible disorders, such as obstruction, should be excluded, and hypovolemia should be corrected with volume replacement. Cardiac output should be maintained.

B. In critically ill patients, a pulmonary artery catheter should be used for evaluation and monitoring.

C. Extracellular fluid volume expansion. Infusion of a 1-2 liter crystalloid fluid bolus may confirm suspected volume-depleted, prerenal azotemia.

D. If the patient remains oliguric despite euvolemia, IV diuretics may be administered. A large single dose of furosemide (100-200 mg) may be administered intravenously to promote diuresis. If urine flow is not improved, the dose of furosemide may be doubled or given in combination with metolazone (Zaroxolyn). Furosemide may be repeated in 2 hours, or a continuous IV infusion of 10-40 mg/hr (max 1000 mg/day) may be used.

E. The dosage or dosing intervals of renally excreted drugs should be modified. Drug levels, blood cell count, electrolytes, creatinine, calcium, and phosphorus levels should be monitored.

F. Hyperkalemia is the most immediately life-threatening complication of renal failure. Serum potassium values greater than 6.5 mEq/L may lead to arrhythmias and cardiac arrest. Potassium should be removed from IV solutions. Hyperkalemia may be treated with sodium polystyrene sulfonate (Kayexalate), 30-60 gm PO/PR every 4-6 hours.

G. Hyperphosphatemia can be controlled with aluminum hydroxide given with meals to bind dietary phosphorus. Antacids that contain magnesium are contraindicated.

H. Fluids. After normal volume has been restored, fluid intake should be reduced to an amount equal to urinary and other losses plus insensible losses of 300-500 mL/day. In oliguric patients, daily fluid intake may need to be restricted to less than 1 L.

I. Nutritional therapy. A renal diet consisting of daily high biologic value protein intake of 0.5 gm/kg/d, sodium 2 g, potassium 40-60 mg/day, and at least 35

kcal/kg of nonprotein calories is recommended. Phosphorus should be restricted to 800 mg/day
  J. **Dialysis.** Indications for dialysis include uremic pericarditis, severe hyperkalemia, pulmonary edema, persistent severe metabolic acidosis (pH less than 7.2), and symptomatic uremia.

References, see page 268.

Hematuria

Hematuria may be a sign of urinary tract malignancy or renal parenchymal disease. Up to 18% of normal persons excrete red blood cells into the urine, averaging 2 RBCs per high-power field (HPF).

I. **Clinical evaluation of hematuria**
  A. Dipstick testing detects hemoglobin and myoglobin; therefore, microscopic examination of the urinary sediment is required before a diagnosis of hematuria can be made.
  B. The patient should be asked about frequency, dysuria, pain, colic, fever, fatigue, anorexia, abdominal, flank, or perineal pain. Exercise, jogging, menstruation, or a history of kidney stones should be sought.
  C. The patient should be examined for hypertension, edema, rash, heart murmurs, or abdominal masses (renal tumor, hydronephrosis from obstruction). Costovertebral-angle tenderness may be a sign of renal calculus or pyelonephritis.
  D. Genitourinary examination may reveal a foreign body in the penile urethra or cervical carcinoma invading the urinary tract. Prostatitis, carcinoma, or benign prostatic hyperplasia may be found.
II. **Laboratory evaluation**
  A. At least one of the following criteria should be met before initiating a workup for hematuria.
    1. More than 3 RBCs/HPF on two of three properly collected clean-catch specimens (abstain from exercise for 48 hours before sampling; not during menses).
    2. One episode of gross hematuria.
    3. One episode of high-grade microhematuria (>100 RBCs HPF)
  B. A properly collected, freshly voided specimen should be examined for red blood cell morphology; the character of the sediment and the presence of proteinuria should be determined.
  C. RBC casts are pathognomonic of glomerulonephritis. WBC casts and granular casts are indicative of pyelonephritis.
  D. Urine culture should be completed to rule out urinary tract infection, which may cause hematuria.
  E. Serum blood urea nitrogen and creatinine levels should be evaluated to rule out renal failure. Impaired renal function is seen more commonly with medical causes of hematuria.
  F. Fasting blood glucose levels should be obtained to rule out diabetes; a complete blood count should be obtained to assess severity of blood loss.
  G. Serum coagulation parameters should be measured to screen for coagulopathy. A skin test for tuberculosis should be completed if risk factors are present. A sickle cell prep is recommended for all African-American

patients.

III. Classification of hematuria
   A. **Medical hematuria** is caused by a glomerular lesion. Plasma proteins are present in the urine out of proportion to the amount of hematuria. Medical hematuria is characterized by glomerular RBCs, which are distorted with crenated membranes and an uneven hemoglobin distribution. Microscopic hematuria and a urine dipstick test of 2+ protein is more likely to have a medical cause.
   B. **Urologic hematuria** is caused by urologic lesions, such as urolithiasis or bladder cancer. It is characterized by minimal proteinuria. Non-glomerular RBCs (disk shaped) and an absence of casts are characteristic.

V. Diagnostic evaluation of medical hematuria
   A. **Renal ultrasound** is used to evaluate kidney size and rule out hydronephrosis or cystic disease.
   B. **24-hour urine.** Creatinine, creatinine clearance and protein should be measured to assess renal failure.
   C. **Immunologic studies** that may suggest a diagnosis include third and fourth complement components, antinuclear antibodies, cryoglobulins, anti-basement membrane antibodies; serum and urine protein electrophoresis (to rule out IgA nephropathy).
   D. **Audiogram** should be obtained if there is a family history of Alport syndrome.
   E. **Skin biopsy** can reveal dermal capillary deposits of IgA in 80% of patients with Berger's disease (IgA nephropathy), which is the most common cause of microhematuria in young adults.

V. Diagnostic evaluation of urologic hematuria
   A. **Intravenous pyelography** is the best screening test for upper tract lesions if the serum creatinine is normal. It is usually contraindicated in renal insufficiency. If renal insufficiency is present, renal ultrasound and cystoscopy with retrograde pyelogram should be used to search for stones or malignancy. If the IVP is normal, cystoscopy with washings for cytology may reveal the cause of bleeding.
   B. **Other tests.** Lesions in the kidney visualized on IVP can be evaluated by renal ultrasound to assess cystic or solid character. CT-guided aspiration of cysts may be considered. Filling defects in the ureter should be evaluated by retrograde pyelogram and ureteral washings.

VI. Idiopathic hematuria
   A. Idiopathic hematuria is a diagnosis of exclusion. Five to 10% of patients with significant hematuria will have no diagnosis. Suspected urologic hematuria with a negative initial workup should be followed every 6-12 months with a urinalysis and urine cytology. An IVP should be done every 2-3 years.
   B. Renal function and proteinuria should be monitored. If renal function declines or if proteinuria exceeds 1 gm/day, renal biopsy is indicated.

References, see page 268.

Hyperkalemia

Body K is 98% intracellular. Only 2% of total body potassium, about 70 mEq, is in the extracellular fluid with the normal concentration of 3.5-5 mEq/L.

Pathophysiology of potassium homeostasis
   A. The normal upper limit of plasma K is 5-5.5 mEq/L, with a mean K level of 4.3.

B. **External potassium balance.** Normal dietary K intake is 1-1.5 mEq/kg in the form of vegetables and meats. The kidney is the primary organ for preserving external K balance, excreting 90% of the daily K burden.

C. **Internal potassium balance**, potassium transfer to and from tissues, is affected by insulin, acid-base status, catecholamines, aldosterone, plasma osmolality, cellular necrosis, glucagon, and drugs.

II. **Clinical disorders of external potassium balance**

A. **Chronic renal failure.** The kidney is able to excrete dietary intake of potassium until the glomerular filtration rate falls below 10 cc/minute or until urine output falls below 1 L/day. Renal failure is advanced before hyperkalemia occurs.

B. **Impaired renal tubular function.** Renal diseases may cause hyperkalemia, and the renal tubular acidosis caused by these conditions may worsen hyperkalemia.

C. **Primary adrenal insufficiency (Addison's disease)** is now a rare cause of hyperkalemia.
   1. **Diagnosis** is indicated by the combination of hyperkalemia and hyponatremia and is confirmed by a low aldosterone and a low plasma cortisol level that does not respond to adrenocorticotropic hormone treatment.
   2. **Treatment** consists of glucocorticoid and mineralocorticoid agents and volume replacement with normal saline.

D. **Drugs** that may cause hyperkalemia include nonsteroidal anti-inflammatory drugs, angiotensin-converting enzyme inhibitors, cyclosporine, and potassium-sparing diuretics. Hyperkalemia is especially common when these drugs are given to patients at risk for hyperkalemia (diabetics, renal failure, hyporeninemic hypoaldosteronism, advanced age).

E. **Excessive potassium intake**
   1. Long-term potassium supplementation results in hyperkalemia most often when an underlying impairment in renal excretion already exists.
   2. Intravenous administration of 0.5 mEq/kg over 1 hour increases serum levels by 0.6 mEq/L. Hyperkalemia often results when infusions of greater than 40 mEq/hour are given.

III. **Clinical disorders of internal potassium balance**

A. **Diabetic patients** are at particular risk for severe hyperkalemia because of renal insufficiency and hyporeninemic hypoaldosteronism.

B. **Systemic acidosis** reduces renal excretion of potassium and moves potassium out of cells, resulting in hyperkalemia.

C. **Endogenous potassium release** from muscle injury, tumor lysis, or chemotherapy may elevate serum potassium.

IV. **Manifestations of hyperkalemia**

A. Hyperkalemia, unless severe, is usually asymptomatic. The effect of hyperkalemia on the heart becomes significant above 6 mEq/L. As levels increase, the initial ECG change is tall peaked T waves. The QT interval is normal or diminished.

B. As K levels rise further, the PR interval becomes prolonged, then the P wave amplitude decreases. The QRS complex widens into a sine wave pattern, with subsequent cardiac standstill.

C. At serum K is >7 mEq/L, muscle weakness may lead to a flaccid paralysis. Sensory abnormalities, impaired speech and respiratory arrest may follow.

V. **Pseudohyperkalemia**

A. Potassium may be falsely elevated by hemolysis during phlebotomy, when K is released from ischemic muscle distal to a tourniquet, and because of erythrocyte fragility disorders.

B. Falsely high laboratory measurement of serum potassium may occur with markedly elevated platelet counts (>10^6 platelet/mm^3) or white blood cell counts (>50,000/mm^3).

VI. Diagnostic approach to hyperkalemia

A. The serum K level should be repeat tested to rule out laboratory error. If significant thrombocytosis or leukocytosis is present, a plasma potassium level should be determined.

B. The 24-hour urine output, urinary K excretion, blood urea nitrogen, and serum creatinine should be measured. Renal K retention is diagnosed when urinary K excretion is less than 20 mEq/day.

C. High urinary K, excretion of >20 mEq/day, is indicative of excessive K intake as the cause.

VII. Renal hyperkalemia

A. If urinary K excretion is low and urine output is in the oliguric range, and creatinine clearance is lower than 20 cc/minute, renal failure is the probable cause. Prerenal azotemia resulting from volume depletion must be ruled out because the hyperkalemia will respond to volume restoration.

B. When urinary K excretion is low, yet blood urea nitrogen and creatinine levels are not elevated and urine volume is at least 1 L daily and renal sodium excretion is adequate (about 20 mEq/day), then either a defect in the secretion of renin or aldosterone or tubular resistance to aldosterone is likely. Low plasma renin and aldosterone levels, will confirm the diagnosis of hyporeninemic hypoaldosteronism. Addison's disease is suggested by a low serum cortisol, and the diagnosis is confirmed with a ACTH (Cortrosyn) stimulation test.

C. When inadequate K excretion is not caused by hypoaldosteronism, a tubular defect in K clearance is suggested. Urinary tract obstruction, renal transplant, lupus, or a medication should be considered.

VIII. Extrarenal hyperkalemia

A. When hyperkalemia occurs along with high urinary K excretion of >20 mEq/day, excessive intake of K is the cause. Potassium excess in IV fluids, diet, or medication should be sought. A concomitant underlying renal defect in K excretion is also likely to be present.

B. Blood sugar should be measured to rule out insulin deficiency; blood pH and serum bicarbonate should be measured to rule out acidosis.

C. Endogenous sources of K, such as tissue necrosis, hypercatabolism, hematoma, gastrointestinal bleeding, or intravascular hemolysis should be excluded.

IX. Management of hyperkalemia

A. Acute treatment of hyperkalemia

1. **Calcium**
   a. If the electrocardiogram shows loss of P waves or widening of QRS complexes, calcium should be given IV; calcium reduces the cell membrane threshold potential.
   b. Calcium gluconate 10% should be given as 2-3 ampules over 5 minutes. In patients with circulatory compromise, 1 ampule of calcium chloride IV should be given over 3 minutes.
   c. If the serum K level is greater than 7 mEq/L, calcium should be given. If digitalis intoxication is suspected, calcium must be given cautiously. Coexisting hyponatremia should be treated with hypertonic saline.

2. **Insulin**
   a. If the only ECG abnormalities are peaked T waves and the serum level is under 7 mEq/L, treatment should begin with insulin (regular insulin,

5-10 U by IV push) with 50% dextrose water (D50W) 50 mL IV push.
   - **b.** Repeated insulin doses of 10 U and glucose can be given every 15 minutes for maximal effect.
3. **Sodium bicarbonate** promotes cellular uptake of K, and it should be given as 1-2 ampules (50-mEq/ampule) IV push.
4. **Potassium elimination measures**
   - **a.** Furosemide (Lasix) 100 mg IV should be given to promote kaliuresis; normal saline may be infused to avoid volume depletion.
   - **b.** Sodium polystyrene sulfonate (Kayexalate) is a cation exchange resin which binds to potassium in the lower GI tract. Dosage is 30-60 gm premixed with sorbitol 20% PO/PR.
   - **c.** Emergent hemodialysis for hyperkalemia is rarely necessary.

References, see page 268.

Hypokalemia

Hypokalemia is characterized by a serum potassium concentration of less than 3.5 mEq/L. Ninety-eight percent of K is intracellular.

I. **Pathophysiology of hypokalemia**
   - A. **Cellular redistribution of potassium.** Hypokalemia may result from the intracellular shift of potassium by insulin, beta-2 agonist drugs, stress induced catecholamine release, thyrotoxic periodic paralysis, and alkalosis-induced shift (metabolic or respiratory).
   - B. **Nonrenal potassium loss**
      1. Gastrointestinal loss can be caused by diarrhea, laxative abuse, villous adenoma, biliary drainage, enteric fistula, clay ingestion, potassium binding resin ingestion, or nasogastric suction.
      2. Sweating, prolonged low potassium diet, hemodialysis and peritoneal dialysis may also cause nonrenal potassium loss.
   - C. **Renal potassium loss**
      1. **Hypertensive high renin states.** Malignant hypertension, renal artery stenosis, renin-producing tumors.
      2. **Hypertensive low renin, high aldosterone states.** Primary hyperaldosteronism (adenoma or hyperplasia).
      3. **Hypertensive low renin, low aldosterone states.** Congenital adrenal hyperplasia (11 or 17 hydroxylase deficiency), Cushing's syndrome or disease, exogenous mineralocorticoids (Florinef, licorice, chewing tobacco), Liddle's syndrome.
      4. **Normotensive states**
         - **a. Metabolic acidosis.** Renal tubular acidosis (type I or II)
         - **b. Metabolic alkalosis (urine chloride <10 mEq/day).** Vomiting
         - **c. Metabolic alkalosis (urine chloride >10 mEq/day).** Bartter's syndrome, diuretics, magnesium depletion, normotensive hyperaldosteronism
      5. **Drugs** associated with potassium loss include amphotericin B, ticarcillin, piperacillin, and loop diuretics.

II. Clinical effects of hypokalemia

A. **Cardiac effects.** The most lethal consequence of hypokalemia is cardiac arrhythmia. Electrocardiographic effects include depressed ST segments, decreased T-wave amplitude, U waves, and a prolonged QT-U interval.

B. **Musculoskeletal effects.** The initial manifestation of K depletion is muscle weakness, which can lead to paralysis. In severe cases, respiratory muscle paralysis may occur.

C. **Gastrointestinal effects.** Nausea, vomiting, constipation, and paralytic ileus may develop.

III. Diagnostic evaluation

A. The 24-hour urinary potassium excretion should be measured.

B. If >20 mEq/day, excessive urinary K loss is the cause. If <20 mEq/d, low K intake, or non-urinary K loss is the cause.

C. In patients with excessive renal K loss and hypertension, plasma renin and aldosterone should be measured to differentiate adrenal from non-adrenal causes of hyperaldosteronism.

D. If hypertension is absent and patient is acidotic, renal tubular acidosis should be considered.

E. If hypertension is absent and serum pH is normal to alkalotic, a high urine chloride (>10 mEq/d) suggests hypokalemia secondary to diuretics or Bartter's syndrome. A low urine chloride (<10 mEq/d) suggests vomiting.

IV. Emergency treatment of hypokalemia

A. **Indications for urgent replacement.** Electrocardiographic abnormalities consistent with severe K depletion, myocardial infarction, hypoxia, digitalis intoxication, marked muscle weakness, or respiratory muscle paralysis.

B. **Intravenous potassium therapy**

1. Intravenous KCL is usually used unless concomitant hypophosphatemia is present, where potassium phosphate is indicated.

2. The maximal rate of intravenous K replacement is 30 mEq/hour. The K concentration of IV fluids should be 80 mEq/L or less if given via a peripheral vein. Frequent monitoring of serum K and constant electrocardiographic monitoring is recommended when depleted potassium levels are being replaced.

V. Non-emergent treatment of hypokalemia

A. Attempts should be made to normalize K levels if <3.5 mEq/L.

B. Oral supplementation is significantly safer than IV. Liquid formulations are preferred due to rapid oral absorption, compared to sustained release formulations, which are absorbed over several hours. Micro-encapsulated and sustained-release forms of KCL are less likely to induce gastrointestinal disturbances than are wax-matrix tablets or liquid preparations.

1. KCL elixir 20-40 mEq qd-tid PO after meals.

2. Micro-K, 10 mEq tabs, 2-3 tabs tid PO after meals (40-100 mEq/d).

References, see page 268.

Hypermagnesemia

Serum magnesium has a normal range of 0.8-1.2 mmol/L. Magnesium homeostasis is regulated by renal and gastrointestinal mechanisms. Hypermagnesemia is usually iatrogenic and is frequently seen in conjunction with renal insufficiency.

I. Clinical evaluation of hypermagnesemia
A. Causes of hypermagnesemia
1. **Renal.** Creatinine clearance <30 mL/minute.
2. **Nonrenal.** Excessive use of magnesium cathartics, especially with renal failure; iatrogenic overtreatment with magnesium sulfate.
3. **Less common causes of mild hypermagnesemia.** Hyperparathyroidism, Addison's disease, hypocalciuric hypercalcemia, and lithium therapy.

B. Cardiovascular manifestations of hypermagnesemia
1. **Lower levels of hypermagnesemia <10 mEq/L.** Delayed interventricular conduction, first-degree heart block, prolongation of the Q-T interval.
2. **Levels greater than 10 mEq/L.** Low grade heart block progressing to complete heart block and asystole occurs at levels greater than 12.5 mmol/L (>6.25 mmol/L).

C. Neuromuscular effects
1. Hyporeflexia occurs at a magnesium level >4 mEq/L (>2 mmol/L); an early sign of magnesium toxicity is diminution of deep tendon reflexes caused by neuromuscular blockade.
2. Respiratory depression due to respiratory muscle paralysis, somnolence and coma occur at levels >13 mEq/L (6.5 mmol/L).
3. Hypermagnesemia should always be considered when these symptoms occur in patients with renal failure, in those receiving therapeutic magnesium, and in laxative abuse.

II. Treatment of hypermagnesemia
A. Asymptomatic, hemodynamically stable patients. Moderate hypermagnesemia can be managed by elimination of intake and maintenance of renal magnesium clearance.
B. Severe hypermagnesemia
1. Furosemide 20-40 mg IV q3-4h should be given as needed. Saline diuresis should be initiated with 0.9% saline, infused at 150 cc/h to replace urine loss.
2. If ECG abnormalities (peaked T waves, loss of P waves, or widened QRS complexes) or if respiratory depression is present, IV calcium gluconate should be given as 1-3 ampules (10% sln, 1 gm per 10 mL amp), added to saline infusate. Calcium gluconate can be infused to reverse acute cardiovascular toxicity or respiratory failure as 15 mg/kg over a 4-hour period.
3. Parenteral insulin and glucose can be given to shift magnesium into cells. Dialysis is necessary for patients who have severe hypermagnesemia.

References, see page 268.

Hypomagnesemia

Magnesium deficiency occurs in up to 11% of hospitalized patients. The most common diagnoses in patients with acute magnesium depletion are malignancy, chronic obstructive pulmonary disease, and alcoholism. The normal range of serum magnesium is 1.5 to 2.0 mEq/L, which is maintained by the kidney, intestine, and bone.

I. Pathophysiology
- **A. Decreased magnesium intake.** Protein-calorie malnutrition, prolonged parenteral (Mg-free) fluid administration, and catabolic illness are common causes of hypomagnesemia.
- **B. Gastrointestinal losses of magnesium** may result from prolonged nasogastric suction, laxative abuse, pancreatitis, extensive small bowel resection, short bowel syndromes, biliary and bowel fistulas, enteropathies, cholestatic liver disease, and malabsorption syndromes.
- **C. Renal losses of magnesium**
  1. Renal loss of magnesium may occur secondary to renal tubular acidosis, glomerulonephritis, interstitial nephritis, or acute tubular necrosis.
  2. Hyperthyroidism, hypercalcemia, and hypophosphatemia may cause magnesium loss.
  3. **Agents that enhance renal magnesium excretion** include alcohol, loop and thiazide diuretics, amphotericin B, aminoglycosides, cisplatin, and pentamidine.
- **D. Alterations in magnesium distribution**
  1. Redistribution of circulating magnesium occurs by extracellular to intracellular shifts, sequestration, hungry bone syndrome, or by acute administration of glucose, insulin, or amino acids.
  2. Magnesium depletion can be caused by large quantities of parenteral fluids and pancreatitis-induced sequestration of magnesium.

II. Clinical manifestations of hypomagnesemia
- **A. Cardiovascular.** Ventricular tachycardia, ventricular fibrillation, atrial fibrillation, multifocal atrial tachycardia, ventricular ectopic beats, hypertension, enhancement of digoxin-induced dysrhythmias, and cardiomyopathies.
- **B. Neuromuscular findings** may include positive Chvostek's and Trousseau's signs, tremors, myoclonic jerks, seizures, and coma.
- **C. ECG changes** include ventricular arrhythmias (extrasystoles, tachycardia) and atrial arrhythmias (atrial fibrillation, supraventricular tachycardia, torsades de pointes). Prolonged PR and QT intervals, ST segment depression, T-wave inversions, wide QRS complexes, and tall T waves may occur.
- **D. Concomitant electrolyte abnormalities** of sodium, potassium, calcium, or phosphate are common.

III. Clinical evaluation
- **A.** Hypomagnesemia is diagnosed when the serum magnesium is less than 0.7-0.8 mmol/L. Symptoms of magnesium deficiency occur when the serum magnesium concentration is less than 0.5 mmol/L. A 24-hour urine collection for magnesium is the first step in the evaluation of hypomagnesemia. Hypomagnesia caused by renal magnesium loss is associated with magnesium excretion that exceeds 24 mg/day.
- **B.** Low urinary magnesium excretion (<1 mmol/day), with concomitant serum hypomagnesemia, suggests magnesium deficiency due to decreased intake, nonrenal losses, or redistribution of magnesium.

IV. Treatment of hypomagnesemia
- **A. Asymptomatic magnesium deficiency**
  1. In hospitalized patients, the daily magnesium requirements can be provided through either a balanced diet, as oral magnesium supplements (0.36-0.46 mEq/kg/day), or 16-30 mEq/day in a parenteral nutrition formulation.
  2. Magnesium oxide is better absorbed and less likely to cause diarrhea than magnesium sulfate. Magnesium oxide preparations include Mag-Ox 400 (240

mg elemental magnesium per 400 mg tablet), Uro-Mag (84 mg elemental magnesium per 400 mg tablet), and magnesium chloride (Slo-Mag) 64 mg/tab, 1-2 tabs bid.

B. Symptomatic magnesium deficiency

1. Serum magnesium ≤0.5 mmol/L requires IV magnesium repletion with electrocardiographic and respiratory monitoring.
2. Magnesium sulfate 1-6 gm in 500 mL of D5W can be infused IV at 1 gm/hr. An additional 6-9 gm of $MgSO_4$ should be provided as intermittent bolus therapy or by continuous infusion over the next 24 hours.

References, see page 268.

Disorders of Water and Sodium Balance

I. Pathophysiology of water and sodium balance

A. Volitional intake of water is regulated by thirst. Maintenance intake of water is the amount of water sufficient to offset obligatory losses.

B. Maintenance water needs

= 100 mL/kg for first 10 kg of body weight
+ 50 mL/kg for next 10 kg
+ 20 mL/kg for weight greater than 20 kg

C. Clinical signs of hyponatremia. Confusion, agitation, lethargy, seizures, and coma. The rate of change of sodium concentration during onset of hyponatremia is more important in causing symptoms than is the absolute concentration of sodium.

D. Pseudohyponatremia

1. A marked elevation of the blood glucose creates an osmotic gradient that pulls water from cells into the extracellular fluid, diluting the extracellular sodium. The contribution of hyperglycemia to hyponatremia can be estimated using the following formula:

   Expected change in serum sodium = (serum glucose - 100) x 0.016
2. Marked elevation of plasma solids (lipids or protein) can also result in erroneous hyponatremia because of laboratory inaccuracy. The percentage of plasma water can be estimated with the following formula:

   % plasma water = 100 - [0.01 x lipids (mg/dL)] - [0.73 x protein (g/dL)]

II. Diagnostic evaluation of hyponatremia

A. Pseudohyponatremia should be excluded by repeat testing, then the cause of the hyponatremia should be determined based on history, physical exam, urine osmolality, serum osmolality, urine, sodium and chloride. An assessment of volume status should determine if the patient is volume contracted, normal volume, or volume expanded.

B. Classification hyponatremic patients based on urine osmolality

1. **Low urine osmolality (50-180 mOsm/L)** indicates primary excessive water intake (psychogenic water drinking).
2. **High urine osmolality (urine osmolality >serum osmolality)**
   a. **High urine sodium (>40 mEq/L) and volume contraction** indicates a renal source of sodium loss and fluid loss (excessive diuretic use, salt-wasting nephropathy, Addison's disease, osmotic diuresis).
   b. **High urine sodium (>40 mEq/L) and normal volume** is most likely caused by water retention due to a drug effect, hypothyroidism, or the syndrome of inappropriate antidiuretic hormone secretion. In SIADH, the

urine sodium level is usually high, but may be low if the patient is on a salt-restricted diet. SIADH is found in the presence of a malignant tumor or a disorder of the pulmonary or central nervous system.

c. **Low urine sodium (<20 mEq/L) and volume contraction,** dry mucous membranes, decreased skin turgor, and orthostatic hypotension indicate an extrarenal source of fluid loss (gastrointestinal disease, burns).

d. **Low urine sodium (<20 mEq/L) and volume-expansion, and edema** is caused by congestive heart failure, cirrhosis with ascites, or nephrotic syndrome. Effective arterial blood volume is decreased. Decreased renal perfusion causes increased reabsorption of water.

III. Treatment of water excess hyponatremia

A. Determine the volume of water excess

Water excess = total body water x [(140/measured sodium) -1]

B. Treatment of asymptomatic hyponatremia.
Water intake should be restricted to 1,000 mL/day. Food alone in the diet contains this much water, so no liquids should be consumed. If an intravenous solution is needed, an isotonic solution of 0.9% sodium chloride (normal saline) should be used. Dextrose should not be used in the infusion because the dextrose is metabolized into water.

C. Treatment of symptomatic hyponatremia

1. If neurologic symptoms of hyponatremia are present, the serum sodium level should be corrected with hypertonic saline. Excessively rapid correction of sodium may result in a syndrome of central pontine demyelination.

2. The serum sodium should be raised at a rate of 1 mEq/L per hour. If hyponatremia has been chronic, the rate should be limited to 0.5 mEq/L per hour. The goal of initial therapy is a serum sodium of 125-130 mEq/L, then water restriction should be continued until the level normalizes.

3. The amount of hypertonic saline needed is estimated using the following formula:

   Sodium needed (mEq) = 0.6 x wt in kg x (desired sodium - measured sodium)

4. Hypertonic 3% sodium chloride contains 513 mEq/L of sodium. The calculated volume required should be administered over the period required to raise the serum sodium level at a rate of 0.5-1 mEq/L per hour.

5. Concomitant administration of furosemide may be required to lessen the risk of fluid overload, especially in the elderly.

IV. Hypernatremia

A. Clinical manifestations of hypernatremia

1. Signs of either volume overload or volume depletion may be prominent.

2. Clinical manifestations include tremulousness, irritability, ataxia, spasticity, mental confusion, seizures, and coma. Symptoms are more likely to occur with acute increases in plasma sodium.

B. Causes of hypernatremia

1. Net sodium gain or net water loss will cause hypernatremia

2. Failure to replace obligate water losses may cause hypernatremia, as in patients unable to obtain water because of an altered mental status or severe debilitating disease.

3. Diabetes Insipidus: If urine volume is high but urine osmolality is low, diabetes insipidus is the most likely cause.

C. Diagnosis of hypernatremia

1. Assessment of urine volume and osmolality are essential in the evaluation of hyperosmolality. The usual renal response to hypernatremia is the excretion of the minimum volume (≤500 mL/day) of maximally concentrated urine (urine osmolality >800 mOsm/kg). These findings suggest extrarenal water loss.

2. Diabetes insipidus generally presents with polyuria and hypotonic urine (urine

osmolality <250 mOsm/kg).

V. Management of hypernatremia

A. Acute treatment of hypovolemic hypernatremia depends on the degree of volume depletion.

1. If there is evidence of hemodynamic compromise (eg, orthostatic hypotension, marked oliguria), fluid deficits should be corrected initially with isotonic saline.

2. Once hemodynamic stability is achieved, the remaining free water deficit should be corrected with 5% dextrose water or 0.45% NaCl.

3. The water deficit can be estimated using the following formula:
   Water deficit = 0.6 x wt in kg x [1 - (140/measured sodium)]

B. The change in sodium concentration should not exceed 1 mEq/liter/hour. Roughly one half of the calculated water deficit can be administered in the first 24 hours, followed by correction of the remaining deficit over the next 1-2 days. The serum sodium concentration and ECF volume status should be evaluated every 6 hours. Excessively rapid correction of hypernatremia may lead to lethargy and seizures secondary to cerebral edema.

C. Maintenance fluid needs from ongoing renal and insensible losses must also be provided. If the patient is conscious and able to drink, water should be given orally or by nasogastric tube.

VI. Mixed disorders

A. **Water excess and saline deficit** occurs when severe vomiting and diarrhea occur in a patient who is given only water. Clinical signs of volume contraction and a low serum sodium are present. Saline deficit is replaced and free water intake restricted until the serum sodium level has normalized.

B. **Water and saline excess** often occurs with heart failure, edema and a low serum sodium. An increase in the extracellular fluid volume, as evidenced by edema, is a saline excess. A marked excess of free water expands the extracellular fluid volume, causing apparent hyponatremia. However, the important derangement in edema is an excess of sodium. Sodium and water restriction and use of furosemide are usually indicated in addition to treatment of the underlying disorder.

C. **Water and saline deficit** is frequently caused by vomiting and high fever and is characterized by signs of volume contraction and an elevated serum sodium. Saline and free water should be replaced in addition to maintenance amounts of water.

References, see page 268.

Endocrinologic Disorders

Diabetic Ketoacidosis

In children under 10 years of age, diabetic ketoacidosis causes 70% of diabetes-related deaths. Diabetic ketoacidosis is defined by hyperglycemia, metabolic acidosis, and ketosis.

I. Clinical presentation
   A. Diabetes is newly diagnosed in 20% of cases of diabetic ketoacidosis. The remainder of cases occur in known diabetics in whom ketosis develops because of a precipitating factor, such as infection or noncompliance with insulin.
   B. Symptoms of DKA include polyuria, polydipsia, fatigue, nausea, and vomiting, developing over 1 to 2 days. Abdominal pain is prominent in 25%.
   C. Physical examination
      1. Patients are typically flushed, tachycardic, and tachypneic. Kussmaul's respiration, with deep breathing and air hunger, occurs when the serum pH is between 7.0 and 7.24.
      2. A fruity odor on the breath indicates the presence of acetone, a by-product of diabetic ketoacidosis.
      3. Fever is seldom present even though infection is common. Hypothermia and hypotension may also occur. Eighty percent of patients with diabetic ketoacidosis have altered mental status. Most are awake but confused; 10% are comatose.
   D. Laboratory findings
      1. Serum glucose level >250 mg/dL
      2. pH <7.35
      3. Bicarbonate level below normal with an elevated anion gap
      4. Presence of ketones in the serum

Indications for Hospital Admission of Patients with Diabetic Ketoacidosis

Glucose >250 mg/dL
Arterial pH <7.35, or venous pH <7.30, or serum bicarbonate <15 mEq/L
Ketonuria, ketonemia, or both

II. Differential diagnosis
   A. Differential diagnosis of ketosis-causing conditions
      1. Alcoholic ketoacidosis does not cause an elevated serum glucose. Alcoholic ketoacidosis occurs with heavy drinking and vomiting.
      2. Starvation ketosis occurs after 24 hours without food and is not usually confused with DKA because glucose and serum pH are normal.
   B. Differential diagnosis of acidosis-causing conditions
      1. Metabolic acidoses are divided into increased anion gap (>14 mEq/L) and normal anion gap (anion gap is determined by subtracting the sum of chloride plus bicarbonate from sodium).
      2. Anion gap acidoses can be caused by any of the ketoacidoses, including DKA, lactic acidosis, uremia, salicylate or methanol poisoning.
      3. Non-anion gap acidoses are associated with a normal glucose level and

absent serum ketones. Non-anion gap acidoses are caused by renal or gastrointestinal electrolyte losses.

C. **Hyperglycemia caused by hyperosmolar nonketotic coma** occurs in patients with type 2 diabetes with severe hyperglycemia. Patients are usually elderly and have a precipitating illness. Glucose level is markedly elevated (>600 mg/dL), osmolarity is increased, and ketosis is minimal.

III. Treatment of diabetic ketoacidosis

A. Fluid resuscitation

1. Fluid deficits average 5 liters or 50 mL/kg. Resuscitation consists of 1 liter of normal saline over the first hour and a second liter over the second and third hours. Thereafter, ½ normal saline should be infused at 250 mL/hr.
2. When the glucose level decreases to 250 mg/dL, 5% dextrose should be added to the replacement fluids to prevent hypoglycemia. If the glucose level declines rapidly, 10% dextrose should be infused along with regular insulin until the anion gap normalizes.

B. Insulin

1. Insulin is infused at 0.1 U/kg per hour. The biologic half life of IV insulin is less than 20 minutes. The insulin infusion should be adjusted each hour so that the glucose level does not exceed 100 mg/dL per hour.
2. When the bicarbonate level is greater than 20 mEq/L and the anion gap is less than 16 mEq/L, the insulin infusion rate may be decreased.

C. Potassium

1. The most common preventable cause of death in patients with DKA is hypokalemia. The typical deficit is between 300 and 600 mEq.
2. Potassium chloride should be started when fluid therapy is started. In most patients, the initial rate of potassium replacement is 20 mEq/h, but hypokalemia requires more aggressive replacement (40 mEq/h).
3. All patients should receive potassium replacement, except for those with renal failure, no urine output, or an initial serum potassium level greater than 6.0 mEq/L.

D. Sodium

1. Patients with diabetic ketoacidosis sometimes have a low serum sodium level because the high level of glucose has a dilutional effect. For every 100 mg/dL that glucose is elevated, the sodium level should be assumed to be higher than the measured value by 1.6 mEq/L.
2. Frequently, patients have an initial serum sodium greater than 150 mEq/L, indicating severe dehydration. For these patients, initial rehydration fluid should consist of ½ normal saline.

E. Phosphate

1. Diabetic ketoacidosis depletes phosphate stores.
2. Serum phosphate level should be checked after 4 hours of treatment. If it is below 1.5 mg/dL, potassium phosphate should be added to the IV solution in place of KCl.

F. Bicarbonate therapy is not required unless the arterial pH value is 7.0 or lower. For a pH of <7.0, intravenous administration of 50 mEq/L of sodium bicarbonate is recommended.

G. Additional therapies

1. **A nasogastric tube** should be inserted in semiconscious patients to protect against aspiration.
2. **Deep vein thrombosis prophylaxis** with subcutaneous heparin should be provided for patients who are elderly, unconscious, or severely hyperosmolar (5,000 U every 12 hours).

IV. Monitoring of therapy

A. **Serum bicarbonate level and anion gap** should be monitored to determine the effectiveness of insulin therapy.

B. **Glucose levels** should be checked at 1-2 hour intervals during IV insulin administration.

C. **Electrolyte levels** should be assessed every 2 hours for the first 6-8 hours, and then q4h. Phosphorus and magnesium levels should be checked after 4 hours of treatment.

D. **Plasma and urine ketones** are helpful in diagnosing diabetic ketoacidosis, but are not necessary during therapy.

V. Determining the underlying cause

A. **Infection** is the underlying cause of diabetic ketoacidosis in 50% of cases. Infection of the urinary tract, respiratory tract, skin, sinuses, ears, or teeth should be sought. Fever is unusual in diabetic ketoacidosis and indicates infection when present. If infection is suspected, antibiotics should be promptly initiated.

B. **Omission of insulin doses** (common in adolescents) is often a precipitating factor.

C. **Myocardial infarction, ischemic stroke, and abdominal catastrophes** may precipitate DKA.

VI. Initiation of subcutaneous insulin

A. When the serum bicarbonate and anion gap levels are normal, subcutaneous regular insulin can be started.

B. Intravenous and subcutaneous administration of insulin should overlap to avoid redevelopment of ketoacidosis. The intravenous infusion may be stopped 1 hour after the first subcutaneous injection of insulin.

C. **Estimation of subcutaneous insulin requirements**

1. Multiply the final insulin infusion rate times 24 hours. Two-thirds of the total dose is given in the morning as two-thirds NPH and one-third regular insulin. The remaining one third of the total dose is given before supper as one-half NPH and one-half regular insulin.

2. Subsequent doses should be adjusted according to the patient's blood glucose response.

References, see page 268.

Diabetes

Up to 4 percent of Americans have diabetes. Vascular disease accounts for over 70 percent of deaths in adults with diabetes.

Classification and pathophysiology

A. **Type 1 diabetes mellitus** primarily occurs in children and adolescents. Patients with type 1 diabetes have an absolute deficiency of endogenous insulin and require exogenous insulin for survival.

B. **Type 2 diabetes** accounts for 90% of individuals with diabetes mellitus, and the incidence increases in frequency with age, obesity and physical inactivity. The initial problem in type 2 diabetes is resistance to the action of insulin at the cellular level.

C. Type 1 and type 2 diabetes are associated with serious micro- and macrovascular complications. Vascular disease is the cause of death in over 70%.

II. Screening

   A. All adults should be screened for diabetes at regular intervals. Factors that confer an increased risk for development of diabetes include impaired glucose tolerance, hypertension, lipid disorders, coronary artery disease, obesity, and physical inactivity.

   B. A fasting plasma glucose test is recommended for screening. A level of 110 to 125 mg/dL is considered to represent "impaired fasting glucose," and a value of greater than or equal to 126 mg/dL, if confirmed on repeat testing, establishes the diagnosis of diabetes. If a patient is found to have a random plasma glucose level over 160 mg/dL, more formal testing with a fasting plasma glucose should be considered.

Criteria for Diagnosis of Diabetes in Nonpregnant Adults

Fasting plasma glucose 126 mg/dL or higher
or
Random plasma glucose 200 mg/dL or higher with symptoms of diabetes
   (fatigue, weight loss, polyuria, polyphagia, polydipsia)
or
Abnormal two-hour 75-g oral glucose tolerance test result, with glucose 200 mg/dL or higher at two hours
Any abnormal test result must be repeated on a subsequent occasion to establish the diagnosis

---

III. Screening for microvascular complications in diabetics

   A. **Retinopathy.** Diabetic retinopathy and macular degeneration are the leading causes of blindness in diabetes. These complications affect nearly all patients with type 1 diabetes and 60% of those with type 2 disease of at least 20 years duration. Adults with diabetes should receive annual dilated retinal examinations beginning at the time of diagnosis.

   B. **Nephropathy**
      1. Diabetes-related nephropathy affects 40% of patients with type 1 disease and 10-20% of those with type 2 disease of 20 or more years duration. Microalbuminuria of 30 to 300 mg/24 hours heralds the onset of nephropathy. Microalbuminuria can be detected with annual urine screening for albumin/creatinine ratio. Abnormal screening test results should be confirmed, and a 24-hour urine sample should be obtained for total microalbuminuria assay and evaluation for creatinine clearance.
      2. The clinical progression of nephropathy can be slowed by (1) administering ACE inhibitors, such as lisinopril (Prinivil) or enalapril (Vasotec), (2) controlling blood pressure to 130-185 mm Hg or lower, (3) promptly treating urinary tract infections, (4) smoking cessation, and (5) limiting protein intake to 0.6 g/kg/day.

   C. **Peripheral neuropathy** affects many patients with diabetes and causes nocturnal or constant pain, tingling and numbness and confers an increased risk for foot infections, foot ulcers, and amputation.
      1. The feet should be evaluated regularly for sensation, pulses and sores. Semmes-Weinstein 10-g monofilament testing should be performed to assess sensation.

   D. **Autonomic neuropathy** is found in many patients with long-standing diabetes. This problem can result in diarrhea, constipation, gastroparesis, vomiting, orthostatic hypotension, and erectile or ejaculatory dysfunction.

IV. Pharmacologic treatment of diabetes

Pharmacotherapy of Diabetes

Agent	Starting dose	Maximum dose	Comments
Sulfonylureas			May cause hypogly-cemia, weight gain. Maximum dose should be used only in combination with insulin therapy
Glipizide (Glucotrol)	5 mg daily	20 mg twice daily	
Glyburide (DiaBeta, Micronase)	2.5 mg daily	10 mg twice daily	
Glimepiride (Amaryl)	1 mg daily	8 mg daily	
Biguanide			Do not use if serum creatinine is greater than 1.4 mg/dL in women or 1.5 mg/dL in men or in the presence of heart failure, chronic obstructive pulmonary disease or liver disease; may cause lactic acidosis
Metformin (Glucophage)	500 mg daily	850 mg three times daily	
Thiazolidinedione			
Pioglitazone (Actos)	15 mg daily	45 mg per day	
Rosiglitazone (Avandia)	4 mg daily	4 mg twice daily	
Alpha-glucosidase inhibitor			Flatulence; start at low dose to minimize side effects; take at meal-times
Acarbose (Precose)	25 mg daily	100 mg three times daily	
Miglitol (Glyset)	25 mg daily	100 mg three times daily	
Meglitamide			Mechanism of action similar to that of sulfonylureas; may cause hypoglycemia; take at mealtimes
Repaglinide (Prandin)	0.5 mg before meals	4 mg three to four times daily	

Routine Diabetes Care

History
Review physical activity, diet, self-monitored blood glucose readings, medications
Assess for symptoms of coronary heart disease
Evaluate smoking status, latest eye examination results, foot care

Physical examination
Weight
Blood pressure
Foot examination
Pulse
Sores or callus
Monofilament test for sensation
Insulin injection sites
Refer for dilated retinal examination annually

Laboratory studies
HbA1c every three to six months
Annual fasting lipid panel
Annual urine albumin/creatinine ratio
Annual serum creatinine

A. **Targets for control.** The American Diabetes Association recommends a glycosylated hemoglobin (HbA$_{1c}$) level of 7 percent or less as the target for glycemic control, with a level persistently over 8 percent serving as a signal to reassess and revise treatment.

B. The agents used to manage type 2 diabetes can be divided into two groups: those that augment the patient's supply of insulin and those that enhance the effectiveness of insulin.

C. **Insulin-augmenting agents**

1. The sulfonylureas and the meglitinides increase the secretion of endogenous insulin, as long as pancreatic beta-cell function remains. Insulin-augmenting agents act by binding to a receptor on the beta cell. Insulin-augmenting agents are ineffective in patients with juvenile-onset type 1 diabetes.

2. Two long-acting sulfonylureas are now available: glimepiride (Amaryl) and extended-release glipizide (Glucotrol XL). The first meglitinide to become available is repaglinide (Prandin).

3. The various insulin-augmenting agents have equivalent therapeutic power but differ in duration of action and site of clearance. Repaglinide and tolbutamide (Orinase) are the most rapid- and short-acting agents, whereas chlorpropamide (Diabinese), extended-release glipizide and glimepiride are the slowest and longest acting agents.

4. At present, glyburide (Micronase), extended-release glipizide (Glucotrol XL) and glimepiride (Amaryl) are the oral antidiabetic agents most widely used. Glyburide is inexpensive; however, for full effectiveness, it must be taken twice daily, and it has an active metabolite that accumulates when renal function declines. Extended-release glipizide and glimepiride are taken once daily, and their clearance depends very little on renal excretion.

D. **Insulin-assisting agents**

1. The insulin-assisting agents include metformin (Glucophage), which is a biguanide; acarbose (Precose) and miglitol (Glyset), which are alpha-glucosidase inhibitors; and pioglitazone (Actos), and rosiglitazone (Avandia), which are thiazolidinediones.

2. Metformin improves the hepatic response to insulin and reduces overnight glucose production and fasting hyperglycemia. At higher dosages, metformin may reduce food intake and help with weight control.

3. Acarbose and miglitol delay the digestion and absorption of complex carbohydrates. Acarbose and miglitol are quite safe, but they often cause flatulence. Neither agent should be used in patients with intestinal disorders.

4. Pioglitazone and rosiglitazone (thiazolidinediones) improve the response of

muscle and adipose tissue to insulin, especially in patients who are extremely obese. Rosiglitazone and pioglitazone have not been reported to have liver toxicity, and less frequent ALT measurements (every two months for the first year) are advised.

5. Metformin is not metabolized and must be excreted by the kidney. Because high blood levels of metformin can cause fatal lactic acidosis, this oral agent cannot be used when the serum creatinine concentration exceeds 1.4 mg per dL in women or 1.5 mg per dL in men. When first taken, metformin often causes nausea or diarrhea.

Comparison of the Clinical Effects of Oral Antihyperglycemic Agents

Class or generic name	Brand name	Effect on glucose level	Average reduction of HbA$_{1c}$ level (%)	Patients best suited for treatment
Acarbose	Precose	Decreases postprandial increase	0.5 to 1	Patients with high postprandial glucose levels
Metformin	Glucophage	Decreases fasting and 24-hour mean levels	1 to 2	Obese patients with recently diagnosed type 2 diabetes
Repaglinide	Prandin	Decreases fasting and postprandial levels	1 to 2	Patients with recently diagnosed type 2 diabetes who have high postprandial glucose levels
Sulfonylureas		Decrease fasting and 24-hour mean levels	1 to 2	Patients with recently diagnosed type 2 diabetes

E. Initiation of treatment

1. The sulfonylureas have fast and predictable effects on glucose levels, few side effects, once-daily dosage and low cost. To minimize the risk of hypoglycemia, the starting dosage of a sulfonylurea should be low. For example, glyburide (DiaBeta, Micronase) should be initiated in a dosage of 1.25 or 2.5 mg once or twice daily, and glimepiride should be started in a dosage of 1 mg once daily. The lowest available dosage of extended-release glipizide is 5 mg per day, which is usually the maximal effective dosage. The starting dosage of repaglinide (Prandin) is 1 mg taken three times daily with meals.

2. The need for low cost or a quick response favors a sulfonylurea. The need for weight control supports the use of metformin. Acarbose is useful for patients with mainly postprandial hyperglycemia. A thiazolidinedione may have a role in patients who are highly insulin resistant.

3. Metformin (Glucophage) can be quite effective in a dosage of 500 mg taken once daily before a major meal or at bedtime. The dosage can be titrated to 850 mg once daily, 500 mg twice daily, or higher.

4. Acarbose (Precose) or miglitol (Glyset) is a better initial choice in patients who have renal impairment and thus cannot use metformin, especially if their fasting glucose level is below 140 mg per dL but their HbA_{1c} concentration is above 7.5 percent (suggesting marked postprandial hyperglycemia).

5. Acarbose and miglitol are best started at a dosage of 25 mg taken once daily with a meal for two weeks. Then the dosage is increased to 25 mg taken twice daily at meals for two more weeks. Finally, the dosage is increased to 25 mg taken three times daily at meals. If necessary, the dosage may be increased to 50 mg with each meal. Gradual titration reduces flatulence.

F. **Combinations of oral agents**
   1. **Sulfonylurea and metformin.** The combination of a sulfonylurea with metformin has been most widely used. When a sulfonylurea alone or metformin alone fails, the other agent can be added in a gradually titrated dosage.
   2. **Sulfonylurea and thiazolidinedione.** The combination of a sulfonylurea plus a thiazolidinedione is also widely used. The starting dosages of pioglitazone and rosiglitazone are 15 mg per day and 4 mg per day, respectively, and both agents can be taken with or without food.

G. **Insulin** should be prescribed for all patients with type 1 diabetes and is beneficial in some individuals with type 2 diabetes. NPH may be injected once per day at bedtime or twice per day, with about two-thirds of the daily dose given before breakfast and one-third given before the evening meal. Insulin therapy may be initiated in patients using oral agents by continuing the oral medications and adding 10 units of NPH insulin at 10 p.m. or bedtime.

References, see page 268.

Hypothyroidism

Hypothyroidism affects two out of every thousand women. It affects about 6-10% of women over the age of 65 and about 2-3% of men.

I. **Clinical evaluation**
   A. The most common cause of hypothyroidism is Hashimoto's thyroiditis, a chronic autoimmune destruction of the thyroid. Other causes of hypothyroidism include radioactive iodine, thyroidectomy, thioamide drugs, and iodine ingestion. Transient hypothyroidism can occur in patients with acute thyroiditis.
   B. **Symptoms of hypothyroidism.** Patients present with cold intolerance, mental slowing, and weight gain. Other symptoms may include constipation, dry skin, menstrual disorders, and muscle cramps.
   C. **Physical examination.** Peripheral edema (pitting and non-pitting), bradycardia, cool dry skin, gravelly voice, hypothermia, brittle hair, and delayed relaxation phase of tendon reflexes.

Differential Diagnosis of Hypothyroidism	
Cause	**Clues to Diagnosis**
Autoimmune thyroiditis (Hashimoto's disease)	Family or personal history of autoimmune thyroiditis or goiter
Iatrogenic: Ablation, medication, surgery	History of thyroidectomy, irradiation with iodine 131, or thioamide drug therapy
Diet (high levels of iodine)	Kelp consumption
Subacute thyroiditis (viral)	History of painful thyroid gland or neck pain
Postpartum thyroiditis	Symptoms of hyperthyroidism followed by hypothyroidism 6 months postpartum

II. Thyroid function tests

A. **Sensitive thyroid stimulating hormone (TSH) assays.** Immunoradiometric assays can detect abnormally low or abnormally high TSH levels. A sensitive TSH assay is the test of choice for screening for hypothyroidism.

B. Assessment of free T_4 concentrations with a free T_4 index or free T_4 assay can confirm the diagnosis and rule out hypothyroidism secondary to pituitary or hypothalamic failure, which causes low levels of TSH and low levels of T_4.

III. Subclinical hypothyroidism

A. Subclinical hypothyroidism is defined as a mildly elevated TSH level (5.1-20 mIU/mL) with a normal or slightly low free T_4 level and no clinical signs of hypothyroidism. It is most prevalent in the elderly and in women.

B. Treatment with levothyroxine (Synthroid) is recommended for all patients with subclinical hypothyroidism.

IV. Euthyroid sick syndrome (ESS)

A. Alterations in thyroid function tests occur in euthyroid patients who have chronic and acute, non-thyroidal illness and catabolic states. Thyroid function tests are abnormal in up to 70% of all hospitalized patients.

B. **Drugs that affect thyroid function testing**
   1. **Amiodarone** induces hypothyroidism and hyperthyroidism and interferes with T_4 metabolism
   2. **Corticosteroids** suppress TSH and block conversion of T_4 to T_3
   3. **Dopamine** can suppresses TSH
   4. **Lithium** induces hypothyroidism by blocking release of T_4 and T_3
   5. **Phenytoin (Dilantin)** interferes with binding of T_4 to plasma proteins, and it may decrease free T_4 level

C. In ESS, the patient with very severe illness may have a low T_4 and normal or low TSH. These patients do not benefit from hormone replacement.

Diagnosis and Management of Hypothyroid Disorders			
TSH (mIU/mL)	Free T4	Diagnosis	Management
High (>20)	Low or borderline	Hypothyroidism	Treatment and monitoring of TSH level
Borderline-high (5.1-20)	Normal or slightly low	Subclinical hypo-thyroidism	Treatment
Normal (0.3-5)	Low	Euthyroid sick syndrome	No treatment
Low (<0.3)	High	Hyperthyroidism	Treatment
Low (<0.3)	Low	Possible pituitary or hypothalamic dysfunction	Evaluation of pituitary and hypothalamus with TRH stimulation test

V. Treatment of hypothyroidism
A. Synthetic levothyroxine (Synthroid, Levoxine) is the therapy of choice for hypothyroidism. Hormone replacement should achieve a normal TSH level. The half-life of levothyroxine is 7 days; therefore, replacement doses should only be adjusted every 5-6 weeks after measuring hormone levels.
B. The starting dose of levothyroxine (Synthroid, Levoxine) is 100 mcg (0.1 mg) per day in young, healthy patients. In elderly patients and in those at risk of coronary artery disease, the initial daily dose should be 25 to 50 mcg; increase slowly every 4-6 weeks, as tolerated, until the optimal dose of 75 to 150 mcg is reached. Manifestations of thyrotoxicity should be excluded before any dosage increase.
C. Periodic monitoring of TSH should be done every 6-12 months for stable patients who do not have symptoms. Overtreatment of hypothyroidism may cause exacerbation of angina, arrhythmias, myocardial infarction, and osteoporosis.

References, see page 268.

Obesity

Obesity is defined as a body mass index (BMI) of 30 kg per m² or more. Overweight is defined as a BMI of 25 to 29.9 kg per m². About 35 percent of American adults (aged 20 years of age or older) are overweight. In addition, 14 percent of children between the ages of 6 and 11, and 12 percent of adolescents between the ages of 12 and 17 are overweight.

I. **Pathophysiology.** The adipocyte has endocrine capabilities and secretes leptin -- a protein product of the *ob* gene -- in response to increased stores of energy. Leptin limits food intake by acting upon the OB receptor in the hypothalamus. In many obese adults, leptin levels are increased, whereas leptin uptake into the central nervous system is low.
II. **Diagnosis of obesity** begins with the determination of BMI. The BMI can be

ascertained by measuring the patient's height and weight and then using a BMI table to find the BMI value.

III. Management

A. For most patients, the initial weight loss objective should be a 10 percent reduction from baseline body weight over a period of about four to six months. After six months, the rate of weight loss often stabilizes or slows.

B. An overweight individual with a BMI of less than 30 kg per m^2 and no health risk factors should have a target, six-month BMI in the range of 20 to 27. A decrease of 300 to 500 kcal per day will produce weight losses of 0.5 to 1 lb (0.22 to .45 kg) per week (10 percent reduction at six months).

C. **Nutrition therapy**

1. A meal plan that creates an energy deficit of 500 to 1,000 kcal per day less than the individual's average daily intake will usually be suitable for weight reduction. Along with caloric reduction, a reduction in total fat consumption should be recommended. Caloric restrictions for the treatment of overweight and obesity can be classified as follows:

   a. Moderate deficit diet (all health risk groups). Women: 1200+ kcal per day; men: 1400+ kcal per day

   b. Low-calorie diet (moderate to extremely high health risk groups). Women: 800 to 1200 kcal per day; men: 800 to 1400+ kcal per day

   c. Very low-calorie diet (high to extremely high-health risk groups). Less than 800 kcal per day.

2. Among patients treated with a moderate deficit diet, weight losses average about 1 lb (0.45 kg) per week. Because even moderate deficit diets may pose nutritional concerns, such as deficiencies in calcium, iron, and folic acid, vitamin and mineral supplementation may be recommended.

D. **Physical activity**

1. Although most weight loss is achieved through decreased caloric intake, physical activity is the primary factor responsible for increased caloric expenditure. Exercise may reduce the desire for foods that are high in fat and also may help to promote dietary compliance.

2. The long-term physical activity goal of most adults should be to perform 30 or more minutes of moderately intensive physical activity such as walking each day.

E. **Behavior modification methods**

1. Stimulus control to detect and respond to environmental cues associated with unhealthy eating habits and physical inactivity (eg, refraining from eating when not hungry).

2. Self-supervision of eating habits and physical activity (eg, keeping a food and activity diary).

3. Positive reinforcement of beneficial lifestyle changes (eg, rewards; social support from family and friends).

4. Stress management (eg, relaxation techniques, meditation, problem-solving strategies).

5. Cognitive restructuring to moderate self-defeating thoughts and emotions (eg, redefining body image and modifying unrealistic goals).

IV. Pharmacologic treatment

A. Pharmacotherapy should be considered only for individuals with high, very high, or extremely high BMI-based health risks:

1. Patients with a BMI of 30 kg per m^2 or more and no attendant risk factors.

2. Patients with a BMI of 27 kg per m^2 or more and one or more obesity-related comorbidities or other diseases.

B. Contraindications to pharmacotherapy include uncontrolled cardiovascular disease, pregnancy, lactation, history of psychiatric disease, and age below 18 years, and concomitant use of monoamine oxidase inhibitors (MAOIs).

C. Responders may exhibit preliminary weight losses of up to 1 lb (0.45 kg) per week; however, weight loss often plateaus or ceases after six to eight months of therapy. Most patients tend to regain weight after discontinuing pharmacotherapy, successful weight maintenance being contingent on significant improvements in dietary habits, physical activity, and behavior.

Anorectic Medication for Obesity Treatment

Medication	Schedule	Trade Name(s)	Dosage (mg)	Common Use
Phentermine	IV		8, 15, 30	Initial dose: 8-15 mg/d Higher dose: 15 mg bid or 30 mg q AM
		Adipex-P	37.5	Initial dose: ½ tablet/d Higher dose: ½ tablet bid or 37.5-mg tablet q AM
		Fastin	30	1 capsule q AM
Phentermine resin	IV	Ionamin	15, 30	Initial dose: 15 mg/d Higher dose: 15 mg bid or 30 mg q AM
Sibutramine	IV	Meridia	5, 10, 15	Initial dose: 5-10 mg/d Higher dose: 15-25 mg/d
Orlistat	IV	Xenical	120	Initial dose: 1 capsule with a fatty meal qd; bid; or tid

D. Phentermine (Fastin, Ionamin)
1. Most side effects of phentermine (eg, headache, nervousness, insomnia, irritability) are associated with central nervous system stimulation, but cardiovascular effects (eg, tachycardia, increased blood pressure, and palpitations) have been reported. Caution should be exercised when prescribing phentermine to individuals who have hypertension. MAOIs are contraindicated during or within two weeks of phentermine.
2. Phentermine should not be used by patients with cardiovascular disease, glaucoma, hyperthyroidism, advanced arteriosclerosis, agitation, or a history of drug abuse..

E. Orlistat (Xenical) is an inhibitor of gastric and pancreatic lipase. Orlistat hinders the breakdown and absorption of dietary fats in the gastrointestinal system, resulting in body weight reduction and decreased serum cholesterol. Orlistat therapy produces greater weight loss than diet alone. The drug may significantly interfere with the uptake of the lipid-soluble vitamins A, E, and beta-carotene and/or antihypertensive agents, oral contraceptives, and lipid-lowering agents. Adverse effects of orlistat include abdominal pain, diarrhea, fecal incontinence, oily stools, nausea, vomiting, and flatulence.

F. Sibutramine (Merida) is a reuptake inhibitor of both serotonin and norepinephrine. Sibutramine increases satiety after the onset of eating. Weight loss with sibutramine is dose-related. Sibutramine produces weight loss of 3 to 5 kg with 10 mg and 4 to 6 kg with 15 mg of sibutramine.

1. The most common side effects observed during treatment with sibutramine are headache, dry mouth, constipation, and insomnia. The most concerning side effect is hypertension. The mean increase in blood pressure is about 2 mm Hg systolic and diastolic at the 15-mg dose. At the 15-mg dose, approximately 13% of subjects experience an increase of at least 15 mm Hg systolic blood pressure.

2. Sibutramine is available in 5-, 10-, and 15-mg doses given once per day. The recommended starting dose is 10 mg/d. The 15-mg dose can be used in subjects who do not respond adequately to 10 mg, and the 5-mg dose can be used in those who do not tolerate the 10-mg dose.

Contraindications and Cautions for Treatment with Sibutramine

Contraindications

Anorexia nervosa
Hypersensitivity to sibutramine or any ingredients
Patients taking monoamine oxidase inhibitors
Patients taking other centrally acting appetite suppressants
Patients taking other serotoninergic drugs
Coronary heart disease
Congestive heart failure
Stroke
Arrhythmia
Uncontrolled hypertension
Severe hepatic or renal disease
Pregnancy or lactation

Use with Caution

Age <18 or >65
History of seizures
Patients taking other drugs that may raise blood pressure (decongestants)
Patients taking other centrally acting drugs

G. Phenylpropanolamine (Acutrim, Dexatrim) and a blend of Chinese herbs (Dianixx) are the only over-the-counter products marketed as appetite suppressant medicines. Chromium salts and hydroxycitric acid have also been promoted as weight-loss agents. There is little scientific evidence to support the efficacy of any of these agents.

Surgical Therapy

A. Surgical therapy should be considered in patients with severe obesity meeting the following criteria:

1. A BMI of 40 kg per m² or more and have failed in attempts at medical treatment, or

2. A BMI of 35 kg per m² or more with coexisting morbidities or other complicating risk factors.

B. The Roux-en-Y gastric bypass (RYGB) and vertical banded gastroplasty (VBG) are the two operative procedures most frequently employed for obesity. These techniques have been recommended because of safety and efficacy. In the

RYGB procedure, the distal stomach is resected, and the remaining gastric pouch is anastomosed to a Roux-en-Y segment of the jejunum. In the VBG procedure, a prosthetic band (usually silicone or polypropylene plastic) is positioned on the stomach.

C. RYGB and VBG can produce impressive weight losses (40 to 75 percent reductions in excess body weight), and both techniques are generally well tolerated. In addition, weight loss surgery may reduce obesity-related comorbidities, such as hypertension, type 2 diabetes mellitus, and sleep apnea.

References, see page 268.

Rheumatic and Hematologic Disorders

Osteoarthritis

Osteoarthritis is the most common joint disorder. Radiographic evidence of this disease is present in the majority of persons by 65 years of age. Approximately 11 percent of persons more than 64 years of age have osteoarthritis of the knee.

Clinical evaluation

A. The typical patient with osteoarthritis is middle-aged or elderly and complains of pain in the knee, hip, hand or spine. Most often, the patient has pain and stiffness in and around the affected joint, along with some limitation of function. The symptoms are often insidious in onset.

B. Pain typically worsens with use of the affected joint and is alleviated with rest. Pain at rest or nocturnal pain is a feature of severe osteoarthritis. Morning stiffness lasting less than 30 minutes is common. (Morning stiffness with rheumatoid arthritis lasts longer than 45 minutes.)

C. Patients with osteoarthritis of the hip may complain of problems with gait. The pain may be felt in the area of the buttock, groin, thigh or knee. Hip stiffness is common, particularly after inactivity. Physical signs of osteoarthritis of the hip include restriction of internal rotation and abduction of the affected hip.

Clinical Features of Osteoarthritis

Symptoms
Joint pain
Morning stiffness lasting less than 30 minutes
Joint instability or buckling
Loss of function
Signs
Bony enlargement at affected joints
Limitation of range of motion
Crepitus on motion
Pain with motion
Malalignment and/or joint deformity
Pattern of joint involvement
Axial: cervical and lumbar spine
Peripheral: distal interphalangeal joint, proximal interphalangeal joint, first carpometacarpal joints, knees, hips

---

D. Patients with osteoarthritis of the knee often complain of instability or buckling, especially when they are descending stairs or stepping off curbs.

E. Involvement of the lower cervical spine may cause neck symptoms, and involvement of the lumbar spine may cause pain in the lower back. Osteophytes of the vertebrae can narrow the foramina and compress nerve roots, causing radicular symptoms, of pain, weakness and numbness.

F. Physical examination should include an assessment of the affected joints, surrounding soft tissue and bursal areas. Crepitus, which is felt on passive range of motion, is a frequent sign of osteoarthritis of the knee.

G. Patients with erosive osteoarthritis may have signs of inflammation in the interphalangeal joints of the hands. This inflammation can be mistaken for

rheumatoid arthritis, which causes similar proximal interphalangeal joi
swelling. The presence of a hot, erythematous, markedly swollen joint sugges
a septic joint or gout, pseudogout or hydroxyapatite arthritis.

H. Radiographic features and laboratory findings
1. Radiographs can usually confirm the diagnosis of osteoarthritis, although th
findings are nonspecific. The cardinal radiographic features of the diseas
are a loss of joint space and the presence of osteophytes.
2. Routine blood tests are normal in patients with osteoarthritis. Analysis
synovial fluid usually reveals a white blood cell count of less than 2,000 p
mm^3.

II. Treatment
A. Exercise. The goals of an exercise program are to maintain range of motio
muscle strength and general health. All patients with osteoarthritis of the kne
should perform quadriceps-strengthening exercises daily. Patients may also I
referred to aerobic exercise programs such as fitness walking or swimming

---

Management of Osteoarthritis of the Knee

- Nonpharmacologic treatment (eg, patient education and support, exercise,
weight loss, joint protection) *plus*
- Acetaminophen (Tylenol) in a dosage of (1-2 tab) q6h up to 4 g per day to
control pain

- Add topical capsaicin cream (eg, ArthriCare) applied four times daily, if
needed.
- If joint effusion is present, consider aspiration and intra-articular injection of a
corticosteroid, such as 40 mg of triamcinolone (Aristocort).
- If more pain or symptom control is needed, add an NSAID in a low dosage,
such as 400 mg of ibuprofen (eg, Advil) taken four times daily, or a
nonacetylated salicylate such as choline magnesium trisalicylate (Trilisate) or
salsalate (Disalcid).
- If more pain or symptom control is needed, use the full dosage of an NSAID,
plus misoprostol (Cytotec) or a proton pump inhibitor if the patient is at risk
for upper gastrointestinal tract bleeding or ulcer disease, or substitute a
cyclo-oxygenase-2 inhibitor for the NSAID; some patients may benefit from
intra-articular injections of a hyaluronic acid-like product.
- If the response is inadequate, consider referring the patient for joint lavage,
arthroscopic debridement, osteotomy or joint replacement.

B. Assistive devices. Many patients with osteoarthritis of the hip and knee a
more comfortable wearing shoes with good shock-absorbing properties
orthoses. The use of a cane can reduce hip loading by 20 to 30 percent.
C. Weight management. There is an association between obesity a
osteoarthritis of the knee. Therefore, primary preventive strategies may inclu
measures to avoid weight gain, or to achieve weight loss in overweig
patients.
D. Supplements. Glucosamine sulfate and chondroitin sulfate cannot I
recommended for use in the treatment of osteoarthritis.
E. Opioid-containing analgesics, including codeine and propoxyphene (Darvo
can be used for short periods to treat exacerbations of pain.
F. Nonsteroidal anti-inflammatory drugs (NSAIDs).
1. Acetaminophen alone can control pain in a substantial number of patie

with osteoarthritis. In patients requiring NSAID therapy, concurrent use of acetaminophen may allow the NSAID dosage to be reduced, thereby limiting toxicity.

2. The risk of NSAID-induced renal and hepatic toxicity is increased in older patients and in patients with preexisting renal or hepatic insufficiency. Thus, it is important to monitor renal and liver function. Nonacetylated salicylates such as choline magnesium trisalicylate (Trilisate) and salsalate (Disalcid) cause less renal toxicity.

3. In patients requiring chronic NSAID treatment, misoprostol (Cytotec), a synthetic prostaglandin E_1 analog, helps to prevent gastric ulcers. Omeprazole (Prilosec), a proton pump inhibitor, appears to be as effective as misoprostol in healing NSAID-induced ulcers and erosions, and it has the advantage of once-daily dosing. Histamine-H_2 blockers such as ranitidine (Zantac) can prevent duodenal ulcers in patients receiving chronic NSAID therapy; however, ranitidine is ineffective in preventing gastric ulcers.

Commonly Used NSAIDs

Product	Dosage Form	Dose
Ibuprofen (Motrin)	300, 400, 600, 800 mg tablets	400/600/800 mg tid-qid
Naproxen (Naprosyn)	250, 375, 500 mg tablets	250/375/500 mg bid
Naproxen (EC-Naprosyn)	375, 500 mg tablets	375/500 mg bid
Etodolac (Lodine)	200, 300 mg capsule, 400 mg tablet	200/300/400 mg bid-tid
Fenoprofen (Nalfon)	200, 300 mg pulvule 600 mg tablet	300-600 mg tid-qid
Ketoprofen (Orudis)	25, 50, 75 mg capsule	50 mg qid 75 mg tid
Flurbiprofen (Ansaid)	50, 100 mg tablet	50/100 mg bid-tid
Tolmetin (Tolectin)	200, 600 mg tablet 400 mg capsule	200/400/600 mg bid-tid in divided doses
Diclofenac sodium (Voltaren)	25, 50, 75 mg tablet	50 mg bid-tid 75 mg bid
Oxaprozin (DayPro)	600 mg tablet	600-1200 mg qd
Piroxicam (Feldene)	10, 20 mg tablet	20 mg qd
Ketoprofen extended release (Oruvail)	200 mg capsule	200 mg qd
Nabumetone (Relafen)	500, 750 mg tablet	1000-2000 mg qd

G. **Cyclo-oxygenase-2 inhibitors**

1. The presently available NSAIDs work through nonspecific inhibition of cyclo-oxygenase 1 and 2 (COX-1 and COX-2). COX-1 is expressed in gastric and renal tissues, whereas COX-2 is only inducible part of the inflammatory response. COX-2 inhibitors are as effective as NSAIDs in the treatment of osteoarthritis.

2. **Celecoxib (Celebrex)** alleviates pain and reduces inflammation but does not induce gastric ulcers or affect platelet function. The risk of gastrointestinal bleeding is low. The most common side effects of are dyspepsia diarrhea and abdominal pain. Dosage is 200 mg per day administered as a single dose or as 100 mg bid.

3. **Rofecoxib (Vioxx)** is a COX-2 inhibitor given as 25-50 mg qd.

H. **Local analgesics.** Capsaicin (eg, ArthriCare), a pepper-plant derivative, has been shown to be better than placebo in relieving the pain of osteoarthritis Capsaicin cream, 0.025 percent, applied four times daily is effective in the management of pain caused by osteoarthritis. Capsaicin cream is available over the counter in concentrations of 0.025, 0.075 and 0.25 percent.

I. **Intra-articular corticosteroid injections.** Patients with a painful flare of osteoarthritis of the knee may benefit from intra-articular injection of a corticosteroid such as methylprednisolone (Medrol) or triamcinolone (Aristocort). When a joint is painful and swollen, short-term pain relief can be achieved with aspiration of joint fluid followed by intra-articular injection of a corticosteroid.

J. **Sodium hyaluronate (Hyalgan) and hylan G-F 20 (Synvisc)** intra-articular injections are at least as effective as continuous NSAID therapy.

K. **Surgery.** Patients whose symptoms are not adequately controlled with medical therapy and who have moderate to severe pain and functional impairment are candidates for orthopedic surgery. Osteoarthritis of the knee that is complicated by internal derangement may be treated with arthroscopic debridement or joint lavage. Total joint arthroplasty usually markedly improves quality of life.

References, see page 268.

Low Back Pain

Approximately 90 percent of adults experience back pain at some time in life, and 50 percent of persons in the working population have back pain every year.

I. **Evaluation of low back pain**

A. A comprehensive history and physical examination can identify the small percentage of patients with serious conditions such as infection, malignancy rheumatologic diseases and neurologic disorders. The possibility of referred pain from other organ systems should also be considered.

B. The history and review of systems include patient age, constitutional symptoms and the presence of night pain, bone pain or morning stiffness. The patient should be asked about the occurrence of visceral pain, claudication, numbness weakness, radiating pain, and bowel and bladder dysfunction.

C. Specific characteristics and severity of the pain, a history of trauma, previous therapy and its efficacy, and the functional impact of the pain on the patient's work and activities of daily living should be assessed.

History and Physical Examination in the Patient with Acute Low Back Pain

History
Onset of pain (eg, time of day, activity)
Location of pain (eg, specific site, radiation of pain)
Type and character of pain (sharp, dull)
Aggravating and relieving factors
Medical history, including previous injuries
Psychosocial stressors at home or work
"Red flags": age greater than 50 years, fever, weight loss
Physical examination
Informal observation (eg, patient's posture, expressions, pain behavior)
Comprehensive general physical examination, with attention to specific areas as indicated by the history
Neurologic evaluation
Back examination
    Palpation
    Range of motion or painful arc
    Stance
    Gait
    Mobility (test by having the patient sit, lie down and stand up)
    Straight leg raise test

D. The most common levels for a herniated disc are L4-5 and L5-S1. The onset of symptoms is characterized by a sharp, burning, stabbing pain radiating down the posterior or lateral aspect of the leg, to below the knee. Pain is generally superficial and localized, and is often associated with numbness or tingling. In more advanced cases, motor deficit, diminished reflexes or weakness may occur.

E. If a disc herniation is responsible for the back pain, the patient can usually recall the time of onset and contributing factors, whereas if the pain is of a gradual onset, other degenerative diseases are more probable than disc herniation.

F. Rheumatoid arthritis often begins in the appendicular skeleton before progressing to the spine. Inflammatory arthritides, such as ankylosing spondylitis, cause generalized pain and stiffness that are worse in the morning and relieved somewhat throughout the day.

G. Cauda equina syndrome. Only the relatively uncommon central disc herniation provokes low back pain and saddle pain in the S1 and S2 distributions. A central herniated disc may also compress nerve roots of the cauda equina, resulting in difficult urination, incontinence or impotence. If bowel or bladder dysfunction is present, immediate referral to a specialist is required for emergency surgery to prevent permanent loss of function.

Differential Diagnosis of Acute Low Back Pain					
Disease or condition	Patient age (years)	Location of pain	Quality of pain	Aggravating or relieving factors	Signs
Back strain	20 to 40	Low back, buttock, posterior thigh	Ache, spasm	Increased with activity or bending	Local tenderness, limited spinal motion
Acute disc herniation	30 to 50	Low back to lower leg	Sharp, shooting or burning pain, paresthesia in leg	Decreased with standing; increased with bending or sitting	Positive straight leg raise test, weakness, asymmetric reflexes
Osteoarthritis or spinal stenosis	>50	Low back to lower leg; often bilateral	Ache, shooting pain, "pins and needles" sensation	Increase with walking, especially up an incline; decreased with sitting	Mild decrease in extension of spine; may have weakness or asymmetric reflexes
Spondylolisthesis	Any age	Back, posterior thigh	Ache	Increased with activity or bending	Exaggeration of the lumbar curve, palpable "step off" (defect between spinous processes), tight hamstrings
Ankylosing spondylitis	15 to 40	Sacroiliac joints, lumbar spine	Ache	Morning stiffness	Decreased back motion, tenderness over sacroiliac joints
Infection	Any age	Lumbar spine, sacrum	Sharp pain, ache	Varies	Fever, percussive tenderness; may have neurologic abnormalities or decreased motion
Malignancy	>50	Affected bone(s)	Dull ache, throbbing pain; slowly progressive	Increased with recumbency or cough	May have localized tenderness, neurologic signs or fever

II. **Physical and neurologic examination of the lumbar spine**

A. **External manifestations of pain,** including an abnormal stance, should be noted. The patient's posture and gait should be examined for sciatic list, which is indicative of disc herniation. The spinous processes and interspinous ligaments should be palpated for tenderness.

B. **Range of motion** should be evaluated. Pain during lumbar flexion suggests discogenic pain, while pain on lumbar extension suggests facet disease. Ligamentous or muscular strain can cause pain when the patient bends contralaterally.

C. **Motor, sensory and reflex function** should be assessed to determine the affected nerve root level. Muscle strength is graded from zero (no evidence of contractility) to 5 (complete range of motion against gravity, with full resistance).

D. **Specific movements and positions that reproduce the symptoms** should be documented. The upper lumbar region (L1, L2 and L3) controls the iliopsoas muscles, which can be evaluated by testing resistance to hip flexion. While seated, the patient should attempt to raise each thigh while the physician's hands are placed on the leg to create resistance. Pain and weakness are indicative of upper lumbar nerve root involvement. The L2, L3 and L4 nerve roots control the quadriceps muscle, which can be evaluated by manually trying to flex the actively extended knee. The L4 nerve root also controls the tibialis anterior muscle, which can be tested by heel walking.

E. **The L5 nerve root** controls the extensor hallucis longus, which can be tested with the patient seated and moving both great toes in a dorsiflexed position against resistance. The L5 nerve root also innervates the hip abductors, which are evaluated by the Trendelenburg test. This test requires the patient to stand on one leg; the physician stands behind the patient and puts his or her hands on the patient's hips. A positive test is characterized by any drop in the pelvis on the opposite side and suggests either L5 nerve root pathology.

F. **Cauda equina syndrome** can be identified by unexpected laxity of the anal sphincter, perianal or perineal sensory loss, or major motor loss in the lower extremities.

G. **Nerve root tension signs** are evaluated with the straight-leg raising test in the supine position. The physician raises the patient's legs to 90 degrees. Normally, this position results in only minor tightness in the hamstrings. If nerve root compression is present, this test causes severe pain in the back of the affected leg and can reveal a disorder of the L5 or S1 nerve root.

H. **The most common sites for a herniated lumbar disc** are L4-5 and L5-S1, resulting in back pain and pain radiating down the posterior and lateral leg, to below the knee.

I. **A crossed straight-leg raising test** may suggest nerve root compression. In this test, straight-leg raising of the contralateral limb reproduces more specific but less intense pain on the affected side. In addition, the femoral stretch test can be used to evaluate the reproducibility of pain. The patient lies in either the prone or the lateral decubitus position, and the thigh is extended at the hip, and the knee is flexed. Reproduction of pain suggests upper nerve root (L2, L3 and L4) disorders.

Indications for Radiographs in the Patient with Acute Low Back Pain

History of significant trauma
Neurologic deficits
Systemic symptoms
Temperature greater than 38°C (100.4°F)
Unexplained weight loss
Medical history
    Cancer
    Corticosteroid use
    Drug or alcohol abuse
Ankylosing spondylitis suspected

Waddell Signs: Nonorganic Signs Indicating the Presence of a Functional Component of Back Pain

Superficial, nonanatomic tenderness
Pain with simulated testing (eg, axial loading or pelvic rotation)
Inconsistent responses with distraction (eg, straight leg raises while the patient is sitting)
Nonorganic regional disturbances (eg, nondermatomal sensory loss)
Overreaction

Location of Pain and Motor Deficits in Association with Nerve Root Involvement

Disc level	Location of pain	Motor deficit
T12-L1	Pain in inguinal region and medial thigh	None
L1-2	Pain in anterior and medial aspect of upper thigh	Slight weakness in quadriceps; slightly diminished suprapatellar reflex
L2-3	Pain in anterolateral thigh	Weakened quadriceps; diminished patellar or suprapatellar reflex
L3-4	Pain in posterolateral thigh and anterior tibial area	Weakened quadriceps; diminished patellar reflex
L4-5	Pain in dorsum of foot	Extensor weakness of big toe and foot
L5-S1	Pain in lateral aspect of foot	Diminished or absent Achilles reflex

J. **Laboratory tests**
    1. Evaluation may include a complete blood count, determination of erythrocyte sedimentation rate.
    2. **Radiographic evaluation**. Plain-film radiography is rarely useful in the

initial evaluation of patients with acute-onset low back pain. Plain-film radiographs are normal or demonstrate changes of equivocal clinical significance in more than 75 percent of patients with low back pain. Views of the spine uncover useful information in fewer than 3 percent of patients. Anteroposterior and lateral radiographs should be considered in patients who have a history of trauma, neurologic deficits, or systemic symptoms.

3. **Magnetic resonance imaging and computed tomographic scanning**
    a. Magnetic resonance imaging (MRI) and computed tomographic (CT) scanning often demonstrate abnormalities in "normal" asymptomatic people. Thus, positive findings in patients with back pain are frequently of questionable clinical significance.
    b. MRI uses no ionizing radiation and is better at imaging soft tissue (eg, herniated discs, tumors). CT scanning provides better imaging of cortical bone (eg, osteoarthritis). MRI has the ability to demonstrate disc damage, including anular tears and edema. MRI can reveal bulging and degenerative discs in asymptomatic persons. MRI or CT studies should be considered in patients with worsening neurologic deficits or a suspected systemic cause of back pain such as infection or neoplasm. These imaging studies may also be appropriate when referral for surgery is a possibility.

4. **Bone scintigraphy** or bone scanning, can be useful when radiographs of the spine are normal but the clinical findings are suspicious for osteomyelitis, bony neoplasm or occult fracture.

5. **Physiologic assessment**. Electrodiagnostic assessments such as needle electromyography and nerve conduction studies are useful in differentiating peripheral neuropathy from radiculopathy or myopathy. Electrodiagnostic studies may not add much if the clinical findings are not suggestive of radiculopathy or peripheral neuropathy.

III. Management of acute low back pain
A. Pharmacologic Therapy
1. The mainstay of pharmacologic therapy for acute low back pain is acetaminophen or a nonsteroidal anti-inflammatory drug (NSAID). If no medical contraindications are present, a two- to four-week course of medication at anti-inflammatory levels is suggested.
2. Naproxen (Naprosyn) 500 mg followed by 250 mg PO tid-qid prn [250, 375,500 mg].
3. Naproxen sodium (Aleve) 200 mg PO tid prn.
4. Naproxen sodium (Anaprox) 550 mg, followed by 275 mg PO tid-qid prn.
5. Ibuprofen (Motrin, Advil) 800 mg, then 400 mg PO q4-6h prn.
6. Diclofenac (Voltaren) 50 mg bid-tid or 75 mg bid.
7. Adequate gastrointestinal prophylaxis, using a histamine H_2 antagonist or misoprostol (Cytotec), should be prescribed for patients who are at risk for peptic ulcer disease.
8. Rofecoxib (Vioxx) and celecoxib (Celebrex) are NSAIDs with selective cyclo-oxygenase-2 inhibition. These agents have fewer gastrointestinal side effects.
9. Celecoxib (Celebrex) is given as 200 mg qd or 100 mg bid.
10. Rofecoxib (Vioxx) is given as 25-50 mg qd.
11. For relief of acute pain, short-term use of a narcotic may be considered.

B. Rest. Two to three days of bed rest in a supine position may be recommended for patients with acute radiculopathy. Sitting raises intradiscal pressures and can theoretically worsen disc herniation and pain. Activity modification is recommended for patients with nonneurogenic pain. With activity restriction,

the patient avoids painful arcs of motion and tasks that exacerbate the back pain.

C. **Physical therapy modalities**

   1. Superficial heat, ultrasound (deep heat), cold packs and massage are useful for relieving symptoms in the acute phase after the onset of low back pain. These modalities provide analgesia and muscle relaxation. However, their use should be limited to the first two to four weeks after the injury.

   2. No convincing evidence has demonstrated the long-term effectiveness of lumbar traction and transcutaneous electrical stimulation in relieving symptoms or improving functional outcome.

D. **Corsets** (lumbosacral orthoses, braces, back supports and abdominal binders) for a short period (a few weeks) may be indicated in patients with osteoporotic compression fractures.

E. **Aerobic exercise** has been reported to improve or prevent back pain. Exercise programs that facilitate weight loss, trunk strengthening and the stretching of musculotendinous structures appear to be most helpful in alleviating low back pain. Exercises should promote the strengthening of muscles that support the spine.

F. **Trigger point injections** can provide extended relief for localized pain sources. An injection of 1 to 2 mL of 1 percent lidocaine (Xylocaine) without epinephrine is usually administered. Epidural steroid injection therapy has been reported to be effective in patients with lumbar disc herniation with radiculopathy.

G. **Indications for herniated disc surgery.** While most patients with a herniated disc may be effectively treated conservatively. Indications for referral include the following: (1) cauda equina syndrome, (2) progressive neurologic deficit, (3) profound neurologic deficit and (4) severe and disabling pain refractory to four to six weeks of conservative treatment.

References, see page 268.

Gout

Gout comprises a heterogeneous group of disorders characterized by deposition of uric acid crystals in the joints and tendons. Gout has a prevalence of 5.0 to 6.6 cases per 1,000 men and 1.0 to 3.0 cases per 1,000 women.

I. **Clinical features**

A. **Asymptomatic hyperuricemia** is defined as an abnormally high serum urate level, without gouty arthritis or nephrolithiasis. Hyperuricemia is defined as a serum urate concentration greater than 7 mg/dL. Hyperuricemia predisposes patients to both gout and nephrolithiasis, but therapy is generally not warranted in the asymptomatic patient.

B. **Acute gout** is characterized by the sudden onset of pain, erythema, limited range of motion and swelling of the involved joint. The peak incidence of acute gout occurs between 30 and 50 years of age. First attacks are monoarticular in 90 percent. In more than one-half of patients, the first metatarsophalangeal joint is the initial joint involved, a condition known as podagra. Joint involvement includes the metatarsophalangeal joint, the instep/forefoot, the ankle, the knee, the wrist and the fingers.

C. **Intercritical gout** consists of the asymptomatic phase of the disease following recovery from acute gouty arthritis.

D. **Recurrent gouty arthritis.** Approximately 60 percent of patients have a second attack within the first year, and 78 percent have a second attack within two years.

E. **Chronic tophaceous gout.** Tophi are deposits of sodium urate that are large enough to be seen on radiographs and may occur at virtually any site. Common sites include the joints of the hands or feet, the helix of the ear, the olecranon bursa, and the Achilles tendon.

II. Diagnosis

A. Definitive diagnosis of gout requires aspiration and examination of synovial fluid for monosodium urate crystals. Monosodium urate crystals are identified by polarized light microscopy.

B. If a polarizing microscope is not available, the characteristic needle shape of the monosodium urate crystals, especially when found within white blood cells, can be identified with conventional light microscopy. The appearance resembles a toothpick piercing an olive.

III. Treatment of gout

A. **Asymptomatic hyperuricemia.** Urate-lowering drugs should not be used to treat patients with asymptomatic hyperuricemia. If hyperuricemia is identified, associated factors such as obesity, hypercholesterolemia, alcohol consumption and hypertension should be addressed.

B. **Acute gout**

1. NSAIDs are the preferred therapy for the treatment of acute gout. Indomethacin (Indocin), ibuprofen (Motrin), naproxen (Naprosyn), sulindac (Clinoril), piroxicam (Feldene) and ketoprofen (Orudis) are effective. More than 90 percent of patients have a resolution of the attack within five to eight days.

Drugs Used in the Management of Acute Gout

Drug	Dosage	Side effects/comments
NSAIDS		
Indomethacin (Indocin) Naproxen (Naprosyn) Ibuprofen (Motrin) Sulindac (Clinoril) Ketoprofen (Orudis)	25 to 50 mg four times daily 500 mg two times daily 800 mg four times daily 200 mg two times daily 75 mg four times daily	Contraindicated with peptic ulcer disease or systemic anticoagulation; side effects include gastropathy, nephropathy, liver dysfunction, and reversible platelet dysfunction; may cause fluid overload in patients with heart failure
Corticosteroids		
Oral	Prednisone, 0.5 mg per kg on day 1, taper by 5.0 mg each day thereafter	Fluid retention; impaired wound healing
Intramuscular	Triamcinolone acetonide (Kenalog), 60 mg intramuscularly, repeat in 24 hours if necessary	May require repeat injections; risk of soft tissue atrophy
Intra-articular	Large joints: 10 to 40 mg Small joints: 5 to 20 mg	Preferable route for monoarticular involvement

Drug	Dosage	Side effects/comments
ACTH	40 to 80 IU intramuscularly; repeat every 8 hours as necessary	Repeat injections are commonly needed; requires intact pituitary-adrenal axis; stimulation of mineralocorticoid release may cause volume overload
Colchicine	0.5 to 0.6 mg PO every hour until relief or side effects occur, or until a maximum dosage of 6 mg is reached	Dose-dependent gastrointestinal side effects; improper intravenous dosing has caused bone marrow suppression, renal failure and death

2. **Corticosteroids**
   a. **Intra-articular, intravenous, intramuscular or oral corticosteroids** are effective in acute gout. In cases where one or two joints are involved, intra-articular injection of corticosteroid can be used.
   b. **Intramuscular triamcinolone acetonide** (60 mg) is as effective as indomethacin in relieving acute gouty arthritis. Triamcinolone acetonide is especially useful in patients with contraindications to NSAIDs.
   c. **Oral prednisone** is an option when repeat dosing is anticipated. Prednisone, 0.5 mg per kg on day 1 and tapered by 5 mg each day is very effective.
3. **Colchicine** is effective in treating acute gout; however, 80 percent of patients experience gastrointestinal side effects, including nausea, vomiting and diarrhea. Intravenous colchicine is available but is highly toxic and not recommended.

C. **Treatment of intercritical gout**
   1. Prophylactic colchicine (from 0.6 mg to 1.2 mg) should be administered at the same time urate-lowering drug therapy is initiate. Colchicine should be used for prophylaxis only with concurrent use of urate-lowering agents. Colchicine is used for prophylaxis until the serum urate concentration is at the desired level and the patient has been free from acute gouty attacks for three to six months.
   2. **Urate-lowering agents**
      a. After the acute gouty attack is treated and prophylactic therapy is initiated, sources of hyperuricemia should be eliminated to lower the serum urate level without the use of medication.
      b. Medications that may aggravate the patient's condition (eg, diuretics) should be discontinued; purine-rich foods and alcohol consumption should be curtailed, and the patient should gradually lose weight, if obese.

Purine Content of Foods and Beverages

High
Avoid: Liver, kidney, anchovies, sardines, herring, mussels, bacon, codfish, scallops, trout, haddock, veal, venison, turkey, alcoholic beverages
Moderate
May eat occasionally: Asparagus, beef, bouillon, chicken, crab, duck, ham, kidney beans, lentils, lima beans, mushrooms, lobster, oysters, pork, shrimp, spinach

---

3. **24-hour urine uric acid excretion measurement** is essential to identify the

most appropriate urate-lowering medication and to check for significant preexisting renal insufficiency.

a. Uricosuric agents should be used in most patients with gout because most are "underexcretors" of uric acid. Inhibitors of uric acid synthesis are more toxic and should be reserved for use in "overproducers" of urate (urine excretion >800 mg in 24 hours).

b. Urate-lowering therapy should not be initiated until the acute attack has resolved, since they may exacerbate the attack.

Urate-Lowering Drugs for the Treatment of Gout and Hyperuricemia			
Drug	Dosage	Indications	Side effects/comments
Probenecid (Benemid)	Begin with 250 mg twice daily, gradually titrating upward until the serum urate level is <6 mg per dL; maximum: 3 g per day	Recurrent gout may be combined with allopurinol in resistant hyperuricemia	Uricosuric agent; creatinine clearance must be >60 mL per minute; therapeutic effect reversed by aspirin therapy; avoid concurrent daily aspirin use; contraindicated in urolithiasis; may precipitate gouty attack at start of therapy; rash or gastrointestinal side effects may occur
Allopurinol (Zyloprim)	Begin with 50 to 100 mg daily, gradually titrating upward until the serum urate level is <6 mg per dL; typical dosage: 200 to 300 mg daily	Chronic gouty arthritis; secondary hyperuricemia related to the use of cytolytics in the treatment of hematologic malignancies; gout complicated by renal disease or renal calculi	Inhibits uric acid synthesis; side effects include rash, gastrointestinal symptoms, headache, urticaria and interstitial nephritis; rare, potentially fatal hypersensitivity syndrome

4. **Probenecid (Benemid)** is the most frequently used uricosuric medication. Candidates for probenecid therapy must have hyperuricemia attributed to underexcretion of urate (ie, <800 mg in 24 hours), a creatinine clearance of >60 mL/minute and no history of nephrolithiasis. Probenecid should be initiated at a dosage of 250 mg twice daily and increased as needed, up to 3 g per day, to achieve a serum urate level of less than 6 mg per dL. Side effects include precipitation of an acute gouty attack, renal calculi, rash, and gastrointestinal problems.

5. **Allopurinol (Zyloprim)** is an inhibitor of uric acid synthesis. Allopurinol is initiated at a dosage of 100 mg per day and increased in increments of 50 to 100 mg per day every two weeks until the urate level is <6 mg per dL. Side effects include rash, gastrointestinal problems, headache, urticaria and interstitial nephritis. A hypersensitivity syndrome associated with fever, bone marrow suppression, hepatic toxicity, renal failure and a systemic hypersensitivity vasculitis is rare.

References, see page 268.

Rheumatoid Arthritis

Rheumatoid arthritis (RA) is a chronic, polyarticular, symmetric, inflammatory disease that affects about 2.5 million people in the United States. The disease has a predilection for small proximal joints, although virtually every peripheral joint in the body can be involved. RA strikes women, usually of childbearing age, three times more often than it does men. This process causes the immune system to attack the synovium of various joints, leading to synovitis.

I. Clinical manifestations

A. RA is a chronic, symmetric polyarthritis. The polyarthritis is often deforming. About 80% of patients describe a slowly progressive onset over weeks or months.

B. Inflammatory features

1. The joints in RA are swollen, tender, slightly warm, and stiff. Synovial fluid is cloudy and has an increased number of inflammatory white blood cells.
2. Patients with RA usually have profound and prolonged morning stiffness. Fatigue, anemia of chronic disease, fever, vasculitis, pericarditis, and myocarditis, are common.

C. Joint involvement. RA may begin in one or two joints, but it almost invariably progresses to affect 20 or more. In some cases, joint involvement is nearly symmetric. Initially, the disease typically involves the metacarpophalangeal, proximal interphalangeal, wrist, and metatarsophalangeal joints, either alone or in combination with others.

D. Proliferative/erosive features. The inflamed synovial tissue evolves into a thickened, boggy mass known as a pannus. Pannus can eat through joint cartilage and into adjacent bone.

E. Joint deformity. Deformities of RA are more likely to be the result of damage to ligaments, tendons, and joint capsule.

II. Diagnosis

A. RA is a clinical diagnosis. The presence of arthritis excludes the many forms of soft tissue rheumatism (eg, tendinitis, bursitis). The degree of inflammation excludes osteoarthritis and traumatic arthritis. Polyarticular involvement of the appropriate joints makes the spondyloarthropathies unlikely. The pannus is often palpable as a rubbery mass of tissue around a joint.

B. Laboratory tests

1. **Rheumatoid factor** helps to confirm the diagnosis of RA. Rheumatoid factor serves as a marker for RA, but it is not reliable because 1-2% of the normal population have rheumatoid factor. Chronic infections, other inflammatory conditions and malignancies may trigger formation of rheumatoid factor. Conversely, 15% of patients with RA are seronegative for rheumatoid factor.

C. Radiography. Typical erosions around joint margins help confirm the diagnosis of RA.

III. Treatment of rheumatoid arthritis

A. Nonsteroidal anti-inflammatory drugs (NSAIDs) do not alter the course of the disease and have been shown to be as toxic as many of the slow-acting antirheumatic agents that modify disease. Therefore, combination therapy early in the course of RA has become the standard approach.

B. Hydroxychloroquine (Plaquenil) sulfate and sulfasalazine (Azulfidine EN-tabs) are often used in combination with methotrexate (Rheumatrex Dose Pack) and cytotoxic agents.

Selected slow-acting and immunosuppressive antirheumatic drugs used in treatment of rheumatoid arthritis

Drug	Type of agent or mechanism of action	Delivery method	Dose	Side effects
Methotrexate (Rheumatrex Dose Pack)	Folate antagonist	PO or SC	5-20 mg/wk	Marrow suppression, mucositis, hepatotoxicity, pulmonary disease, susceptibility to infection
Cyclosporine (Neoral)	Inhibits interferon-gamma and TNF-alpha	PO	2-4 mg/kg daily	Marrow suppression, renal toxicity, hyperuricemia, susceptibility to infection
Azathioprine (Imuran)	Purine antagonist	PO	50-250 mg/day	Marrow suppression, GI intolerance, hepatotoxicity, susceptibility to infection
Chlorambucil (Leukeran)	Alkylating agent	PO	2-8 mg/day	Marrow suppression (particularly thrombocytopenia), tumors, susceptibility to infection
Cyclophosphamide (Cytoxan, Neosar)	Alkylating agent	PO	25-150 mg/day	Marrow suppression, hemorrhagic cystitis, transitional cell carcinoma and other tumors, susceptibility to infection
Leflunomide (Arava)	Pyrimidine antagonist	PO	100 mg/day for 3 days, then 20 mg/day	Diarrhea, dyspepsia, rash, alopecia, hepatotoxicity, marrow suppression
Infliximab (Remicade)	Chimeric (mouse/human) TNF-alpha antibody	IV	10 mg/kg infusions sporadically	Susceptibility to infection, autoimmune phenomenon, diarrhea, rash, infusion reactions
Etanercept (Enbrel)	TNFR:Fc fusion protein inhibits TNF-alpha	SC	25 mg twice/wk	Injection site reactions, upper respiratory tract infections; theoretically, sepsis or tumors

C. Methotrexate is the "gold standard" of RA therapy. In addition to being efficacious, methotrexate is surprisingly well tolerated. Potential toxic effects of methotrexate include bone marrow suppression, hepatotoxicity, interstitial pneumonitis, pulmonary fibrosis, increased susceptibility to infection, and pseudo-sun sensitivity.

D. Cytotoxic agents. Azathioprine (Imuran), chlorambucil (Leukeran), and cyclophosphamide (Cytoxan, Neosar) have been found to be helpful in treatment of recalcitrant RA. However, the usefulness of these agents is limited by toxic side effects.

E. Leflunomide
  1. Leflunomide (Arava) is the first antipyrimidine agent to be used in treatment of RA. Because the drug is teratogenic in animals, its use is contraindicated in pregnant women and women of childbearing age who are not using reliable contraception.
  2. Efficacy studies have shown that 60% of patients improve with leflunomide therapy, as demonstrated by decreases in the number of swollen and tender joints and by improvement on global assessments. Leflunomide is an effective oral alternative to patients who do not respond to or cannot tolerate methotrexate therapy.

F. Inhibitors of TNF-alpha
  1. The inflammatory and destructive processes characteristic of RA are mediated, in part, by TNF-alpha cytokines released from macrophages and lymphocytes..
  2. **Infliximab (Remicade).** Patients with RA have shown definite clinical improvement after intravenous administration of this agent, which contains chimeric (mouse/human) monoclonal antibodies to TNF-alpha. These antibodies bind circulating TNF-alpha. Joint swelling and tenderness, grip strength, duration of morning stiffness improve significantly.
  3. **Etanercept (Enbrel)** is the first efficacious biologic antirheumatic therapeutic agent. Joint swelling and tenderness, morning stiffness, erythrocyte sedimentation rate, general pain level, and assessments of disease activity improve significantly. Etanercept combined with methotrexate produces a synergistic effect.

References, see page 268.

Deep Venous Thrombosis

Deep venous thrombosis (DVT) has an incidence of 1 case per 1,000 persons. Fifty percent of venous thrombi of the lower extremity will embolize to the lung if not treated.

I. Risk factors for deep venous thrombosis
  A. Venous stasis risk factors include prolonged immobilization, stroke, myocardial infarction, heart failure, obesity, varicose veins, anesthesia, and age >65 years old.
  B. Endothelial injury risk factors include surgery, trauma, central venous access catheters, pacemaker wires, previous thromboembolic event.
  C. Hypercoagulable state risk factors include malignant disease and high estrogen level (pregnancy, oral contraceptives).
  D. Hematologic disorders. Polycythemia, leukocytosis, thrombocytosis, antithrombin III deficiency, protein C deficiency, protein S deficiency, antiphospholipid syndrome, and inflammatory bowel disease.

II. Signs and symptoms of deep venous thrombosis
  A. The disorder may be asymptomatic or the patient may complain of pain, swelling "heaviness," aching, or the sudden appearance of varicose veins. Risk factors

for DVT may be absent.

B. DVT may manifest as a unilaterally edematous limb with a erythrocyanotic appearance, dilated superficial veins, elevated skin temperature, or tenderness in the thigh or calf. Absence of clinical signs does not preclude the diagnosis.

C. A swollen, tender leg with a palpable venous "cord" in the popliteal fossa strongly suggests popliteal DVT. Marked discrepancy in limb circumference supports the diagnosis of DVT, but most patients do not have measurable swelling. The clinical diagnosis of DVT is correct only 50% of the time; therefore, diagnostic testing is mandatory when DVT is suspected.

III. Diagnostic testing

A. Ultrasonography. Color-flow Duplex scanning is the imaging test of choice for patients with suspected DVT. This test is noninvasive and widely available. The Doppler component evaluates blood flow for proximal obstruction, and the addition of color flow technology provides accurate images. The color-flow duplex scan can detect 95-99% of acute thrombi above the knee. Ultrasound can also distinguish other causes of leg swelling, such as tumor, popliteal cyst, abscess, aneurysm, or hematoma. Pain, edema, dyspnea, and a history of DVT are most predictive of positive scans.

B. When results of duplex scanning are positive, these techniques are adequately specific to diagnose DVT. Results that do not support the clinical impression should be investigated with venography.

C. Contrast venography. When ultrasound techniques fail to demonstrate a thrombus, venography is the diagnostic "gold standard" for patients at high clinical risk. The test is negative if contrast medium is seen throughout the deep venous system. Venography can cause iatrogenic venous thrombosis in 4%, and allergic contrast reactions occur in 3% of patients.

D. MRI may have an accuracy comparable to that of contrast venography, and it may soon replace contrast venography as the "gold standard" of venous imaging.

IV. Treatment of deep venous thrombosis

A. Pulmonary embolism (PE) and phlegmasia dolens are life-threatening conditions. If either diagnosis is clinically obvious, heparin should be started prior to imaging studies. Hypotensive patients with these conditions require rapid crystalloid infusion and thrombolytics.

B. Patients with suspected DVT require objective testing, preferably with duplex scanning. If venous thrombosis is confirmed, anticoagulation should be initiated unless contraindicated. Patients with absolute contraindications to heparin require vena cava interruption.

C. Heparin

1. Heparin activates antithrombin III to prevent conversion of fibrinogen to fibrin. Significant bleeding occurs in about 10% of patients, and complications occur at the rate of 1-2% per day. Thrombocytopenia develops in 3%, usually, after 3-5 days.

Management of Deep Venous Thrombosis

Superficial Venous Thrombosis
- Use duplex scan to screen for involvement of deep system
- Elevation, nonsteroidal anti-inflammatory drugs

Deep Venous Thrombosis
- Begin warfarin on the first hospital day
- Low-molecular-weight heparin--more effective and safer than standard heparin

Phlegmasia Dolens
- Enoxaparin
- Heparin 80 U/kg load, 18 U/kg/hr drip
- Thrombolysis for severe disease in young adults
- Vena cava filter if thrombosis in presence of adequate anticoagulation

2. The heparin drip must be continued for 4-5 days. When IV heparin is used, the patient should be admitted to the hospital and the activated PTT should be checked in six hours. An adequate response is 1.5-2.5 times control. Absolute contraindications to heparin include active internal bleeding, malignant hypertension, CNS neoplasm, recent and significant trauma or surgery, and/or a history of heparin-induced thrombocytopenia. Relative contraindications include recent GI bleed or hemorrhagic stroke.

Heparin Weight-Based Nomogram

Initial dose = 80 U/kg bolus, then infuse18 U/kg/h

On Repeat PTT in 6 hours
PTT less than 40 s--rebolus with 80 U/kg, increase drip by 4 U/kg/h
PTT 40-60 s--rebolus with 40 U/kg, increase drip by U/kg/h
PTT 60-80 s--no change
PTT 80-100 s--decrease drip by 2 U/kg/h
PTT greater than 100--hold drip for 1 hour, then decrease drip by 3 U/kg/h

D. **Warfarin (Coumadin).** After starting heparin or another anticoagulation agent (ie, Low Molecular Weight Heparin [LMWH]), the warfarin (Coumadin) 10 mg by mouth should be initiated. By initiating warfarin on the first hospital day, the patient may be discharged in 4-5 days, by which time the INR will usually be in the 2.0-3.0 range. After discharge, most patients will require three months of anticoagulant therapy

E. **Low molecular weight heparins (LMWH)**
1. LMWH has improved antithrombotic effects and has fewer adverse effects than heparin. LMWH has reduced thromboembolic complications, bleeding and mortality when compared to unfractionated heparin. LMWH can be given subcutaneously once or twice a day without need for coagulation tests; therefore, home treatment for DVT is possible.

Exclusions for Home Treatment for DVT

Medical Exclusions
Concurrent Pulmonary Embolism (PE)
Serious co-morbid condition
Cancer, infection, stroke
Prior DVT or PE
Contraindications to anticoagulation
Familial bleeding disorder
Known deficiency of Antithrombin III, Protein C, Protein S Pregnancy
Social Exclusions
No phone
Lives far from hospital
Unable to understand instructions or comply with follow-up
Family or patient resistance to home therapy

Low Molecular Weight Heparin Protocol

Subcutaneous enoxaparin 1 mg/kg q12hours for a minimum of five days and achieving INR of 2-3 (from warfarin therapy)
Warfarin to be started on first day of therapy
INR should be monitored during outpatient treatment
Warn patients to return immediately for shortness of breath, hemorrhage, or clinical decomposition

2. Because LMWH primarily inhibits factor X-a and has little effect on thrombin or platelet aggregation, there are fewer hemorrhagic complications. LMWH usually does not elevate the PTT. LMWH is valued for its antithrombotic effect and lack of anticoagulant effect.
3. **Enoxaparin (Lovenox)** is the *only* LMWH currently approved for treatment of DVT. The dose of enoxaparin for inpatient treatment of DVT, with or without PE is 1 mg/kg q12hours SQ or 1.5 mg/kg SQ qd. The dose of enoxaparin for *outpatient* therapy of deep venous thrombosis *without* pulmonary embolism is 1 mg/kg q12hours SQ.
4. Enoxaparin should be administered for at least five days, and warfarin can be started on the same day as the LMWH or the day after. Blood should be drawn daily to monitor the prothrombin time for the first few days; the International Normalized Ration (INR) should be between 2.0 and 3.0 for two consecutive days before the LMWH is stopped.

eferences, see page 268.

ulmonary Embolism

proximately 300,000 Americans suffer pulmonary embolism each year. Among those whom the condition is diagnosed, 2 percent die within the first day and 10 percent ve recurrent pulmonary embolism; the death rate among the latter group is 45 rcent.

I. **Diagnosis of pulmonary embolism**
   A. Pulmonary embolism should suspected in any patient with new cardiopulmonary symptoms or signs and significant risk factors. If no other satisfactory explanation can be found in a patient with findings suggestive of pulmonary embolism, the workup for PE must be pursued to completion.
   B. **Signs and symptoms of pulmonary embolism.** Pleuritic chest pain, unexplained shortness of breath, tachycardia, hypoxemia, hypotension, hemoptysis, cough, syncope. The classic triad of dyspnea, chest pain, and hemoptysis is seen in only 20% of patients. The majority of patients have only a few subtle symptoms or are asymptomatic.
   C. Patients with massive pulmonary emboli may experience sudden onset of precordial pain, dyspnea, syncope, or shock. Other findings include distended neck veins, cyanosis, diaphoresis, pre-cordial heave, loud P2, right ventricular S3, or murmur of tricuspid insufficiency.
   D. Deep venous thrombosis may manifest as an edematous limb with an erythrocyanotic appearance, dilated superficial veins, and elevated skin temperature.

Frequency of Symptoms and Signs in Pulmonary Embolism

Symptoms	Frequency (%)	Signs	Frequency (%)
Dyspnea	84	Tachypnea (>16/min)	92
Pleuritic chest pain	74	Rales	58
Apprehension	59	Accentuated S2	53
Cough	53	Tachycardia	44
Hemoptysis	30	Fever (>37.8°C)	43
Sweating	27	Diaphoresis	36
Non-pleuritic chest pain	14	S3 or S4 gallop	34
Syncope		Thrombophlebitis	32

Conditions That Can Cause Acute Respiratory Symptoms

Acute bronchitis	Pericarditis
Acute myocardial infarction	Pneumonia
Asthma	Pneumothorax
Cardiogenic shock	Pulmonary edema
Congestive heart failure	Pulmonary embolism
Exacerbation of chronic obstructive pulmonary disease	Septic shock

II. **Risk factors for pulmonary embolism**
   A. **Venous stasis.** Prolonged immobilization, hip surgery, stroke, myocardial infarction, heart failure, obesity, varicose veins, anesthesia, age >65 years of
   B. **Endothelial injury.** Surgery, trauma, central venous access catheters, pacemaker wires, previous thromboembolic event.
   C. **Hypercoagulable state.** Malignant disease, high estrogen level (oral contraceptives).
   D. **Hematologic disorders.** Polycythemia, leukocytosis, thrombocytosis, antithrombin III deficiency, protein C deficiency, protein S deficiency, antiphospholipid syndrome, inflammatory bowel disease, factor 5 Leiden defect

III. Diagnostic evaluation

A. Chest radiographs are nonspecific and insensitive, and findings are normal in up to 40 percent of patients with pulmonary embolism. Abnormalities may include an elevated hemidiaphragm, focal infiltrates, atelectasis, and small pleural effusions.

B. Electrocardiography is nonspecific and often normal. The most common abnormality is sinus tachycardia. ST-segment or T-wave changes are also common findings. Occasionally, acute right ventricular strain causes tall peaked P waves in lead II, right axis deviation, right bundle branch block, or atrial fibrillation.

C. Blood gas studies. There is no level of arterial oxygen that can rule out pulmonary embolism. Most patients with pulmonary embolism have a normal arterial oxygen.

D. Ventilation-perfusion scan

1. Patients with a clearly normal perfusion scan do not have a pulmonary embolism, and less than 5 percent of patients with near-normal scan have a pulmonary embolism. A high-probability scan has a 90 percent probability of a pulmonary embolism.

2. **A low-probability V/Q scan** can exclude the diagnosis of pulmonary embolism only if the patient has a clinically low probability of pulmonary embolism.

3. **Intermediate V/Q scans** are not diagnostic and usually indicate the need for further diagnostic testing. One-third of patients with intermediate scans have a pulmonary embolism.

E. Venous imaging

1. If the V/Q scan is nondiagnostic, a workup for deep venous thrombosis (DVT) should be pursued using duplex ultrasound. The identification of DVT in a patient with signs and symptoms suggesting pulmonary embolism proves the diagnosis of pulmonary embolism. A deep venous thrombosis can be found in 80% of cases of pulmonary emboli.

2. Inability to demonstrate the existence of a DVT does not significantly lower the likelihood of pulmonary embolism because clinically asymptomatic DVT may not be detectable.

3. Patients with a nondiagnostic V/Q scan and no demonstrable site of DVT should proceed to pulmonary angiography.

F. Angiography. Contrast pulmonary arteriography is the "gold standard" for the diagnosis of pulmonary embolism. False-negative results occur in 2-10% of patients. Angiography carries a low risk of complications (minor 5%, major nonfatal 1%, fatal 0.5%).

IV. Management of acute pulmonary embolism in stable patients

A. Oxygen should be initiated for all patients.

B. Heparin anticoagulation

1. Heparin therapy should be started as soon as the diagnosis of pulmonary embolism is suspected. Full dose heparin can be given immediately after major surgery.

2. **Heparin administration.** 5,000 u (80 U/kg IVP, then 1,300 u (18 U/kg/h) IV infusion. Obtain aPTT in 6 hours, and adjust dosage based on the table below to maintain the aPTT between 60-85 seconds. Contraindications to heparin include active internal bleeding and recent and significant trauma.

Heparin Maintenance Dose Adjustment				
aPTTs	Bolus Dose	Stop infusion (min)	Rate Change, mL/h*	Repeat aPTT
<50	5000 U	0	+3 (increase by 150 U/h)	6 h
50-59	0	0	+2 (increase by 100 U/h)	6 h
60-85	0	0	0 (no change)	next AM
86-95	0	0	-1 (decrease by 50 U/h)	next AM
96-120	0	30	-2 (decrease by 100 U/h)	6 h
>120	0	60	-3 (decrease by 150 U/h)	6 h

*50 U/mL

3. Platelet count should be monitored during heparin therapy; thrombocytopeni develops in up to 5%. Heparin may rarely induce hyperkalemia, whic resolves spontaneously upon discontinuation.
4. **Warfarin (Coumadin)** may be started as soon as the diagnosis of pulmona embolism is confirmed and heparin has been initiated. Starting dose is 10 m PO qd for 3 days. The dose is then adjusted to keep the Internation. Normalized Ratio (INR) at 2.0 to 3.0. The typical dosage is 2.0-7.5 mg PO q Heparin and warfarin regimens are overlapped for 3 to 5 days until the INR 2.0-3.0, then heparin is discontinued.
5. Therapy with warfarin is generally continued for 3-6 months. In patients wit an ongoing risk factor or following a second episode of DVT, lifelor anticoagulation with warfarin may be necessary.
6. **Low-molecular-weight heparin (LMWH).** LMWH is as effective a unfractionated heparin for DVT or uncomplicated pulmonary embolism. It doe not require dosage adjustment and may allow for earlier hospital discharg Enoxaparin (Lovenox) 1 mg/kg SQ q12h.

V. **Management of acute pulmonary embolism in unstable patients**
   A. Patients with pulmonary embolism who have severe hypoxemia or any degre of hypotension are considered to be in unstable condition.
   B. **Heparin and oxygen** should be started immediately.
   C. **Fluid and pharmacologic management.** In acute cor pulmonale, gent pharmacologic preload reduction with furosemide unloads the congeste pulmonary circuit and reduces right ventricular pressures. Hydralazin isoproterenol, or norepinephrine may be required. Pulmonary artery pressu monitoring may be helpful.
   D. **Thrombolysis**
      1. Unstable patients (systolic <90 mmHg) with proven pulmonary embolis require immediate clot lysis by thrombolytic therapy. Tissue plasminog activator (Activase) is recommended because it is the fastest-acti

thrombolytic agent.
   2. **Contraindications to thrombolytics**
      a. **Absolute contraindications.** Active bleeding, cerebrovascular accident or surgery within the past 2 months, intracranial neoplasms.
      b. **Relative contraindications.** Recent gastrointestinal bleeding, uncontrolled hypertension, recent trauma (cardiopulmonary resuscitation), pregnancy.
   3. **Alteplase (tPA, Activase).** 100 mg by peripheral IV infusion over 2 hr. Heparin therapy should be initiated after cessation of the thrombolytic infusion. Heparin is started without a loading dose when the activated partial thromboplastin time is 1.5 times control rate at 18 U/kg/hr.

VI. **Emergency thoracotomy.** Emergency surgical removal of embolized thrombus is reserved for instances when there is an absolute contraindication to thrombolysis or when the patient's condition has failed to improve after thrombolysis. Cardiac arrest from pulmonary embolism is an indication for immediate thoracotomy.

References, see page 268.

Gynecologic Disorders

Osteoporosis

Osteoporosis is a common cause of skeletal fractures. Bone loss accelerates during menopause due to a decrease in estrogen production. Approximately 20% of women have osteoporosis in their seventh decade of life, 30% of women in their eighth decade of life, and 70% of women older than 80 years.

I. Diagnosis
  A. Risk factors for osteoporosis include female gender, increasing age, family history, Caucasian or Asian race, estrogen deficient state, nulliparity, sedentarism, low calcium intake, smoking, excessive alcohol or caffeine consumption, and use of glucocorticoid drugs. Patients who have already sustained a fracture have a markedly increased risk of sustaining further fractures.
  B. Bone density testing. Bone density is the strongest predictor of fracture risk. Bone density can be assessed by dual X-ray absorptiometry.

Indications for Bone Density Testing
Estrogen-deficient women at clinical risk for osteoporosis
Individuals with vertebral abnormalities
Individuals receiving, or planning to receive, long-term glucocorticoid therapy
Individuals with primary hyperparathyroidism
Individuals being monitored to assess the response of an osteoporosis drug

II. Prevention and treatment strategies
  A. A balanced diet including 1000-1500 mg of calcium, weight bearing exercise, and avoidance of alcohol and tobacco products should be encouraged. Daily calcium supplementation (1000-1500 mg) along with 400-800 IU vitamin D should be recommended.
  B. Estrogen therapy is recommended for most females. Females who are not willing or incapable of receiving estrogen therapy and have osteopenic bone densities may consider alendronate and raloxifene. After the age of 65, a bone density test should be performed to decide if pharmacologic therapy should be considered to prevent or treat osteoporosis.

Drugs for Osteoporosis			
Drug	Dosage	Indication	Comments
Estrogen	0.625 mg qd with medroxypro-gesterone (Provera), 2.5 mg qd	Prevention and Treatment	Recommended for most menopausal females

Drug	Dosage	Indication	Comments
Raloxifene (Evista)	60 mg PO QD	Prevention	No breast or uterine tissue stimulation. Decrease in cholesterol similar to estrogen.
Alendronate (Fosamax)	5 mg PO QD 10 mg PO QD	Prevention Treatment	Take in the morning with 2-3 glasses of water, at least 30 min before any food, beverages, or medication. Reduction in fracture risk.
Calcitonin	200 IU QD (nasal) 50-100 IU QD SQ	Treatment	Modest analgesic effect. Not indicated in the early post-menopausal years.
Calcium	1000-1500 mg/day	Prevention/ Treatment	Calcium alone may not prevent osteoporosis
Vitamin D	400-800 IU QD	Prevention/ Treatment	May help reduce hip fracture incidence

C. Estrogen replacement therapy
   1. Postmenopausal women without contraindications should consider ERT. Contraindications include a family or individual history of breast cancer; estrogen dependent neoplasia; undiagnosed genital bleeding or a history of or active thromboembolic disorder.
   2. ERT should be initiated at the onset of menopause. Conjugated estrogens, at a dose of 0.625 mg per day, result in increases in bone density of 5%.
   3. **Bone density assessment** at regular intervals (possibly every 3-5 years) provides density data to help determine if continuation of ERT may be further recommended. If ERT is discontinued and no other therapies are instituted, serial bone density measurements should be continued to monitor bone loss.
   4. ERT doubles the risk of endometrial cancer in women with an intact uterus. This increased risk can be eliminated by the addition of medroxyprogesterone (Provera), either cyclically (12-14 days/month) at a dose of 5-10 mg, or continuously at a dose of 2.5 mg daily.
   5. Other adverse effects related to ERT are breast tenderness, weight gain, headaches, and libido changes.
D. Selective estrogen receptor modulators
   1. Selective estrogen receptor modulators (SERMs) act as estrogen analogs. Tamoxifen is approved for the prevention of breast cancer in patients with a strong family history of breast cancer. Tamoxifen prevents bone loss at the spine.
   2. **Raloxifene (Evista)**
      a. **Raloxifene** is approved for the prevention of osteoporosis. When used at 60 mg per day, raloxifene demonstrates modest increases (1.5-2% in 24 months) in bone density. This increase in density is half of that seen in those patients receiving ERT. Raloxifene has a beneficial effect on the lipid profile similar to that seen with estrogen.
      b. Raloxifene lacks breast stimulation properties, and it may provide a protective effect against breast cancer, resulting in a 50-70% reduction in

breast cancer risk.
   c. Minor side effects include hot flashes and leg cramps. Serious side effects include an increased risk of venous thromboembolism.
E. **Bisphosphonates – alendronate (Fosamax)**
   1. Alendronate is an oral bisphosphonate approved for the treatment and prevention of osteoporosis. Alendronate exerts its effect on bone by inhibiting osteoclasts.
   2. The dose for prevention of osteoporosis is 5 mg per day. This dose results in significant increases in densities of 2-3.5%, similar to those observed in ERT. The dose for treatment of osteoporosis is 10 mg per day. Alendronate provides a 50% reduction in fracture risk.
   3. Patients should take the pill in the morning with 2-3 glasses of water, at least 30 minutes before any food or beverages. No other medication should be taken at the same time, particularly calcium preparations. Patients should not lie down after taking alendronate to avoid gastroesophageal reflux. Contraindicates include severe renal insufficiency and hypocalcemia.

References, see page 268.

Management of the Abnormal Pap Smear

Cervical cancer has an incidence of about 15,700 new cases each year (representing 6% of all cancers), and 4,900 women die of the disease each year. Those at increased risk of preinvasive disease include patients with human-papilloma virus (HPV) infection, those infected with HIV, cigarette smokers, those with multiple sexual partners, and those with previous preinvasive or invasive disease.

I. **Screening for cervical cancer**
   A. Regular Pap smears are recommended for all women who are or have been sexually active and who have a cervix.
   B. Testing should begin when the woman first engages in sexual intercourse. Adolescents whose sexual history is thought to be unreliable should be presumed to be sexually active at age 18.
   C. Pap smears should be performed at least every 1 to 3 years. Testing is usually discontinued after age 65 in women who have had regular normal screening tests. Women who have had a hysterectomy, including removal of the cervix for reasons other than cervical cancer or its precursors, do not require Pap testing.
II. **Management of minor Pap smear abnormalities**
   A. **Satisfactory, but limited by few (or absent) endocervical cells**
      1. Endocervical cells are absent in up to 10% of Pap smears before menopause and up to 50% postmenopausally.
      2. **Management.** The Pap smear is usually either repeated annually or recall women with previously abnormal Pap smears.
   B. **Unsatisfactory for evaluation**
      1. Repeat Pap smear midcycle in 6-12 weeks.
      2. If atrophic smear, treat with estrogen cream for 6-8 weeks, then repeat Pap smear.
   C. **Benign cellular changes**
      1. **Infection--candida**. Most cases represent asymptomatic colonization. Treatment should be offered for symptomatic cases. The Pap should be repeated at the usual interval.

2. **Infection–Trichomonas**. If wet preparation is positive, treat with metronidazole (Flagyl), then continue annual Pap smears.

3. **Infection--predominance of coccobacilli consistent with shift in vaginal flora.** This finding implies bacterial vaginosis, but it is a non-specific finding. Diagnosis should be confirmed by findings of a homogeneous vaginal discharge, positive amine test, and clue cells on saline suspension.

4. **Infection-herpes simplex virus**. Pap smear has a poor sensitivity, but good specificity, for HSV. Positive smears usually are caused by asymptomatic infection. The patient should be informed of pregnancy risks and the possibility of transmission. Treatment is not necessary, and the Pap should be repeated as for a benign result.

5. **Inflammation on Pap smear**
   a. **Mild inflammation** on an otherwise normal smear does not need further evaluation.
   b. **Moderate or severe inflammation** should be evaluated with a saline preparation, KOH preparation, and gonorrhea and Chlamydia tests. If the source of infection is found, treatment should be provided, and a repeat Pap smear should be done every 6 to 12 months. If no etiology is found, the Pap smear should be repeated in 6 months.
   c. **Persistent inflammation** may be infrequently the only manifestation of high-grade squamous intraepithelial lesions (HGSIL) or invasive cancer; therefore, persistent inflammation is an indication for colposcopy.

6. **Atrophy with inflammation** is common in post-menopausal women or in those with estrogen-deficiency states. Atrophy should be treated with vaginal estrogen for 4-6 weeks, then repeat Pap smear.

III. Managing cellular abnormalities

A. **Atypical squamous cells of undetermined significance (ASCUS).** On retesting, 25%-60% of patients will have LSIL or HSIL, and 15% will demonstrate HSIL. In a low-risk patient, it is reasonable to offer the option of repeating the cervical smears every 4 months for the next 2 years--with colposcopy, endocervical curettage (ECC) and directed biopsy if findings show progression or the atypical cells have not resolved. Alternatively, the patient can proceed immediately with colposcopy, ECC, and directed biopsy. In a high-risk patient (particularly when follow-up may be a problem), it is advisable to proceed with colposcopy, ECC, and directed biopsy.

B. **Low-grade squamous intraepithelial lesion (LSIL).** The smear will revert to normal within 2 years in 30%-60% of patients. Another 25% have, or will progress to, moderate or severe dysplasia (HSIL). With a low-risk patient, cervical smears should be repeated every 4 months for 2 years; colposcopy, ECC, and directed biopsy are indicated for progression or nonresolution. In the high-risk patient, prompt colposcopy, ECC, and directed biopsy are recommended.

The Bethesda system

Adequacy of the specimen
  Satisfactory for evaluation
  Satisfactory for evaluation but limited by... Specify reason
  Unsatisfactory for evaluation: Specify reason
General categorization (optional)
  Within normal limits
  Benign cellular changes: See descriptive diagnoses
  Epithelial cell abnormality: See descriptive diagnoses
Descriptive diagnoses
  Benign cellular changes
  Infection
  Trichomonas vaginalis
  Fungal organisms morphologically consistent with Candida spp
  Predominance of coccobacilli consistent with shift in vaginal flora
  Bacteria morphologically consistent with Actinomyces spp
  Cellular changes associated with herpes simplex virus
  Other
  Reactive changes
  Inflammation (includes typical repair)
  Atrophy with inflammation (atrophic vaginitis)
  Radiation
  Intrauterine contraceptive device
Epithelial cell abnormalities
Squamous cell
  Atypical squamous cells of undetermined significance (ASCUS): Qualify
  Low-grade squamous intraepithelial lesion (LSIL) compassing HPV; mild dysplasia/CIN 1
  High-grade squamous intraepithelial lesions (HSIL) encompassing moderate and severe dysplasia, CIS/CIN 2 and CIN
  Squamous cell carcinoma
Glandular cell
  Endometrial cells, cytologically benign, in a postmenopausal woman
  Atypical glandular cells of undetermined significance (AGUS): Qualify
  Endocervical adenocarcinoma
  Endometrial adenocarcinoma
  Extrauterine adenocarcinoma
  Adenocarcinoma, not otherwise specified
Other malignant neoplasms: Specify

C. **High-grade squamous intraepithelial lesions (HSIL),** moderate-to-severe dysplasia, CIS 1, CIN 2, and CIN 3 Colposcopy, ECC, and directed biopsies are recommended.

D. **Atypical glandular cells of undetermined significance (AGUS).** One-third of those for whom the report "favors reactive" will actually have dysplasia. For this reason, colposcopy, ECC (or cytobrush), and directed biopsies are recommended. If glandular neoplasia is suspected or persistent AGUS does not correlate with ECC findings, cold-knife conization perhaps with dilatation and curettage (D&C) is indicated. D&C with hysteroscopy is the treatment of choice for AGUS endometrial cells.

E. **Squamous cell carcinoma** should be referred to a gynecologist or oncologist experienced in its treatment.

IV. Management of glandular cell abnormalities

A. Endometrial cells on Pap smear. When a Pap smear is performed during menstruation, endometrial cells may be present. However, endometrial cells on a Pap smear performed during the second half of the menstrual cycle or in a post-menopausal patient may indicate the presence of polyps, hyperplasia, or endometrial adenocarcinoma. An endometrial biopsy should be considered in these women.

B. Atypical glandular cells of undetermined significance (AGUS). Colposcopically directed biopsy and endocervical curettage is recommended in all women with AGUS smears, and abnormal endometrial cells should be investigated by endometrial biopsy, fractional curettage, or hysteroscopy.

C. Adenocarcinoma. This diagnosis requires endocervical curettage, cone biopsy, and/or endometrial biopsy.

V. Colposcopically directed biopsy

A. Liberally apply a solution of 3-5% acetic acid to cervix, and inspect cervix for abnormal areas (white epithelium, punctation, mosaic cells, atypical vessels). Biopsies of any abnormal areas should be obtained under colposcopic visualization. Record location of each biopsy. Monsel solution may be applied to stop bleeding.

B. Endocervical curettage is done routinely during colposcopy, except during pregnancy.

VI. Treatment based on cervical biopsy findings

A. Benign cellular changes (infection, reactive inflammation). Treat the infection, and repeat the smear every 4-6 months; after 2 negatives, repeat yearly.

B. Squamous intraepithelial lesions
  1. Women with SIL should be treated on the basis of the histological biopsy diagnosis. Patients with CIN I require no further treatment because the majority of these lesions resolve spontaneously. Patients with CIN II or CIN III require treatment to prevent development of invasive disease.
  2. These lesions are treated with cryotherapy, laser vaporization, or loop electric excision procedure (LEEP).

References, see page 268.

Sexually Transmissible Infections

Approximately 12 million patients are diagnosed with a sexually transmissible infection (STI) annually in the United States. Sequella of STIs include infertility, chronic pelvic pain, ectopic pregnancy, and other adverse pregnancy outcomes.

Diagnosis and Treatment of Bacterial Sexually Transmissible Infections

Organism	Diagnostic Methods	Recommended Treatment	Alternative
Chlamydia trachomatis	Direct fluorescent antibody, enzyme immunoassay, DNA probe, cell culture, DNA amplification	Doxycycline 100 mg PO 2 times a day for 7 days or Azithromycin (Zithromax) 1 g PO	Ofloxacin (Floxin) 300 mg PO 2 times a day for 7 days or erythromycin base 500 mg PO 4 times a day for 7 days or erythromycin ethylsuccinate 800 mg PO 4 times a day for 7 days.
Neisseria gonorrhoeae	Culture DNA probe	Ceftriaxone (Rocephin) 125 mg IM or Cefixime 400 mg PO or Ciprofloxacin (Cipro) 500 mg PO or Ofloxacin (Floxin) 400 mg PO plus Doxycycline 100 mg 2 times a day for 7 days or azithromycin 1 g PO	Single IM dose of ceftizoxime 500 mg, cefotaxime 500 mg, cefotetan 1 g, and cefoxitin (Mefoxin) 2 g with probenecid 1 g PO; or enoxacin 400 mg PO, lomefloxacin 400 mg PO, or norfloxacin 800 mg PO
Treponema pallidum	Clinical appearance Dark-field microscopy Nontreponemal test: rapid plasma reagin, VDRL Treponemal test: MHA-TP, FTA-ABS	Primary and secondary syphilis and early latent syphilis (<1 year duration): benzathine penicillin G 2.4 million units IM in a single dose.	Penicillin allergy in patients with primary, secondary, or early latent syphilis (<1 year of duration): doxycycline 100 mg PO 2 times a day for 2 weeks.

Diagnosis and Treatment of Viral Sexually Transmissible Infections

Organism	Diagnostic Methods	Recommended Treatment Regimens
Herpes simplex virus	Clinical appearance Cell culture confirmation	First episode: Acyclovir (Zovirax) 400 mg PO 5 times a day for 7-10 days, or famciclovir (Famvir) 250 mg PO 3 times a day for 7-10 days, or valacyclovir (Valtrex) 1 g PO 2 times a day for 7-10 days. Recurrent episodes: acyclovir 400 mg PO 3 times a day for 5 days, or 800 mg PO 2 times a day for 5 days or famciclovir 125 mg PO 2 times a day for 5 days, or valacyclovir 500 mg PO 2 times a day for 5 days Daily suppressive therapy: acyclovir 400 mg PO 2 times a day, or famciclovir 250 mg PO 2 times a day, or valacyclovir 250 mg PO 2 times a day, 500 mg PO 1 time a day, or 1000 mg PO 1 time a day

Organism	Diagnostic Methods	Recommended Treatment Regimens
Human papilloma virus	Clinical appearance of condyloma papules Cytology	External warts: Patient may apply podofilox 0.5% solution or gel 2 times a day for 3 days, followed by 4 days of no therapy, for a total of up to 4 cycles, or imiquimod 5% cream at bedtime 3 times a week for up to 16 weeks. Cryotherapy with liquid nitrogen or cryoprobe, repeat every1-2 weeks; or podophyllin, repeat weekly; or TCA 80-90%, repeat weekly; or surgical removal. Vaginal warts: cryotherapy with liquid nitrogen, or TCA 80-90%, or podophyllin 10-25%
Human immunodeficiency virus	Enzyme immunoassay Western blot (for confirmation) Polymerase chain reaction	Antiretroviral agents

Treatment of Pelvic Inflammatory Disease		
Regimen	Inpatient	Outpatient
A	Cefotetan (Cefotan) 2 g IV q12h; or cefoxitin (Mefoxin) 2 g IV q6h plus doxycycline 100 mg IV or PO q12h.	Ofloxacin (Floxin) 400 mg PO bid for 14 days plus metronidazole 500 mg PO bid for 14 days.
B	Clindamycin 900 mg IV q8h plus gentamicin loading dose IV or IM (2 mg/kg of body weight), followed by a maintenance dose (1.5 mg/kg) q8h.	Ceftriaxone (Rocephin) 250 mg IM once; or cefoxitin 2 g IM plus probenecid 1 g PO; or other parenteral third-generation cephalosporin (eg, ceftizoxime, cefotaxime) plus doxycycline 100 mg PO bid for 14 days.

I. **Chlamydia trachomatis**
   A. Chlamydia trachomatis is the most prevalent STI in the United States. Chlamydia infections are most common in women age 15-19 years.
   B. Routine screening of asymptomatic, sexually active adolescent females undergoing pelvic examination is recommended. Annual screening should be done for women age 20-24 years who are either inconsistent users of barrier contraceptives or who acquired a new sex partner or had more than one sexual partner in the past 3 months.

II. **Gonorrhea.** Gonorrhea has an incidence of 800,000 cases annually. Routine screening for gonorrhea is recommended among women at high risk of infection, including prostitutes, women with a history of repeated episodes of gonorrhea, women under age 25 years with two or more sex partners in the past year, and women with mucopurulent cervicitis.

III. **Syphilis**
   A. Syphilis has an incidence of 100,000 cases annually. The rates are highest in the South, among African Americans, and among those in the 20- to 24-year-old age group.

B. Prostitutes, persons with other STIs, and sexual contacts of persons with active syphilis should be screened.

V. Herpes simplex virus and human papillomavirus
   A. An estimated 200,000-500,000 new cases of herpes simplex occur annually in the United States. New infections are most common in adolescents and young adults.
   B. Human papillomavirus affects about 30% of young, sexually active individuals.

References, see page 268.

Vaginitis

Vaginitis is the most common gynecologic problem encountered by primary care physicians. It may result from bacterial infections, fungal infection, protozoan infection, contact dermatitis, atrophic vaginitis, or allergic reaction.

Pathophysiology
A. Vaginitis results from alterations in the vaginal ecosystem, either by the introduction of an organism or by a disturbance that allows normally present pathogens to proliferate.
B. Antibiotics may cause the overgrowth of yeast. Douching may alter the pH level or selectively suppress the growth of endogenous bacteria.

Clinical evaluation of vaginal symptoms
A. The type and extent of symptoms, such as itching, discharge, odor, or pelvic pain should be determined. A change in sexual partners or sexual activity, changes in contraception method, medications (antibiotics), and history of prior genital infections should be sought.
B. **Physical examination**
   1. Evaluation of the vagina should include close inspection of the external genitalia for excoriations, ulcerations, blisters, papillary structures, erythema, edema, mucosal thinning, or mucosal pallor.
   2. The color, texture, and odor of vaginal or cervical discharge should be noted.
C. **Vaginal fluid pH** can be determined by immersing pH paper in the vaginal discharge. A pH level greater than 4.5 often indicates the presence of bacterial vaginosis or Trichomonas vaginalis.
D. **Saline wet mount**
   1. One swab should be used to obtain a sample from the posterior vaginal fornix, obtaining a "clump" of discharge. Place the sample on a slide, add one drop of normal saline, and apply a coverslip.
   2. Coccoid bacteria and clue cells (bacteria-coated, stippled, epithelial cells) are characteristic of bacterial vaginosis.
   3. Trichomoniasis is confirmed by identification of trichomonads--mobile, oval flagellates. White blood cells are prevalent.
E. **Potassium hydroxide (KOH) preparation**
   1. Place a second sample on a slide, apply one drop of 10% potassium hydroxide (KOH) and a coverslip. A pungent, fishy odor upon addition of KOH--a positive whiff test--strongly indicates bacterial vaginosis.
   2. The KOH prep may reveal Candida in the form of thread-like hyphae and budding yeast.
F. **Screening for STDs.** Testing for gonorrhea and chlamydial infection should be

completed for women with a new sexual partner, purulent cervical discharge or cervical motion tenderness.

III. **Differential diagnosis**
   A. The most common cause of vaginitis is bacterial vaginosis, followed by Candida albicans. The prevalence of trichomoniasis has declined in recent years.
   B. Common nonvaginal etiologies include contact dermatitis from spermicidal creams, latex in condoms, or douching. Any STD can produce vaginal discharge.

Clinical Manifestations of Vaginitis	
Candidal Vaginitis	Nonmalodorous, thick, white, "cottage cheese-like" discharge that adheres to vaginal walls Presence of hyphal forms or budding yeast cells on wet-mount Pruritus Normal pH (<4.5)
Bacterial Vaginosis	Thin, dark or dull grey, homogeneous, malodorous discharge that adheres to the vaginal walls Elevated pH level (>4.5) Positive KOH (whiff test) Clue cells on wet-mount microscopic evaluation
Trichomonas Vaginalis	Copious, yellow-gray or green, homogeneous or frothy, malodorous discharge Elevated pH level (>4.5) Mobile, flagellated organisms and leukocytes on wet-mount microscopic evaluation Vulvovaginal irritation, dysuria
Atrophic Vaginitis	Vaginal dryness or burning

IV. **Bacterial Vaginosis**
   A. Bacterial vaginosis develops when a shift in the normal vaginal ecosystem causes replacement of the usually predominant lactobacilli with mixed bacterial flora. Bacterial vaginosis is the most common type of vaginitis. It is found in 10-25% of patients in gynecologic clinics.
   B. There is usually little itching, no pain, and the symptoms tend to have an indolent course. A malodorous fishy vaginal discharge is characteristic.
   C. There is usually little or no inflammation of the vulva or vaginal epithelium. The vaginal discharge is thin, dark or dull grey, and homogeneous.
   D. A wet-mount will reveal clue cells (epithelial cells stippled with bacteria), an abundance of bacteria, and the absence of homogeneous bacilli (lactobacilli).
   E. **Diagnostic criteria** (3 of 4 criterial present)
      1. pH >4.0
      2. Clue cells
      3. Positive KOH whiff test
      4. Homogeneous discharge.
   F. **Treatment regimens**
      1. **Topical (intravaginal) regimens**
         a. Metronidazole gel (MetroGel) 0.75%, one applicatorful (5 g) bid 5 days.
         b. Clindamycin cream (Cleocin) 2%, one applicatorful (5 g) qhs for 7 nights. Topical therapies have a 90% cure rate.

2. **Oral metronidazole (Flagyl)**
   a. Oral metronidazole is equally effective as topical therapy, with a 90% cure rate.
   b. Dosage is 500 mg bid or 250 mg tid for 7 days. A single 2-g dose is slightly less effective (69-72%) and causes more gastrointestinal upset. Alcohol products should be avoided because nausea and vomiting (disulfiram reaction) may occur.
3. Routine treatment of sexual partners is not necessary, but it is sometimes helpful for patients with frequent recurrences.
4. **Persistent cases** should be reevaluated and treated with clindamycin, 300 mg PO bid for 7 days along with treatment of sexual partners.
5. **Pregnancy.** Clindamycin is recommended, either intravaginally as a daily application of 2% cream or PO, 300 mg bid for 7 days. After the first trimester, oral or topical therapy with metronidazole is acceptable.

V. **Candida Vulvovaginitis**
A. Candida is the second most common diagnosis associated with vaginal symptoms. It is found in 25% of asymptomatic women. Fungal infections account for 33% of all vaginal infections.
B. Patients with diabetes mellitus or immunosuppressive conditions such as infection with the HIV are at increased risk for candidal vaginitis. Candidal vaginitis occurs in 25-70% of women after antibiotic therapy.
C. The most common symptom is pruritus. Vulvar burning and an increase or change in consistency of the vaginal discharge may be noted.
D. **Physical examination**
   1. Candidal vaginitis causes a nonmalodorous, thick, adherent, white vaginal discharge that appears "cottage cheese-like."
   2. The vagina is usually hyperemic and edematous. Vulvar erythema may be present.
E. The normal pH level is not usually altered with candidal vaginitis. Microscopic examination of vaginal discharge diluted with saline (wet-mount) and 10% KOH preparations will reveal hyphal forms or budding yeast cells. Some yeast infections are not detected by microscopy because there are relatively few numbers of organisms. Confirmation of candidal vaginitis by culture is not recommended. Candida on Pap smear is not a sensitive finding because the yeast is a constituent of the normal vaginal flora.
F. **Treatment of candida vulvovaginitis**
   1. For severe symptoms and chronic infections, a 7-day course of treatment is used, instead of a 1- or 3-day course. If vulvar involvement is present, a cream should be used instead of a suppository.
   2. Most C. albicans isolates are susceptible to either clotrimazole or miconazole. An increasing number of nonalbicans Candida species are resistant to the OTC antifungal agents and require the use of prescription antifungal agents. Greater activity has been achieved using terconazole, butoconazole, tioconazole, ketoconazole, and fluconazole.

Antifungal Medications		
Medication	**How Supplied**	**Dosage**
Prescription Agents Oral Agents		
Fluconazole (Diflucan)	150-mg tablet	1 tablet PO 1 time
Ketoconazole (Nizoral)	200 mg	1 tablet PO bid for 5 days
Prescription Topical Agents		
Butoconazole (Femstat)	2% vaginal cream [28 g]	1 vaginally applicatorful qhs for 3 nights
Clotrimazole (Gyne-Lotrimin)	500-mg tablet	1 tablet vaginally qhs 1 time
Miconazole (Monistat 3)	200-mg vaginal suppositories	1 suppository vaginally qhs for 3 nights
Tioconazole (Vagistat)	6.5% cream [5 g]	1 applicatorful vaginally qhs 1 time
Terconazole (Terazol 3)	Cream: 0.4% [45 gm]	One applicatorful intravaginally qhs x 7 days
	Cream: 0.8% [20 g]	One applicatorful intravaginally qhs x 3 days
	Vag suppository: 80 mg [3]	One suppository intravaginally qhs x 3 days
Over-the-Counter Agents		
Clotrimazole (Gyne-Lotrimin)	1% vaginal cream [45 g] 100-mg vaginal tablets	1 applicatorful vaginally qhs for 7-14 nights 1 tablet vaginally qhs for 7-14 days
Miconazole (Monistat 7)	2% cream [45 g]	1 applicatorful vaginally qhs for 7 days
	100-mg vaginal suppository	1 suppository vaginally qhs for 7 days

3. Ketoconazole, 200-mg oral tablets twice daily for 5 days, is effective treating resistant and recurrent candidal infections. Effectiveness is resul from the elimination of the rectal reservoir of yeast.
4. Resistant infections also may respond to vaginal boric acid, 600 mg in siz 0 gelatin capsules daily for 14 days.
5. Treatment of male partners is usually not necessary but may be considere if the partner has yeast balanitis or is uncircumcised.
6. **During pregnancy**, butoconazole (Femstat) should be used in the 2nd 3rd trimester. Miconazole or clotrimazole may also be used.

G. **Resistant or recurrent cases**
   1. Recurrent infections should be reevaluated. Repeating topical therapy f a 14- to 21-day course may be effective. Oral regimens have the potenti

for eradicating rectal reservoirs.

2. Cultures are helpful in determining whether a non-candidal species is present. Patients with recalcitrant disease should be evaluated for diabetes and HIV.

Trichomonas vaginalis

A. Trichomonas, a flagellated anaerobic protozoan, is a sexually transmitted disease with a high transmission rate. Non-sexual transmission is possible because the organism can survive for a few hours in a moist environment.

B. A copious, yellow-gray or green homogeneous discharge is present. A foul odor, vulvovaginal irritation, and dysuria is common. The pH level is usually greater than 4.5.

C. The diagnosis of trichomonal infection is made by examining a wet-mount preparation for mobile, flagellated organisms and an abundance of leukocytes. Occasionally the diagnosis is reported on a Pap test, and treatment is recommended.

D. **Treatment of Trichomonas vaginalis**

1. Metronidazole (Flagyl), 2 g PO in a single dose for both the patient and sexual partner, or 500 mg PO bid for 7 days.

2. Topical therapy with topical metronidazole is not recommended because the organism may persist in the urethra and Skene's glands. Screening for coexisting sexually transmitted diseases should be completed.

3. **Recurrent or recalcitrant infections**

   a. If patients are compliant but develop recurrent infections, treatment of their sexual partners should be confirmed.

   b. Cultures should be performed. In patients with persistent infection, a resistant trichomonad strain may require high dosages of metronidazole of 2.5 g/d, often combined with intravaginal metronidazole for 10 days.

Other diagnoses causing vaginal symptoms

A. One-third of patients with vaginal symptoms will not have laboratory evidence of bacterial vaginosis, Candida, or Trichomonas. Other causes of the vaginal symptoms include cervicitis, allergic reactions, and vulvodynia.

B. Atrophic vaginitis should be considered in postmenopausal patients if the mucosa appears pale and thin and wet-mount findings are negative.

1. Oral estrogen (Premarin) 0.625 mg qd should provide relief.

2. Estradiol vaginal cream 0.01% may be effective as 2-4 g daily for 1-2 weeks, then 1 g, one to three times weekly.

3. Conjugated estrogen vaginal cream (Premarin) may be effective as 2-4 g daily (3 weeks on, 1 week off) for 3-6 months.

C. **Allergy and chemical irritation**

1. Patients should be questioned about use of substances that cause allergic or chemical irritation, such as deodorant soaps, laundry detergent, vaginal contraceptives, bath oils, perfumed or dyed toilet paper, hot tub or swimming pool chemicals, and synthetic clothing.

2. Topical steroids and systemic antihistamines can help alleviate the symptoms.

*references, see page 268.

Breast Cancer Screening

Breast cancer is the most common form of cancer in women. There are 200,000 new cases of breast cancer each year, resulting in 47,000 deaths per year. The lifetime risk of breast cancer is one in eight for a woman who is age 20. For patients under age 60, the chance of being diagnosed with breast cancer is 1 in about 400 in a given year.

I. **Pathophysiology**
   A. The etiology of breast cancer remains unknown, but two breast cancer genes have been cloned–the BRCA-1 and the BRCA-2 genes. Only 10% of all of the breast cancers can be explained by mutations in these genes.
   B. Estrogen stimulation is an important promoter of breast cancer, and, therefore, patients who have a long history of menstruation are at increased risk. Early menarche and late menopause are risk factors for breast cancer. Late age at birth of first child or nulliparity also increase the risk of breast cancer.
   C. Family history of breast cancer in a first degree relative and history of benign breast disease also increase the risk of breast cancer. The use of estrogen replacement therapy or oral contraceptives slightly increases the risk of breast cancer. Radiation exposure and alcoholic beverage consumption also increase the risk of breast cancer.

Recommended Intervals for Breast Cancer Screening Studies			
	Age <40 yr	**40-49 yr**	**50-75 yr**
Breast Self-Examination	Monthly by age 30	Monthly	Monthly
Professional Breast Examination	Every 3 yr, ages 20-39	Annually	Annually
Mammography, Low Risk Patient		Annually	Annually
Mammography, High Risk Patient	Begin at 35 yr	Annually	Annually

II. **Diagnosis and evaluation**
   A. **Clinical evaluation of a breast mass** should assess duration of the lesion, associated pain, relationship to the menstrual cycle or exogenous hormone use, and change in size since discovery. The presence of nipple discharge and its character (bloody or tea-colored, unilateral or bilateral, spontaneous or expressed) should be assessed.
   B. **Menstrual history.** The date of last menstrual period, age of menarche, age of menopause or surgical removal of the ovaries, regularity of the menstrual cycle, previous pregnancies, age at first pregnancy, and lactation history should be determined.
   C. **History of previous breast biopsies,** breast cancer, or cyst aspiration should be investigated. Previous or current oral contraceptive and hormone replacement therapy and dates and results of previous mammograms should be ascertained.
   D. **Family history** should document breast cancer in relatives and the age at which family members were diagnosed.

III. Physical examination

A. The breasts should be inspected for asymmetry, deformity, skin retraction, erythema, peau d'orange (indicating breast edema), and nipple retraction, discoloration, or inversion.

B. Palpation

1. The breasts should be palpated while the patient is sitting and then supine with the ipsilateral arm extended. The entire breast should be palpated systematically.
2. The mass should be evaluated for size, shape, texture, tenderness, fixation to skin or chest wall. The location of the mass should be documented with a diagram in the patient's chart. The nipples should be expressed to determine whether discharge can be induced. Nipple discharge should be evaluated for single or multiple ducts, color, and any associated mass.
3. The axillae should be palpated for adenopathy, with an assessment of size of the lymph nodes, their number, and fixation. The supraclavicular and cervical nodes should also be assessed.

IV. Breast imaging

A. Mammography

1. **Screening mammography** is performed in the asymptomatic patients and consists of two views. Patients are not examined by a mammographer. Screening mammography reduces mortality from breast cancer and should usually be initiated at age 40.
2. **Diagnostic mammography** is performed after a breast mass has been detected. Patients usually are examined by a mammographer, and films are interpreted immediately and additional views of the lesion are completed. Mammographic findings predictive of malignancy include spiculated masses with architectural distortion and microcalcifications. A normal mammography in the presence of a palpable mass does not exclude malignancy.

B. Ultrasonography is used as an adjunct to mammography to differentiate solid from cystic masses. It is the primary imaging modality in patients younger than 30 years old.

V. Methods of breast biopsy

A. Stereotactic core needle biopsy. Using a computer-driven stereotactic unit, the lesion is localized in three dimensions, and an automated biopsy needle obtains samples. The sensitivity and specificity of this technique are 95-100% and 94-98%, respectively.

B. Palpable masses. Fine-needle aspiration biopsy (FNAB) has a sensitivity ranging from 90-98%. Nondiagnostic aspirates require surgical biopsy.

1. The skin is prepped with alcohol and the lesion is immobilized with the nonoperating hand. A 10 mL syringe, with a 18 to 22 gauge needle, is introduced in to the central portion of the mass at a 90° angle. When the needle enters the mass, suction is applied by retracting the plunger, and the needle is advanced. The needle is directed into different areas of the mass while maintaining suction on the syringe.
2. Suction is slowly released before the needle is withdrawn from the mass. The contents of the needle are placed onto glass slides for pathologic examination.

C. Impalpable lesions

1. **Needle localized biopsy**
   a. Under mammographic guidance, a needle and hookwire are placed into the breast parenchyma adjacent to the lesion. The patient is taken to the operating room along with mammograms for an excisional breast biopsy.
   b. The skin and underlying tissues are infiltrated with 1% lidocaine with

epinephrine. For lesions located within 5 cm of the nipple, a periareolar incision may be used or use a curved incision located over the mass and parallel to the areola. Incise the skin and subcutaneous fat, then palpate the lesion and excise the mass.

c. After removal of the specimen, a specimen x-ray is performed to confirm that the lesion has been removed. The specimen can then be sent fresh for pathologic analysis.

d. Close the subcutaneous tissues with a 4-0 chromic catgut suture, and close the skin with 4-0 subcuticular suture.

References, see page 268.

Amenorrhea

Amenorrhea may be associated with infertility, endometrial hyperplasia, or osteopenia. It may be the presenting sign of an underlying metabolic, endocrine, congenital, or gynecologic disorder.

I. **Pathophysiology of amenorrhea**
  A. Amenorrhea may be caused by failure of the hypothalamic-pituitary-gonadal axis, by absence of end organs, or by obstruction of the outflow tract.
  B. **Menses** usually occur at intervals of 28 days, with a normal range of 18-40 days.
  C. **Amenorrhea** is defined as the absence of menstruation for 3 or more months in a women with past menses (secondary amenorrhea) or by the absence of menarche by age 16 in girls who have never menstruated (primary amenorrhea). Pregnancy is the most common cause of amenorrhea.

II. **Clinical evaluation of amenorrhea**
  A. **Menstrual history** should include the age of menarche, last menstrual period, and previous menstrual pattern. Diet, medications, and psychologic stress should be assessed.
  B. **Galactorrhea**, previous radiation therapy, chemotherapy, or recent weight gain or loss may provide important clues.
  C. **Prolonged, intense exercise**, often associated with dieting, can lead to amenorrhea. Symptoms of decreased estrogen include hot flushes and night sweats.
  D. **Physical examination**
    1. **Breast development and pubic hair distribution** should be assessed because they demonstrate exposure to estrogens and sexual maturity. Galactorrhea is a sign of hyperprolactinemia.
    2. **Thyroid gland** should be palpated for enlargement and nodules. Abdominal striae in a nulliparous woman suggests hypercortisolism (Cushing's syndrome).
    3. **Hair distribution** may reveal signs of androgen excess. The absence of both axillary and pubic hair in a phenotypically normal female suggests androgen insensitivity.
    4. **External genitalia and vagina** should be inspected for atrophy from estrogen deficiency or clitoromegaly from androgen excess. An imperforate hymen or vaginal septum can block the outflow tract.
    5. **Palpation of the uterus and ovaries** assures their presence and detects abnormalities.

III. Diagnostic approach to amenorrhea

A. Menstrual flow requires an intact hypothalamic-pituitary-ovarian axis, a hormonally responsive uterus, and an intact outflow tract. The evaluation should localize the abnormality to either the uterus, ovary, anterior pituitary, or hypothalamus.

B. **Step one--exclude pregnancy.** Pregnancy is the most common cause of secondary amenorrhea, and it must be excluded with a pregnancy test.

C. **Step two--exclude hyperthyroidism and hyperprolactinemia**

1. **Hypothyroidism and hyperprolactinemia** can cause amenorrhea. These disorders are excluded with a serum thyroid-stimulating hormone (TSH) and prolactin.

2. **Hyperprolactinemia.** Prolactin inhibits the secretion of gonadotropin-releasing hormone. One-third of women with no obvious cause of amenorrhea have hyperprolactinemia. Mildly elevated prolactin levels should be confirmed by repeat testing and review the patient's medications. Hyperprolactinemia requires an MRI to exclude a pituitary tumor.

Drugs Associated with Amenorrhea	
Drugs that Increase Prolactin	Antipsychotics Tricyclic antidepressants Calcium channel blockers
Drugs with Estrogenic Activity	Digoxin, marijuana, oral contraceptives
Drugs with Ovarian Toxicity	Chemotherapeutic agents

D. **Step three--assess estrogen status**

1. **The progesterone challenge test** is used to determine estrogen status and determine the competence of the uterine outflow tract.

2. Medroxyprogesterone (Provera) 10 mg is given PO qd for 10 consecutive days. Uterine bleeding within 2-7 days after completion is considered a positive test. A positive result suggests chronic anovulation, rather than hypothalamic-pituitary insufficiency or ovarian failure, and a positive test also confirms the presence of a competent outflow tract.

3. A negative test indicates either an incompetent outflow tract, nonreactive endometrium, or inadequate estrogen stimulation.

   a. An abnormality of the outflow tract should be excluded with a regimen of conjugated estrogens (Premarin), 1.25 mg daily on days 1 through 21 of the cycle. Medroxyprogesterone (Provera) 10 mg is given on the last 5 days of the 21-day cycle. (A combination oral contraceptive agent can also be used.)

   b. Withdrawal bleeding within 2-7 days of the last dose of progesterone confirms the presence of an unobstructed outflow tract and a normal endometrium, and the problem is localized to the hypothalamic-pituitary axis or ovaries.

4. In patients who have had prolonged amenorrhea, an endometrial biopsy should be considered before withdrawal bleeding is induced. Biopsy can reveal endometrial hyperplasia.

E. **Step four--evaluation of hypoestrogenic amenorrhea**

1. Serum follicle-stimulating hormone (FSH) and luteinizing hormone (LH) levels should be measured to localize the problem to the ovary, pituitary or

hypothalamus.
2. **Ovarian failure**
   a. An FSH level greater than 50 mIU/mL indicates ovarian failure.
   b. Ovarian failure is considered "premature" when it occurs in women less than 40 years of age.
3. **Pituitary or hypothalamic dysfunction**
   a. A normal or low gonadotropin level is indicative of pituitary or hypothalamic failure. An MRI is the most sensitive study to rule out a pituitary tumor.
   b. If MRI does not reveal a tumor, a defect in pulsatile GnRH release from the hypothalamus is the probable cause.

IV. Management of chronic anovulation
A. Adequate estrogen and anovulation is indicated by withdrawal bleeding with the progesterone challenge test.
B. Often there is a history of weight loss, psychosocial stress, or excessive exercise. Women usually have a normal or low body weight and normal secondary sex characteristics.
   1. Reducing stress and assuring adequate nutrition may induce ovulation. These women are at increased risk for endometrial cancer because of the hyperplastic effect of unopposed estrogen.
   2. Progesterone (10 mg/day for the first 7-10 days of every month) is given to induce withdrawal bleeding. If contraception is desired, a low-dose oral contraceptive should be used.

V. Management of hypothalamic dysfunction
A. Amenorrheic women with a normal prolactin level, a negative progesterone challenge, with low or normal gonadotropin levels, and with a normal sella turcica imaging are considered to have hypothalamic dysfunction.
B. Hypothalamic amenorrhea usually results from psychologic stress, depression, severe weight loss, anorexia nervosa, or strenuous exercise.
C. Hypoestrogenic women are at risk for osteoporosis and cardiovascular disease. Oral contraceptives are appropriate in young women. Women not desiring contraception should take estrogen, 0.625 mg, with medroxyprogesterone (Provera) 2.5 mg, every day of the month. Calcium and vitamin D supplementation are also recommended.

VI. Management of disorders of the outflow tract or uterus--intrauterine adhesions (Asherman syndrome)
A. Asherman syndrome is the most common outflow-tract abnormality that causes amenorrhea. This disorder should be considered if amenorrhea develops following curettage or endometritis.
B. Hysterosalpingography will detect adhesions. Therapy consists of hysteroscopy and lysis of adhesions.

VII. Management of disorders of the ovaries
A. Ovarian failure is suspected if menopausal symptoms are present. Women with premature ovarian failure who are less than 30 years of age should undergo karyotyping to rule out the presence of a Y chromosome. If a Y chromosome is detected, testicular tissue should be removed.
B. Patients with ovarian failure should be prescribed estrogen 0.625 mg with progesterone 2.5 mg daily with calcium and vitamin D.

VIII. Disorders of the anterior pituitary
A. Prolactin-secreting adenoma are excluded by MRI of the pituitary.
B. Cabergoline (Dostinex) or bromocriptine (Parlodel) are used for most adenomas;

surgery is considered later.

References, see page 268.

Abnormal Vaginal Bleeding

Menorrhagia (excessive bleeding) is most commonly caused by anovulatory menstrual cycles. Occasionally it is caused by thyroid dysfunction, infections or cancer.

I. Pathophysiology of normal menstruation
   A. In response to gonadotropin-releasing hormone from the hypothalamus, the pituitary gland synthesizes follicle-stimulating hormone (FSH) and luteinizing hormone (LH), which induce the ovaries to produce estrogen and progesterone.
   B. During the follicular phase, estrogen stimulation causes an increase in endometrial thickness. After ovulation, progesterone causes endometrial maturation. Menstruation is caused by estrogen and progesterone withdrawal.
   C. Abnormal bleeding is defined as bleeding that occurs at intervals of less than 21 days, more than 36 days, lasting longer than 7 days, or blood loss greater than 80 mL.

II. Clinical evaluation of abnormal vaginal bleeding
   A. A menstrual and reproductive history should include last menstrual period, regularity, duration, frequency; the number of pads used per day, and intermenstrual bleeding.
   B. Stress, exercise, weight changes and systemic diseases, particularly thyroid, renal or hepatic diseases or coagulopathies, should be sought. The method of birth control should be determined.
   C. Pregnancy complications, such as spontaneous abortion, ectopic pregnancy, placenta previa and abruptio placentae, can cause heavy bleeding. Pregnancy should always be considered as a possible cause of abnormal vaginal bleeding.

III. Puberty and adolescence--menarche to age 16
   A. Irregularity is normal during the first few months of menstruation; however, soaking more than 25 pads or 30 tampons during a menstrual period is abnormal.
   B. Absence of premenstrual symptoms (breast tenderness, bloating, cramping) is associated with anovulatory cycles.
   C. Fever, particularly in association with pelvic or abdominal pain may, indicate pelvic inflammatory disease. A history of easy bruising suggests a coagulation defect. Headaches and visual changes suggest a pituitary tumor.
   D. Physical findings
      1. Pallor not associated with tachycardia or signs of hypovolemia suggests chronic excessive blood loss secondary to anovulatory bleeding, adenomyosis, uterine myomas, or blood dyscrasia.
      2. Fever, leukocytosis, and pelvic tenderness suggests PID.
      3. Signs of impending shock indicate that the blood loss is related to pregnancy (including ectopic), trauma, sepsis, or neoplasia.
      4. Pelvic masses may represent pregnancy, uterine or ovarian neoplasia, or a pelvic abscess or hematoma.
      5. Fine, thinning hair, and hypoactive reflexes suggest hypothyroidism.
      6. Ecchymoses or multiple bruises may indicate trauma, coagulation defects, medication use, or dietary extremes.

E. Laboratory tests

1. CBC and platelet count and a urine or serum pregnancy test should be obtained.
2. Screening for sexually transmitted diseases, thyroid function, and coagulation disorders (partial thromboplastin time, INR, bleeding time) should be completed.
3. **Endometrial sampling** is rarely necessary for those under age 20.

F. Treatment of infrequent bleeding

1. Therapy should be directed at the underlying cause when possible. If the CBC and other initial laboratory tests are normal and the history and physical examination are normal, reassurance is usually all that is necessary.
2. Ferrous gluconate, 325 mg bid-tid, should be prescribed.

G. Treatment of frequent or heavy bleeding

1. Treatment with nonsteroidal anti-inflammatory drugs (NSAIDs) improves platelet aggregation and increases uterine vasoconstriction. NSAIDs are the first choice in the treatment of menorrhagia because they are well tolerated and do not have the hormonal effects of oral contraceptives.
   a. Mefenamic acid (Ponstel) 500 mg tid during the menstrual period.
   b. Naproxen (Anaprox, Naprosyn) 500 mg loading dose, then 250 mg tid during the menstrual period.
   c. Ibuprofen (Motrin, Nuprin) 400 mg tid during the menstrual period.
   d. Gastrointestinal distress is common. NSAIDs are contraindicated in renal failure and peptic ulcer disease.
2. Iron should also be added as ferrous gluconate 325 mg tid.

H. Patients with hypovolemia or a hemoglobin level below 7 g/dL should be hospitalized for hormonal therapy and iron replacement.

1. Hormonal therapy consists of estrogen (Premarin) 25 mg IV q6h until bleeding stops. Thereafter, oral contraceptive pills should be administered q6h x 7 days, then taper slowly to one pill qd.
2. If bleeding continues, IV vasopressin (DDAVP) should be administered. Hysteroscopy may be necessary, and dilation and curettage is a last resort. Transfusion may be indicated in severe hemorrhage.
3. Iron should also be added as ferrous gluconate 325 mg tid.

IV. Primary childbearing years--ages 16 to early 40s

A. Contraceptive complications and pregnancy are the most common causes of abnormal bleeding in this age group. Anovulation accounts for 20% of cases.

B. Adenomyosis, endometriosis, and fibroids increase in frequency as a woman ages, as do endometrial hyperplasia and endometrial polyps. Pelvic inflammatory disease and endocrine dysfunction may also occur.

C. Laboratory tests

1. CBC and platelet count, Pap smear, and pregnancy test.
2. Screening for sexually transmitted diseases, thyroid-stimulating hormone, and coagulation disorders (partial thromboplastin time, INR, bleeding time).
3. If a non-pregnant woman has a pelvic mass, ultrasonography or hysterosonography (with uterine saline infusion) is required.

D. Endometrial sampling

1. Long-term unopposed estrogen stimulation in anovulatory patients can result in endometrial hyperplasia, which can progress to adenocarcinoma; therefore in perimenopausal patients who have been anovulatory for an extended interval, the endometrium should be biopsied.
2. Biopsy is also recommended before initiation of hormonal therapy for women over age 30 and for those over age 20 who have had prolonged bleeding.
3. Hysteroscopy and endometrial biopsy with a Pipelle aspirator should be done

on the first day of menstruation (to avoid an unexpected pregnancy) or any-time if bleeding is continuous.

E. Treatment

1. Medical protocols for anovulatory bleeding (dysfunctional uterine bleeding) are similar to those described above for adolescents.

2. **Hormonal therapy**

   a. In women who do not desire immediate fertility, hormonal therapy may be used to treat menorrhagia.

   b. A 21-day package of oral contraceptives is used. The patient should take one pill three times a day for 7 days. During the 7 days of therapy, bleeding should subside, and, following treatment, heavy flow will occur. After 7 days off the hormones, another 21-day package is initiated, taking one pill each day for 21 days, then no pills for 7 days.

   c. Alternatively, medroxyprogesterone (Provera), 10-20 mg per day for days 16 through 25 of each month, will result in a reduction of menstrual blood loss. Pregnancy will not be prevented.

   d. Patients with severe bleeding may have hypotension and tachycardia. These patients require hospitalization, and estrogen (Premarin) should be administered IV as 25 mg q4-6h until bleeding slows (up to a maximum of four doses). Oral contraceptives should be initiated concurrently as described above.

3. Iron should also be added as ferrous gluconate 325 mg tid.

4. Surgical treatment can be considered if childbearing is completed and medical management fails to provide relief.

V. Premenopausal, perimenopausal, and postmenopausal years--age 40 and over

A. Anovulatory bleeding accounts for about 90% of abnormal vaginal bleeding in this age group. However, bleeding should be considered to be from cancer until proven otherwise.

B. History, physical examination and laboratory testing are indicated as described above. Menopausal symptoms, personal or family history of malignancy and use of estrogen should be sought. A pelvic mass requires an evaluation with ultrasonography.

C. Endometrial carcinoma

1. In a perimenopausal or postmenopausal woman, amenorrhea preceding abnormal bleeding suggests endometrial cancer. Endometrial evaluation is necessary before treatment of abnormal vaginal bleeding.

2. Before endometrial sampling, determination of endometrial thickness by transvaginal ultrasonography is useful because biopsy is often not required when the endometrium is less than 5 mm thick.

D. Treatment

1. Cystic hyperplasia or endometrial hyperplasia without cytologic atypia is treated with depo-medroxyprogesterone, 200 mg IM, then 100 to 200 mg IM every 3 to 4 weeks for 6 to 12 months. Endometrial hyperplasia requires repeat endometrial biopsy every 3 to 6 months.

2. Atypical hyperplasia requires fractional dilation and curettage, followed by progestin therapy or hysterectomy.

3. If the patient's endometrium is normal (or atrophic) and contraception is a concern, a low-dose oral contraceptive may be used. If contraception is not needed, estrogen and progesterone therapy should be prescribed.

4. **Surgical management**

   a. **Vaginal or abdominal hysterectomy** is the most absolute curative treatment.

   b. **Dilatation and curettage** can be used as a temporizing measure to stop

bleeding.
  c. Endometrial ablation and resection by laser, electrodiathermy "rollerball," or excisional resection are alternatives to hysterectomy.

References, see page 268.

Menopause

The average age of menopause is 51 years, with a range of 41-55. Menopause occurs before age 40 in about 5% of women. An elevated follicle-stimulating hormone (FSH) level greater than 40 mIU/mL.

I. **Pharmacologic therapy for symptoms of menopause**
  A. **Vasomotor instability.** A hot flush is a flushed or blushed feeling of the face, neck and upper chest. The most severe hot flushes usually occur at night. Estrogen therapy can reduce hot flushes.
  B. **Psychologic symptoms.** Mood swings, depression and concentration difficulties are associated with menopause. Estrogen improves mood or dysphoria associated with menopause.
  C. **Urogenital symptoms.** Declining estrogen levels lead to atrophy of the urogenital tissues and vaginal thinning and shortening, resulting in dyspareunia and urethral irritation. Urinary tract infections and urinary incontinence may develop. Estrogen treatment (oral or intravaginal) reduces these problems
II. **Pharmacologic management of long-term risks**
  A. **Coronary artery disease**. Physiologic effects of estrogen, such as arterial vasodilatation, increased high-density lipoprotein (HDL) cholesterol levels and decreased low-density lipoprotein (LDL) cholesterol levels, are likely to reduce cardiovascular risk.
  B. **Osteoporosis**. More than 250,000 hip fractures occur annually. Estrogen deficiency is the primary cause of osteoporosis, although many other secondary causes for osteoporosis exist (eg, poor diet, glucocorticoid excess). Thus, women at risk for osteoporosis should be considered candidates for HRT.

Minimum Effective Dosages of Estrogens for Prevention of Osteoporosis	
Formulation	**Minimum effective dosage**
Conjugated estrogen Premarin (0.3, 0.625, 0.9, 1.25, 2.5 mg)	0.625 mg
Micronized estradiol Estrace (0.5, 1.0, 2.0 mg)	1.0 mg

Esterified estrogen
    Estratab (0.3, 0.625, 2.5 mg)
    Menest (0.3, 0.625, 1.25, 2.5 mg)
	0.625 mg

Estropipate
    Ogen (0.625, 1.25, 2.5 mg)
    Ortho-Est (0.625, 1.25 mg)
	1.25 mg

Transdermal estradiol
    Climara (0.05, 0.1 mg)
    Estraderm (0.05, 0.1 mg)
	0.05 mg

Combination preparations	
Combipatch	0.05 mg estradiol/0.14 mg norethindrone
Estratest	1.25 mg esterified estrogen/2.5 mg methyltestosterone
Estratest HS	0.625 mg esterified estrogen/1.25 mg methyltestosterone
Premphase	0.625 mg conjugated estrogen (14 tablets) and 0.625 mg conjugated estrogen/5 mg medroxyprogesterone (14 tablets in sequence)
Prempro	0.625 mg conjugated estrogen/2.5 mg or 5.0 mg medroxyprogesterone. Take one tab daily.
Vaginal preparations	
Micronized estradiol cream (Estrace)	0.01% or 0.1 mg per g (42.5 g/tube)
Estropipate cream (Ogen)	1.5 mg per g (42.5 g/tube)
Conjugated estrogen cream (Premarin)	0.625 mg per g (42.5 g/tube)
Estradiol vaginal ring (Estring)	7.5 µg per 24 hours every 90 days

III. **Hormone replacement therapy administration and regimens**
   A. The benefits of HRT in reducing the risks of hip fracture outweigh the risk of breast cancer in nearly all women. However, long-term HRT is not recommended for women at high risk for breast cancer.
   B. Effective doses of estrogen for the prevention of osteoporosis are: 0.625 mg of conjugated estrogen, 0.5 mg of micronized estradiol, and 0.3 mg of esterified estrogen.
   C. In those women with a uterus, a progestin should be given continuously (2.5 mg of medroxyprogesterone per day) or in a sequential fashion (5-10 mg of medroxyprogesterone (Provera) for 12-14 days each month). The most common HRT regimen consists of estrogen with or without progestin. The oral route of administration is preferable because of the hepatic effect on HDL cholesterol levels.

Relative and Absolute Contraindications for Hormone Replacement Therapy

Absolute contraindications	**Relative contraindications**
Estrogen-responsive breast cancer	Chronic liver disease
Endometrial cancer	Severe hypertriglyceridemia
Undiagnosed abnormal vaginal bleeding	Endometriosis
Active thromboembolic disease	Previous thromboembolic disease
History of malignant melanoma	Gallbladder disease

    D. Estrogen cream. 1/4 of an applicator(0.6 mg) daily for 1-2 weeks, then 2-3 times/week will usually relieve urogenital symptoms. This regimen is used concomitantly with oral estrogen.

    E. Adverse effects attributed to HRT include breast tenderness, breakthrough bleeding and thromboembolic disorders.

    F. Bisphosphonates inhibit osteoclast activity. Alendronate (Fosamax) is effective in increasing BMD and reducing fractures by 40 percent. To prevent esophagitis, alendronate should be taken in an upright position with a full glass of water 30 minutes before eating. Alendronate is indicated for osteoporosis in women who have a contraindication to estrogen.

    G. Raloxifene (Evista), a selective estrogen receptor modulator has been FDA-labeled for prophylactic treatment of osteoporosis. This agent offers an alternative to traditional HRT. The modulator increases bone density (although only one-half as effectively as estrogen) and reduces total and LDL cholesterol levels.

IV. Complementary therapies

    A. Adequate dietary calcium intake is essential, and supplementation is helpful if dietary sources are inadequate. Total calcium intake should approximate 1,500 mg per day, which usually requires supplementation.

    B. Vitamin D supplementation (400 to 800 IU per day) is recommended for women who do not spend 30 minutes per day in the sun.

    C. Treatment of low libido consists of micronized testosterone cream (1 mg/mL) applied to the inner surface of both forearms daily. Start with 1 mg/day and increase to 2.5 mg/day if necessary. Androgens are known to increase libido and protect bone mass.

References, see page 268.

Urologic Disorders

Erectile Dysfunction

Erectile dysfunction is defined as the persistent inability to achieve or maintain penile erection sufficient for sexual intercourse. Between the ages of 40 and 70 years, the probability of complete erectile dysfunction triples from 5.1 percent to 15 percent.

I. **Physiology of erection**
   A. Penile erection is mediated by the parasympathetic nervous system, which when stimulated causes arterial dilation and relaxation of the cavernosal smooth muscle. The increased blood flow into the corpora cavernosa in association with reduced venous outflow results in penile rigidity.
   B. Nitric oxide is a chemical mediator of erection. This substance is released from nerve endings and vascular endothelium, causing smooth muscle relaxation, resulting in venous engorgement and penile tumescence.

Causes of Erectile Dysfunction and Diagnostic Clues			
Cause	History	Physical Examination	Possible laboratory findings
Vascular	Coronary artery disease; hypertension; claudication; dyslipidemia; smoking	Decreased pulses; bruits; elevated blood pressure; cool extremities	Abnormal lipid profile Abnormal penile-brachial pressure index
Diabetes mellitus	Diabetes; polyuria; polydipsia; polyphagia	Peripheral neuropathy; retinopathy; obesity	Abnormal fasting blood glucose Elevated glycosylated hemoglobin Proteinuria Glycosuria Hypertriglyceridemia
Hypogonadism	Decreased libido; fatigue	Bilateral testicular atrophy; scant body hair; gynecomastia	Decreased free testosterone Increased LH Increased FSH
Hyperprolactinemia	Decreased libido; galactorrhea; visual complaints; headache	Bitemporal hemianopsia	Elevated prolactin Abnormal CT or MRI scans of pituitary gland
Hypothyroidism	Fatigue; cold intolerance	Goiter; myxedema; dry skin; coarse hair	Increased TSH Decreased free T_4
Hyperthyroidism	Heat intolerance; weight loss; diaphoresis; palpitations	Lid lag; exophthalmos; hyperreflexia; tremor; tachycardia	Decreased TSH Increased free T_4

Cause	History	Physical Examination	Possible laboratory findings
Cushing's syndrome	Easy bruising; weight gain; corticosteroid use	Truncal obesity; "moon face"; "buffalo hump"; striae	Elevated overnight dexamethasone suppression test
Alcoholism	Excessive alcohol use; social, economic or occupational consequences of alcohol abuse; withdrawal symptoms	Positive screen; thin body habitus; palmar erythema; spider telangiectasias; gynecomastia; tremor	Abnormal hepatic transaminases Decreased albumin Macrocytic anemia
Neurologic	Spinal cord injury; nerve injury (prostate surgery); stroke; peripheral neuropathy; incontinence; multiple sclerosis; Parkinson's disease	Motor or sensory deficits; aphasia; gait abnormality; abnormal bulbocavernosus reflex; tremor	
Mechanical	Genital trauma or surgery; Peyronie's disease; congenital abnormalities	Fibrous penile plaques or chordae	None
Psychogenic	Nocturnal erections; sudden onset; history of depression; anhedonia; poor relationship with partner; anxiety; life crisis	Sad or withdrawn affect; tearful; psychomotor retardation; depression	Nocturnal penile tumescence (stamp test; Snap-Gauge)
Pharmacologic	Inquire about all prescription and nonprescription drugs		

II. History and physical examination

A. The history should include the frequency and duration of symptoms, the presence or absence of morning erections, and the quality of the relationship with the sexual partner. The sudden onset of erectile dysfunction in association with normal morning erections or a poor relationship suggests psychogenic impotence. Chronic disease such as atherosclerosis, hypertension or diabetes mellitus should be sought. Decreased libido and symptoms of hypothyroidism should be evaluated.

B. Common pharmacologic causes of erectile dysfunction include antihypertensive drugs, most notably the centrally acting agents, beta-blockers and diuretics. Antipsychotic and antidepressant drugs are also frequently implicated. Excessive alcohol intake, heroin use and cigarette smoking are common causes.

C. **Physical examination.** Signs of hypogonadism, such as gynecomastia or the loss of axillary and pubic hair, should be noted. The size and consistency of the testes should be noted. The penis should be examined for fibrosis and plaques indicative of Peyronie's disease. The bulbocavernosus and cremasteric reflexes should be assessed. The bulbocavernosus reflex is elicited by squeezing the glans penis while observing for contraction of the external anal sphincter.

Agents That May Cause Erectile Dysfunction	

Antidepressants
  Monoamine oxidase inhibitors
  Selective serotonin reuptake
  inhibitors
  Tricyclic antidepressants
Antihypertensives
  Beta blockers
  Centrally acting alpha agonists
  Diuretics
Antipsychotics
Anxiolytics
	Miscellaneous
	  Cimetidine (Tagamet)
	  Corticosteroids
	  Finasteride (Proscar)
	  Gemfibrozil (Lopid)
	Drugs of abuse
	  Alcohol
	  Anabolic steroids
	  Heroin
	  Marijuana

I. Laboratory tests

A. A urinalysis, complete blood count and basic chemistry panel will help to rule out most metabolic and renal diseases. In elderly men, thyroid-stimulating hormone level should be measured to rule out thyroid dysfunction. A free testosterone level should be obtained in all men aged 50 and older and in those younger than 50 who have symptoms or signs of hypogonadism (eg, decreased libido, testicular atrophy, reduced amount of body hair).

B. The prolactin level should be measured if the free testosterone level is low, the patient has a substantial loss of libido, or if a prolactinoma is suspected on the basis of a history of headache with visual field cuts. Luteinizing hormone level is reserved for use in distinguishing primary from secondary hypogonadism in men with low testosterone levels.

J. Treatment strategies

Newer Pharmacologic Agents for Erectile Dysfunction				
Drug	Efficacy	Ease of use	Side effects	Comment
Intracavernosal alprostadil (Caverject)	Significantly greater than placebo	Injected into penis	Penile pain; hematoma; priapism	Method of delivery may limit compliance
Transurethral alprostadil (MUSE)	Significantly greater than placebo	Inserted into urethra doses of 500 µg	Penile pain	Method of delivery may limit compliance
Sildenafil (Viagra)	Significantly greater than placebo	Taken orally one hour before anticipated intercourse	Headache; flushing; dyspepsia	Avoid use with nitrates

A. **Transurethral alprostadil** provides the same significant improvement in erectile function as injectable alprostadil with a better tolerated method of delivery. Successful and satisfactory intercourse occurs in 65%. The most common reported side effect is penile pain. Dosage is initially 125 to 250 µg, with adjustment up or down as indicated. Few patients respond to less than 500 mg. The drug is available in 125-, 250-, 500- and 1,000-µg suppositories. Transurethral alprostadil should not be used during sexual intercourse with a pregnant woman.

B. **Sildenafil (Viagra)** inhibits the conversion of cGMP to guanosine monophosphate in the corpus cavernosum. Sildenafil is effective in men with erectile dysfunction of organic, psychogenic or combined causes.

   1. The most common side effects of sildenafil are headache, flushing and dyspepsia. A small percentage of patients report an alteration in color perception.
   2. Sildenafil is contraindicated in patients taking nitrates because of the potential for sudden severe hypotension.
   3. Erection appropriate for intercourse is attained in 72% of the men receiving 25 mg, 80 percent of those receiving 50 mg, and 85 percent of men those given 100 mg of sildenafil.
   4. Sildenafil should initially be prescribed at 50 mg to be taken one hour before anticipated intercourse. The dose can be increased to 100 mg if needed. Sildenafil should not be used more than once a day.

Side Effects of Sildenafil (Viagra)		
Side effect	Placebo (%)	Sildenafil, 50 mg (%)
Headache	6	21
Flushing	1	27
Dyspepsia	1	11
Rhinitis	2	3
Change in perception of color	<1	6

C. **Intracavernosal alprostadil (Caverject)** has success rates of 67 to 85 percent. When injected directly into the corpus cavernosum, alprostadil (prostaglandin E_1) produces an erection within several minutes. The usual dose is between 5 and 40 µg per injection. Patients usually start at 2.5 µg and titrate up in 5-µg increments for effect, with a maximum dose of 60 µg.

D. **Testosterone cypionate** (200 mg IM q 2 weeks) or testosterone patches may be beneficial if the serum-free testosterone is low (<9 ng/dL). Older males (>50 years) are at risk for development of prostate cancer. A careful rectal examination and PSA testing is recommended prior to institution of, and during testosterone therapy.

E. **Vacuum constriction devices (VCD)** are an effective treatment alternative for erectile dysfunction. The design involves a plastic cylinder that is placed on the penis with negative pressure created. A constriction band is placed at the base of the penis. Almost every patient can be a candidate for these devices. Contraindications include penile angulation deformity, prior history of priapism, and anticoagulants.

F. **Surgical treatment** of erectile dysfunction consists of placement of a penile prosthesis. Devices available include semirigid or inflatable prostheses. An occasionally indicated treatment option is vascular surgery.

References, see page 268.

Benign Prostatic Hyperplasia

I. **Clinical evaluation**
A. Between the ages of 70 and 79, the 4-year risk of urinary retention in men with BPH is about 8.7%. Other significant sequelae of BPH include detrusor instability, infection, stone formation, bladder diverticula, and upper tract dilation with renal insufficiency. As many as 7% of men with acute urinary retention subsequently have myotonic bladder, which often requires intermittent catheterization.

B. **Obstructive symptoms**, such as nocturia, a slow urine stream, intermittency, and double voiding, are generally evaluated through focused history taking, and a digital rectal examination, with or without serum PSA testing.

C. **Symptoms of BPH** may be obstructive, which are secondary to bladder outlet obstruction or impaired bladder contractility, or irritative, which result from decreased vesicle compliance and increased bladder instability. Obstructive symptoms include a weak stream, hesitancy (prolonged time between the attempt to urinate and actual urinary flow), abdominal straining, terminal dribbling, an intermittent stream, and retention; irritative symptoms are frequency, nocturia, urgency, and pain during urination.

D. **Irritative symptoms**, such as dysuria, strangury, and hematuria, require cystoscopic examination to exclude bladder cancer, stone formation, carcinoma in situ, and interstitial cystitis.

E. **Physical examination** should include a digital rectal examination, looking for any palpable nodules and induration or irregularities, and a focused neurologic examination to rule out a neurologic cause of symptoms.

F. **Laboratory assessment.** Urinalysis and a serum creatinine assay are useful to ascertain there is no infection, hematuria, or decreased renal function. Measurement of PSA to detect prostate cancer is optional.

. **Medical treatment options for BPH**
A. Watchful waiting is a valid course of action for men who are relatively less symptomatic. If the patient has moderate or severe symptoms, however, medical therapy may include alpha-adrenergic receptor blockers and 5-alpha-reductase inhibitors.

B. Alpha-adrenergic receptor blockers, including doxazosin (Cardura), prazosin (Minipress), and terazosin (Hytrin), inhibit alpha-adrenergic-mediated contraction of smooth muscle in the prostate. They rapidly improve symptoms by reducing smooth muscle tone.

C. Adverse effects of alpha-blockers include dizziness and postural hypotension and asthenia, both of which affect 7% of patients. These antihypertensive agents may be particularly useful for managing BPH in the hypertensive patient.

D. Therapy for BPH with terazosin (Hytrin) is usually begun with a daily dosage of 1 mg hs. Dosage is raised to 2 mg, 5 mg, and 10 mg. Clinical response may not be seen for 4-6 weeks, even at the 10-mg dosage. Doxazosin is usually given at dosages of 0.5 mg qd.

E. **Tamsulosin (Flomax)**, a more specific alpha-adrenergic blocker, preferentially binds to the alpha-adrenergic receptor sites in the urinary tract, but not as strongly to alpha-adrenergic receptor sites in cardiovascular tissue. Dosage is 0.4 mg qd, given about 30 minutes after the same meal each day. The adverse effect profile associated with tamsulosin is milder than that seen with other alpha-adrenergic blocking agents, with postural hypotension and syncope occurring only rarely. Because of its selectivity, tamsulosin offers no advantage to the hypertensive patient with BPH, however.

Starting dosages of alpha-blocking agents for managing benign prostatic hypertrophy

Drug	Starting dosage
Tamsulosin (Flomax)	0.4 mg qd
Terazosin (Hytrin)	1 mg qd, adjusted up to 5 mg qd
Doxazosin mesylate (Cardura)	1 mg qd, adjusted up to 4 mg qd

F. **alpha-reductase inhibitors.** Finasteride (Proscar) shrinks glandular tissue by blocking the conversion of testosterone to dihydrotestosterone. Symptomatic relief may not be apparent for 3-6 months. The daily dosage is 5 mg. The most common adverse affect is decreased libido, which happens in 5% of men. Up to 4% may develop an ejaculatory disorder or impotence.

III. **Surgical treatment options for BPH**
  A. If symptoms persist, and there is gross bleeding, further evaluation is indicated before surgery for BPH.
  B. Transurethral resection of the prostate (TURP), is the most frequently recommended surgical treatment. TURP reduces symptoms in 88% of patients. Long-term complications include retrograde ejaculation in up to 70% of patients, impotence in 13.6%, and incontinence in 1%.

References, see page 268.

Acute Epididymoorchitis

I. **Clinical evaluation of testicular pain**
  A. Epididymoorchitis is indicated by a unilateral painful testicle and a history of unprotected intercourse, new sexual partner, urinary tract infection, dysuria, or discharge. Symptoms may occur following acute lifting or straining.
  B. The epididymis and testicle are painful, swollen, and tender. The scrotum may be erythematosus and warm, with associated spermatic cord thickening or penile discharge.
  C. **Differential diagnosis of painful scrotal swelling**
    1. Epididymitis, testicular torsion, testicular tumor, hernia.
    2. Torsion is characterized by sudden onset, age <20, an elevated testicle, and previous episodes of scrotal pain. The epididymis is usually located anterior

on either side, and there is an absence of evidence of urethritis and UTI.
3. Epididymitis is characterized by fever, laboratory evidence of urethritis or cystitis, and increased scrotal warmth.

II. Laboratory evaluation of epididymoorchitis

A. Epididymoorchitis is indicated by leukocytosis with a left shift; UA shows pyuria and bacteriuria. Midstream urine culture will reveal gram negative bacilli. Chlamydia and Neisseria cultures should be obtained.

B. **Common pathogens**
1. **Younger men.** Epididymoorchitis is usually associated with sexually transmitted organisms such as Chlamydia and gonorrhea.
2. **Older men.** Epididymoorchitis is usually associated with a concomitant urinary tract infection or prostatitis caused by E. coli, proteus, Klebsiella, Enterobacter, or Pseudomonas.

III. Treatment of epididymoorchitis

A. Bed rest, scrotal elevation with athletic supporter, an ice pack, analgesics, and antipyretics are prescribed. Sexual and physical activity should be avoided.

B. **Sexually transmitted epididymitis in sexually active males**
1. Ceftriaxone (Rocephin) 250 mg IM x 1 dose **AND** doxycycline 100 mg PO bid x 10 days **OR**
2. Ofloxacin (Floxin) 300 mg bid x 10 days.
3. Treat sexual partners

C. **Epididymitis secondary to urinary tract infection**
1. TMP/SMX DS bid for 10 days **OR**
2. Ofloxacin (Floxin) 300 mg PO bid for 10 days.

References, see page 268.

Prostatitis and Prostatodynia

I. Acute bacterial prostatitis

A. Acute bacterial prostatitis is characterized by abrupt onset of fever and chills with symptoms of urinary tract infection or obstruction, low back or perineal pain, malaise, arthralgia, and myalgias. Urinary retention may develop.

B. **Physical exam.** The prostate is enlarged, indurated, very tender, and warm. Prostate massage is contraindicated because of possible bacterial dissemination.

C. **Laboratory evaluation**
1. Urine reveals WBCs. Culture reveals gram-negative organisms such as E coli or other Enterobacteriaceae.
2. Nosocomial infections are often associated with a Foley catheter and may be caused by Pseudomonas, enterococci, or S. aureus.

D. **Treatment** of acute prostatitis requires 28 days of antibiotic treatment. Fluoroquinolones are the drugs of choice.
1. Ciprofloxacin (Cipro) 500 mg PO bid.
2. Norfloxacin (Noroxin) 400 mg PO bid.
3. Trimethoprim/SMX (TMP-SMX, Septra) 160/800 mg (1 DS tab) PO bid.
4. Doxycycline (Vibramycin) 100 mg PO bid.

E. **Extremely ill septic patients with high fever**
1. Hospitalization for bed rest, hydration, analgesics, antipyretics, stool softeners.
2. Ampicillin 1 gm IV q4-6h **AND** gentamicin or tobramycin-loading dose of 100-

120 mg IV (1.5-2 mg/kg); then 80 mg-1 mg/kg IV q8h (2-5 mg/kg/d) **OR**
3. Ciprofloxacin (Cipro) 200 mg IV q12h.

II. Chronic bacterial prostatitis
A. Chronic prostatitis is characterized by recurrent urinary tract infections, perineal, low back or suprapubic pain, testicular, or penile pain, voiding dysfunction, post-ejaculatory pain, and intermittent hematospermia.

B. The prostate is usually normal and nontender, but it may occasionally be enlarged and tender.

C. **Laboratory evaluation**
  1. Urinalysis and culture usually shows low grade bacteriuria (E. coli or other Gram negative Enterobacteriaceae, Enterococcus faecalis, S. aureus, coagulase negative staphylococcus).
  2. Microscopic examination of expressed prostatic secretions reveals more than 10-15 WBCs per high-power field.

D. **Long-term treatment (16 weeks)**
  1. A fluoroquinolone is the drug of choice.
  2. Ciprofloxacin (Cipro) 250-500 mg PO bid.
  3. Ofloxacin (Floxin) 200-400 mg PO/IV bid.
  4. Trimethoprim/sulfamethoxazole (TMP-SMZ, Septra) 160/800 mg (1 DS tab) PO bid.
  5. **Suppression** is indicated if recurrent symptomatic infections occur: Fluoroquinolone or TMP/SMX (1 single-strength tab qd).

III. Chronic nonbacterial prostatitis
A. The most common type of prostatitis is nonbacterial. It is eight times more frequent than bacterial prostatitis. It is characterized by perineal, suprapubic or low back pain, and irritative or obstructive urinary symptoms. Symptoms and exam are similar to chronic bacterial prostatitis but with no recurrent UTI history.

B. Cultures are sterile and show no bacteria or uropathogens. Microscopic examination reveals 10-15 WBC's per high-power field.

C. **Treatment (2-4 week trial of antibiotics):**
  1. Doxycycline (100 mg bid) or erythromycin (500 mg qid) may relieve symptoms.
  2. Irritative symptoms may respond to nonsteroidal anti-inflammatory agents, muscle relaxants, anticholinergics, hot sitz baths, normal sexual activity, regular mild exercise, and avoidance of spicy foods and excessive caffeine and alcohol. Serial prostatic massage may be helpful.
  3. The disorder is usually self-limited. In persistent cases, carcinoma of the prostate and interstitial cystitis must be excluded.

IV. Prostatodynia
A. Symptoms are similar to prostatitis, but there are no objective findings suggesting that symptoms arise in the prostate gland. Age ranges between 22-56 years.

B. Symptoms include pain or discomfort in the perineum, groin, testicles, penis and urethra. Irritative or obstructive voiding symptoms are predominant. Stress is often a contributing factor. Tender musculature may be found on rectal examination.

C. **Urine** is normal (no WBC or bacteria), sterile for uropathogen. Urodynamic testing may detect uncoordinated voiding patterns. Cystoscopic examination may be useful.

D. **Treatment**
  1. Alpha-adrenergic blocking agents (terazosin 1-5 mg qd and doxazosin 1-4 mg qd) can be used to relax the bladder neck sphincter. Muscle-relaxing agents such as diazepam (Valium 2-10 mg bid) may provide relief.

2. Nonsteroidal anti-inflammatory agents, sitz baths, normal sexual activity, avoidance of stress, spicy foods, caffeine, and alcohol may be beneficial.

References, see page 268.

Psychiatric Disorders

Depression

The lifetime prevalence of major depression in the United States is 17 percent. In primary care, depression has a prevalence rate of 4.8 to 8.6 percent.

I. **Diagnosis**
    A. The Diagnostic and Statistical Manual of Mental Disorders (DSM-IV) includes nine symptoms in the diagnosis of major depression. These nine symptoms can be divided into two clusters: (1) physical or neurovegetative symptoms and (2) psychologic or psychosocial symptoms. The nine symptoms are: depressed mood plus sleep disturbance; interest/pleasure reduction; guilt feelings or thoughts of worthlessness; energy changes/fatigue; concentration/attention impairment; appetite/weight changes; psychomotor disturbances, and suicidal thoughts.
    B. **Family history** may reveal depression, suicide, or drug or alcohol abuse.
    C. **Suicide risk.** The risk of suicide is higher in depressed patients who are divorced or widowed, elderly, white, male or living alone, and in those with chronic medical illness or psychotic symptoms.

Diagnostic Criteria for Major Depression, DSM IV

Cluster 1: Physical or neurovegetative symptoms
Sleep disturbance
Appetite/weight changes
Attention/concentration problem
Energy-level change/fatigue
Psychomotor disturbance

Cluster 2: Psychologic or psychosocial symptoms
Depressed mood and/or
Interest/pleasure reduction
Guilt feelings
Suicidal thoughts

Note: Diagnosis of major depression requires at least one of the first two symptoms under cluster 2 and four of the remaining symptoms to be present for at least two weeks. Symptoms should not be accounted for by bereavement.

II. **Selection of an antidepressant**
    A. Information about the patient's past medical history and the family history of antidepressant response provides predictive data about future response.
    B. **Target symptoms.** Patients with insomnia, agitation and anxiety may benefit from a sedative anti-depressant in divided doses, with the major dose administered at bedtime.
    C. **Side effect profile.** Cardiac side effects occur with tricyclics, maprotiline and amoxapine. Drugs with limited cardiac side effects are bupropion (Wellbutrin), SSRIs and MAOIs. Tricyclics should be avoided in the treatment of patients with

ischemic heart disease. Tricyclic overdose may cause death as a result of cardiac arrhythmia. In patients with a risk of suicide, the total dosage of prescribed tricyclic antidepressant should be limited to 1,000 mg (500 mg with nortriptyline [Pamelor]).

D. Orthostatic hypotension is frequently caused by tricyclics (the tertiary agents more so than the secondary agents), MAOIs, amoxapine, maprotiline, nefazodone (Serzone) and trazodone (Desyrel). Venlafaxine (Effexor) can cause a sustained elevation of blood pressure.

E. Sedation and weight gain are side effects that may occur with tricyclics and some heterocyclics. Protriptyline (Vivactil), SSRIs, bupropion, venlafaxine and MAOIs are less likely to cause troublesome sedation than other agents. However, nonsedating drugs can be associated with insomnia, agitation and restlessness.

F. Gastrointestinal side effects, such as nausea, vomiting and diarrhea, are most often caused by drugs that block the reuptake of serotonin. Thus, the SSRIs, nefazodone, and venlafaxine are most likely to cause these effects. Smaller increments of dosage increase during the early phase of treatment and administration with food can decrease the effects. These effects are often transitory and may improve after seven to 10 days of treatment.

G. Anticholinergic side effects manifest as dry mouth, constipation, paralytic ileus and urinary retention. They may also cause photophobia and precipitate acute narrow-angle glaucoma. Tricyclics, amoxapine, maprotiline and mirtazapine (Remeron) frequently cause these side effects; the newer antidepressants have much less anticholinergic activity.

H. Sexual dysfunctions

1. Anorgasmia, decreased libido, erectile dysfunction and ejaculatory disturbances are often caused by SSRIs and venlafaxine. Tricyclics, amoxapine, maprotiline and mirtazapine can cause erectile dysfunction. Trazodone can cause priapism.

2. Sexual dysfunction associated with SSRIs may respond to dose reduction or drug holidays. Adjunctive use of buspirone (BuSpar), bupropion (Wellbutrin) or cyproheptadine (Periactin), in dosages of 4 to 12 mg taken one to two hours before coitus, may also be helpful.

Characteristics of Common Antidepressants

Drug	Recommended Dosage	Comments
Selective Serotonin Reuptake Inhibitors (SSRIs)		
Citalopram (Celexa)	Initially 10-20 mg qd (average dose 20 mg/d); maximum 40 mg/d	Minimal sedation, activation, or inhibition of hepatic enzymes, nausea, anorgasmia, headache
Fluoxetine (Prozac)	10-20 mg qd initially, taken in AM	Anxiety, insomnia, agitation, nausea, anorgasmia, erectile dysfunction, headache, anorexia.
Fluvoxamine (LuVox)	50-100 mg qhs; max 300 mg/d [50, 100 mg]	Headache, nausea, sedation, abnormal ejaculation, diarrhea

Drug	Recommended Dosage	Comments
Paroxetine (Paxil)	20 mg/d initially, given in AM; increase in 10-mg/d increments as needed to max of 50 mg/d. [10, 20, 30, 40 mg]	Headache, nausea, somnolence, dizziness, insomnia, abnormal ejaculation, anxiety, diarrhea, dry mouth.
Sertraline (Zoloft)	50 mg/d, increasing as needed to max of 200 mg/d [50, 100 mg]	Insomnia, agitation, dry mouth, headache, nausea, anorexia, sexual dysfunction.
Secondary Amine Tricyclic Antidepressants		
Desipramine (Norpramin, generics)	100-200 mg/d, gradually increasing to 300 mg/d as tolerated.[10, 25, 50, 75, 100, 150 mg]	No sedation; may have stimulant effect; best taken in morning to avoid insomnia.
Nortriptyline (Pamelor)	25 mg tid-qid, max 150 mg/d. [10, 25, 50, 75 mg]	Sedating
Tertiary Amine Tricyclics		
Amitriptyline (Elavil, generics)	75 mg/d qhs-bid, increasing to 150-200 mg/d. [25, 50, 75, 100, 150 mg]	Sedative effect precedes antidepressant effect. High anticholinergic activity.
Clomipramine (Anafranil)	25 mg/d, increasing gradually to 100 mg/d; max 250 mg/d; may be given once qhs [25, 50, 75 mg].	Relatively high sedation, anticholinergic activity, and seizure risk.
Protriptyline (Vivactil)	5-10 mg PO tid-qid; 15-60 mg/d [5, 10 mg]	Useful in anxious depression; nonsedating
Doxepin (Sinequan, generics)	50-75 mg/d, increasing up to 150-300 mg/d as needed [10, 25, 50, 75, 100, 150 mg]	Sedating. Also indicated for anxiety. Contraindicated in patients with glaucoma or urinary retention.
Imipramine (Tofranil, generics)	75 mg/d in a single dose qhs, increasing to 150 mg/d; 300 mg/d. [10, 25, 50 mg]	High sedation and anticholinergic activity. Use caution in cardiovascular disease.
Miscellaneous		
Bupropion (Wellbutrin, Wellbutrin SR)	100 mg bid; increase to 100 mg tid [75, 100 mg] Sustained release: 100-200 mg bid [100, 150 mg]	Agitation, dry mouth, insomnia, headache, nausea, constipation, tremor. Good choice for patients with sexual side effects from other agents; contraindicated in seizure disorders.
Maprotiline (Ludiomil)	75 to 225 in single or divided doses [25, 50, 75 mg].	Delays cardiac conduction; high anticholinergic activity; contraindicated in seizure disorders.
Mirtazapine (Remeron)	15 to 45 PO qd [15, 30 mg]	High anticholinergic activity; contraindicated in seizure disorders.

Drug	Recommended Dosage	Comments
Nefazodone (Serzone)	Start at 100 mg PO bid, increase to 150-300 mg PO bid as needed [100, 150, 200, 250 mg].	Headache, somnolence, dry mouth, blurred vision. Postural hypotension, impotence.
Reboxetine (Vestra)	10 mg per day	Selective norepinephrine reuptake inhibitor. Dry mouth, insomnia, constipation, increased sweating
Trazodone (Desyrel, generics)	150 mg/d, increasing by 50 mg/d every 3-4 d 400 mg/d in divided doses [50, 100, 150, 300 mg]	Rarely associated with priapism. Orthostatic hypotension in elderly. Sedating.
Venlafaxine (Effexor)	75 mg/d in 2-3 divided doses with food; increase to 225 mg/d as needed. [25, 37.5, 50, 75, 100 mg].	Inhibits norepinephrine and serotonin. Hypertension, nausea, insomnia, dizziness, abnormal ejaculation, headache, dry mouth, anxiety.

III. **Mixed serotonin-norepinephrine inhibitors**
   A. **Venlafaxine (Effexor)** is effective in treating severe, melancholic depression that has been unresponsive to other agents. Hypertension has been reported; therefore, this drug is reserved for patients unresponsive to first-line antidepressants.
   B. **Mixed serotonin effects**
      1. **Trazodone (Desyrel)** is very sedating, which can be beneficial for insomnia caused by depression. It is sometimes used along with an SSRI in patients who have difficulty sleeping. It has minimal anticholinergic side effects, but it can cause postural hypotension. It has been associated with priapism.
      2. **Nefazodone (Serzone)** is related to trazodone, but appears to have a more favorable side-effect profile. Sexual dysfunction has not been reported.
IV. **Mixed norepinephrine-dopamine reuptake inhibitors**
   A. **Bupropion (Wellbutrin)** has similar efficacy to SSRIs and TCAs, and efficacy has been shown in patients previously unresponsive to TCAs. Side effects can include agitation and insomnia, psychosis, confusion, and weight loss. Bupropion is contraindicated in patients with seizure disorders.
V. **Adjunct therapy.** Combined treatment may be beneficial in patients with incomplete response to a single antidepressant. A low-dose TCA or trazodone is often used along with an SSRI. Triiodothyronine may increase the efficacy of antidepressants.

References, see page 268.

Generalized Anxiety Disorder

Generalized anxiety disorder (GAD), is characterized by unrealistic or excessive anxiety and worry about two or more life circumstances for at least six months.

I. **Clinical evaluation**
   A. Chronic worry is a prominent feature of GAD as opposed to the intermittent terror that characterizes panic disorder. Patients may report that they "can't stop worrying."

B. Other features of GAD include insomnia, irritability, trembling, dry mouth, and a heightened startle reflex.

C. Symptoms of depression should be sought because 30-50% of patients with anxiety disorders will also have depression. Drugs and alcohol may contribute to anxiety disorders.

II. Medical disorders causing anxiety symptoms

A. **Hyperthyroidism** may also cause anxiety, tachycardia, palpitations, sweating, and dyspnea.

B. **Cardiac rhythm disturbances and mitral valve prolapse** may cause anxiety symptoms.

C. **Substance abuse or dependence** with withdrawal symptoms may resemble anxiety.

D. **Pharmacologic causes of anxiety include** salicylate intoxication, NSAIDs, antihistamine, phenylpropanolamine, pseudo-ephedrine, psychotropics (akathisia), stimulants, selective serotonin reuptake inhibitors. Caffeine, cocaine, amphetamines, theophylline, beta-agonists, steroids, and marijuana can cause anxiety.

III. Laboratory evaluation of anxiety disorders

A. Chemistry profile (glucose, calcium, phosphate), TSH.

B. **Special tests.** Urine drug screen, cortisol, serum catecholamine level.

IV. Treatment of anxiety

A. Caffeinated beverages and excess alcohol should be avoided. Daily exercise and adequate sleep (with the use of medication if necessary) should be advised.

B. **Buspirone (BuSpar)**
   1. Buspirone is a first-line treatment of GAD. Buspirone requires 3-6 weeks at a dosage of 10-20 mg tid for efficacy. It lacks sedative effects, and there is no physiologic dependence or withdrawal syndrome.
   2. Combined benzodiazepine-buspirone therapy may be used for generalized anxiety disorder, with subsequent tapering of the benzodiazepine after 2-4 weeks.
   3. Previous treatment with benzodiazepines or a history of substance abuse decreases the response to buspirone. Buspirone may have some antidepressant effects.

C. **Antidepressants**
   1. Tricyclic antidepressants are widely used to treat anxiety disorders. Their onset of action is much slower than that of the benzodiazepines, but they have no addictive potential and may be more effective. An antidepressant is the agent of choice when depression is present in addition to anxiety.
   2. Sedating antidepressants often have an early effect of promoting better sleep, although 2-3 weeks may pass before a patient experiences an antianxiety benefit. Better sleep usually brings some relief from symptoms, and the patient's functional level begins to improve almost immediately.
   3. Anxious patients benefit from the sedating effects of imipramine (Tofranil), amitriptyline (Elavil), and doxepin (Sinequan). The daily dosage should be at least 50-100 mg.
   4. Desipramine (Norpramin) is useful if sedation is not desired.

D. **Benzodiazepines**
   1. Benzodiazepines almost always relieve anxiety if given in adequate doses, and they have no delayed onset of action. Benzodiazepines should be reserved for patients who have failed to respond to buspirone and antidepressants or who are intolerant to their side effects.
   2. Benzodiazepines are very useful for treating anxiety during the period in which it takes buspirone or antidepressants to exert their effects. Benzodiazepines

should then be tapered after several weeks.

3. Benzodiazepines have few side effects other than sedation. Tolerance to their sedative effects develops, but not to their antianxiety properties.

4. Clonazepam (Klonopin) and diazepam (Valium) have long half-lives; therefor, they are less likely to result in interdose anxiety and are easier to taper.

5. Drug dependency develops if the benzodiazepine is used regularly for more than 2-3 weeks. A withdrawal syndrome occurs in 70% of patients, including intense anxiety, tremulousness dysphoria, sleep and perceptual disturbances and appetite suppression.

6. Patients with depression and anxiety should not receive benzodiazepines because they may worsen depression.

7. Benzodiazepines can be used in conjunction with an antidepressant. Therapy starts with alprazolam and an SSRI or tricyclic antidepressant. Alprazolam is then tapered after 2-3 weeks.

Anti-Anxiety Agent Dosages

Drug	Dosage	Comments
Benzodiazepines		
Alprazolam (Xanax)	0.25-0.5 mg tid; increase by 1 mg/d at 3-4 day intervals to 0.75-4 mg/d [0.25, 0.5, 1, 2 mg]	Intermediate onset. Least sedating drug in class. Strong potential for dependence
Chlordiazepoxide (Librium, generics)	5 mg tid; 15-100 mg/d [5, 10, 25 mg]	Intermediate onset
Clonazepam (Klonopin)	0.5 mg tid; 1.5-20 mg/d [0.5, 1, 2 mg]	Intermediate onset. Long half-life; much less severe withdrawal
Clorazepate (Tranxene, generics)	7.5 mg bid; 15-60 mg/d [3.75, 7.5, 15 mg]	Fast onset
Diazepam (Valium, generics)	2 mg bid; 4-40 mg/d [2, 5, 10 mg]	Very fast onset
Halazepam (Paxipam)	20-40 mg tid-qid; 80-160 mg/d [20, 40 mg]	Intermediate to slow onset
Lorazepam (Ativan, generics)	1 mg bid; 2-6 mg/d [0.5, 1, 2 mg]	Intermediate onset
Oxazepam (Serax, generics)	10 mg tid; 30-120 mg/d [10, 15, 30 mg]	Intermediate to slow onset
Antidepressants		
Buspirone (BuSpar)	10 mg bid; max 60 mg/d; increase to 10 mg tid prn [5, 10, 15 mg dividose]	Antidepressant; nonaddicting, nonsedating. Not for prn usage; requires 2-3 wk to become effective.
Amitriptyline (Elavil, generics)	75 mg/d qhs-bid, increasing to 150-200	Sedating, high anticholinergic activity

Drug	Dosage	Comments
Doxepin (Sinequan, generics)	75 mg qhs or bid, max 300 mg/d [10, 25, 50, 75, 100, 150 mg]	A tricyclic antidepressant with antianxiety effects.

References, see page 268.

Panic Disorder

Panic disorder is characterized by the occurrence of panic attacks--sudden, unexpected periods of intense fear or discomfort. About 15% of the general population experiences panic attacks; 1.6-3.2% of women and 0.4%-1.7% of men have panic disorder.

DSM-IV Criteria for panic attack

A discrete period of intense fear or discomfort in which four or more of the following symptoms developed abruptly and reached a peak within 10 minutes.
 Chest pain or discomfort
 Choking
 Depersonalization or derealization
 Dizziness, faintness, or unsteadiness
 Fear of "going crazy" or being out of control
 Fear of dying
 Flushes or chills
 Nausea or gastrointestinal distress
 Palpitations or tachycardia
 Paresthesias
 Shortness of breath (or feelings of smothering)
 Sweating
 Trembling or shaking

Diagnostic criteria for panic disorder without agoraphobia

Recurrent, unexpected panic attacks
And
At least one attack has been followed by at least 1 month of one (or more) of the following:
Persistent concern about experiencing more attacks
Worry about the meaning of the attack or its consequences (fear of losing control, having a heart attack, or "going crazy")
A significant behavioral change related to the attacks
And
Absence of agoraphobia
And
Direct physiological effects of a substance (drug abuse or medication) or general medical condition has been ruled out as a cause of the attacks
And
The panic attacks cannot be better accounted for by another mental disorder

Clinical evaluation
A. Panic attacks are manifested by the sudden onset of an overwhelming fear,

accompanied by feelings of impending doom, for no apparent reason.

B. The essential criterion for panic attack is the presence of 4 of 13 cardiac, neurologic, gastrointestinal, or respiratory symptoms that develop abruptly and reach a peak within 10 minutes. The physical symptoms include shortness of breath, dizziness or faintness, palpitations, accelerated heart rate, and sweating. Trembling, choking, nausea, numbness, flushes, chills, or chest discomfort are also common, as are cognitive symptoms such as fear of dying or losing control.

C. One third of patients develop agoraphobia, or a fear of places where escape may be difficult, such as bridges, trains, buses, or crowded areas. Medications, substance abuse, and general medical conditions such as hyperthyroidism must be ruled out as a cause of the patient's symptoms.

D. The history should include details of the panic attack, its onset and course, history of panic, and any treatment. Questioning about a family history of panic disorder, agoraphobia, hypochondriasis, or depression is important. Because panic disorder may be triggered by marijuana or stimulants such as cocaine, a history of substance abuse must be identified. A medication history, including prescription, over-the-counter, and herbal preparations, is essential.

E. The patient should be asked about stressful life events or problems in daily life that may have preceded onset of the disorder. The extent of any avoidance behavior that has developed or suicidal ideation, self-medication, or exacerbation of an existing medical disorder should be assessed.

Differential Diagnosis of Panic Attacks	
Medical conditions	**Psychiatric Conditions**
Audio-vestibular dysfunction	Claustrophobia
Caffeinism	Dissociative disorders
Complex partial seizures	Generalized anxiety without panic
Congestive heart failure	Severe depression
Epilepsy	Simple phobia
Hyperthyroidism	Social phobias
Hypoglycemia	Medications
Pheochromocytoma	Acute intoxication or withdrawal from alcohol, caffeine or illicit drugs (amphetamines, cannabis, cocaine)

II. Management

A. Patients should reduce or eliminate caffeine consumption, including coffee and tea, cold medications, analgesics, and beverages with added caffeine. Alcohol use is a particularly insidious problem because patients may use drinking to alleviate the panic.

Pharmacologic treatment of panic disorder

Drug	Dosage range (mg/d)	
	Initial	Therapeutic
SSRIs		
Fluoxetine (Prozac)	5-10	10-60
Fluvoxamine (LuVox)	25-50	25-300
Paroxetine (Paxil)	10-20	20-50
Sertraline (Zoloft)	25-50	50-200
Citalopram (Celexa)	10-20 mg qd	20-40
Benzodiazepines		
Alprazolam (Xanax)	0.5 In divided doses, tid-qid	1-4 In divided doses, tid-qid
Clonazepam (Klonopin)	0.5 In divided doses, bid-tid	1-4 In divided doses, bid-tid
Diazepam (Valium)	2.0 In divided doses, bid-tid	2-20 In divided doses, bid
Lorazepam (Ativan)	0.5 In divided doses, bid-tid	1-4 In divided doses, bid-tid
TCAs		
Amitriptyline (Elavil)	10	10-300
Clomipramine (Anafranil)	25	25-300
Desipramine (Norpramin)	10	10-300
Imipramine (Tofranil)	10	10-300
Nortriptyline (Pamelor)	10	10-300
MAOIs		
Phenelzine (Nardil)	15	15-90
Tranylcypromine (Parnate)	10	10-30

B. **Selective serotonin reuptake inhibitors (SSRIs)** are an effective, well-tolerated alternative to benzodiazepines and TCAs. SSRIs are superior to either imipramine or alprazolam. They lack the cardiac toxicity and anticholinergic effects of TCAs. Fluoxetine (Prozac), fluvoxamine (LuVox), paroxetine (Paxil), sertraline (Zoloft), and citalopram (Celexa) have shown efficacy for the treatment of panic disorder.

C. **Tricyclic antidepressants (TCAs)** have demonstrated efficacy in treating panic. They are, however, associated with a delayed onset of action and side effects--particularly orthostatic hypotension, anticholinergic effects, weight gain, and cardiac toxicity.

D. **Benzodiazepines**

1. Clonazepam (Klonopin), alprazolam (Xanax), and lorazepam (Ativan), are effective in blocking panic attacks. Advantages include a rapid onset of therapeutic effect and a safe, favorable, side-effect profile. Among the drawbacks are the potential for abuse and dependency, worsening of depressive symptoms, withdrawal symptoms on abrupt discontinuation, anterograde amnesia, early relapse on discontinuation, and inter-dose rebound anxiety.

2. Benzodiazepines are an appropriate first-line treatment only when rapid symptom relief is needed. The most common use for benzodiazepines is to stabilize severe initial symptoms until another treatment (eg, an SSRI or

cognitive behavioral therapy) becomes effective.

3. The starting dose of alprazolam is 0.5 mg bid. Approximately 70% of patients will experience a discontinuance reaction characterized by increased anxiety, agitation, and insomnia when alprazolam is tapered. Clonazepam's long duration of effect diminishes the need for multiple daily dosing. Initial symptoms of sedation and ataxia are usually transient.

E. Monoamine oxidase inhibitors (MAOIs). MAOIs such phenelzine sulfate (Nardil) may be the most effective agents for blocking panic attacks and for relieving the depression and concomitant social anxiety of panic disorder. Recommended doses range from 45-90 mg/d. MAOI use is limited by adverse effects such as orthostatic hypotension, weight gain, insomnia, risk of hypertensive crisis, and the need for dietary monitoring. MAOIs are often reserved for patients who do not respond to safer drugs.

F. Beta-blockers are useful in moderating heart rate and decreasing dry mouth and tremor; they are less effective in relieving subjective anxiety.

G. Treatment of refractory patients. Interventions for refractory cases may consist of adding buspirone (BuSpar) to an SSRI, or switching to an MAOI.

H. Behavioral therapy and psychotherapy. Cognitive behavioral therapy teaches patients to master anxiety.

References, see page 268.

Insomnia

Insomnia is the perception by patients that their sleep is inadequate or abnormal. Insomnia may affect as many as 69% of adult primary care patients. The incidence of sleep problems increases with age. Younger persons are apt to have trouble falling asleep, whereas older persons tend to have prolonged awakenings during the night.

I. Causes of insomnia

A. Situational stress concerning job loss or problems often disrupt sleep. Patients under stress may experience interference with sleep onset and early morning awakening. Attempting to sleep in a new place, changes in time zones, or changing bedtimes due to shift work may interfere with sleep.

B. Drugs associated with insomnia include antihypertensives, caffeine, diuretics, oral contraceptives, phenytoin, selective serotonin reuptake inhibitors, protriptyline, corticosteroids, stimulants, theophylline, and thyroid hormone.

C. Psychiatric disorders. Depression is a common cause of poor sleep, often characterized by early morning awakening. Associated findings include hopelessness, sadness, loss of appetite, and reduced enjoyment of formerly pleasurable activities. Anxiety disorders and substance abuse may cause insomnia.

D. Medical disorders. Prostatism, peptic ulcer, congestive heart failure, and chronic obstructive pulmonary disease may cause insomnia. Pain, nausea, dyspnea, cough, and gastroesophageal reflux may interfere with sleep.

E. Obstructive sleep apnea syndrome

1. This sleep disorder occurs in 5-15% of adults. It is characterized by recurrent discontinuation of breathing during sleep for at least 10 seconds. Abnormal oxygen saturation and sleep patterns result in excessive daytime fatigue and drowsiness. Loud snoring is typical. Overweight, middle-aged men are particularly predisposed. Weight loss can be helpful in obese patients.

2. Diagnosis is by polysomnography. Use of hypnotic agents is contraindicated since they increase the frequency and the severity of apneic episodes.

II. Clinical evaluation of insomnia

A. Acute personal and medical problems should be sought, and the duration and pattern of symptoms and use of any psychoactive agents should be investigated. Substance abuse, leg movements, sleep apnea, loud snoring, nocturia, and daytime napping or fatigue should be sought.

B. Consumption of caffeinated beverages, prescribed drugs, over-the-counter medications, and illegal substances should be sought.

III. Behavioral therapy

A. A regular schedule of going to bed, arising, and eating meals should be recommended. Daytime naps should be discouraged. Daily exercise is helpful, but it should not be done in the late evening. Caffeine should not be consumed in the late afternoon or evening.

B. **Stimulus restriction.** Patients are advised to lie in bed only when they are sleepy and not when reading, eating, or watching television. If they do not fall asleep after a few minutes, they should get out of bed and read until they are sleepy.

C. **Sleep restriction** may be helpful. Each night, patients reduce the time in bed 30 minutes until reaching 4 hours per night; thereafter, they may add 15 minutes each night until 85% of time in bed is spent sleeping.

D. **Relaxation therapy** may include abdominal breathing, yoga or meditation, autogenic training, progressive muscle relaxation, and biofeedback.

IV. Pharmacologic management

A. Hypnotics are the primary drugs used in the management of insomnia. These drugs include the benzodiazepines and the benzodiazepine receptor agonists in the imidazopyridine or pyrazolopyrimidine classes.

Recommended dosages, T_{max}, elimination half-life, and receptor selectivity of hypnotic medications commonly used to treat insomnia (Dosages recommended for the elderly are shown in parentheses)

Benzodiazepine hypnotics	Recommended dose, mg	T_{max}	Elimination half-life	Receptor selectivity
Benzodiazepine receptor agonists				
Imidazopyridine				
Zolpidem (Ambien)	5-10 (5)	1.6	2.6	Yes
Pyrazolopyrimidine				
Zaleplon (Sonata)	5-10 (5)	1.0	1.0	Yes
Hypnotic Medications				
Estazolam (ProSom)	1-2 (0.5-1)	2.7	17.1	No
Flurazepam (Dalmane)	15-30 (15)	1.0	47.0-100	No
Triazolam (Halcion)	0.250 (0.125)	1.2	2.6	No
Temazepam (Restoril)	7.5-60 (7.5-20)	0.8	8.4	No
Quazepam (Doral)	7.5-15.0 (7.5)	2.0	73.0	No

Benzodiazepines used as hypnotics				
Alprazolam (Xanax)	0.25-0.50	1.0-2.0	11.2	No
Diazepam (Valium)	2.0-10.0	1.0-4.0	20-200	No
Clonazepam (Klonopin)	0.5-4.0		30-40	No
Lorazepam (Ativan)	2.0-4.0	2.0	18.0	No

B. Zolpidem (Ambien) and zaleplon (Sonata) have the advantage of achieving hypnotic effects with less tolerance and fewer adverse effects.

C. The safety profile of these benzodiazepines and benzodiazepine receptor agonists is good; lethal overdose is rare, except when benzodiazepines are taken with alcohol. Sedative effects may be enhanced when benzodiazepines are used in conjunction with other central nervous system depressants.

D. **Zolpidem (Ambien)** is a benzodiazepine agonist with a short elimination half-life that is effective in inducing sleep onset and promoting sleep maintenance. Zolpidem may be associated with greater residual impairment in memory and psychomotor performance than zaleplon.

E. **Zaleplon (Sonata)** is a benzodiazepine receptor agonist that is rapidly absorbed (T_{MAX} = 1 hour) and has a short elimination half-life of 1 hour. Zaleplon does not impair memory or psychomotor functioning at as early as 2 hours after administration, or on morning awakening. Zaleplon does not cause residual impairment when the drug is given in the middle of the night. Zaleplon can be used at bedtime or after the patient has tried to fall asleep naturally.

F. **Benzodiazepines with long half-lives**, such as flurazepam (Dalmane), may be effective in promoting sleep onset and sustaining sleep. These drugs may have effects that extend beyond the desired sleep period, however, resulting in daytime sedation or functional impairment. Patients with daytime anxiety may benefit from the residual anxiolytic effect of a long-acting benzodiazepine administered at bedtime. Benzodiazepines with intermediate half-lives, such as temazepam (Restoril), facilitate sleep onset and maintenance with less risk of daytime residual effects.

G. **Benzodiazepines with short half-lives**, such as triazolam (Halcion), are effective in promoting the initiation of sleep but may not contribute to sleep maintenance.

H. **Sedating antidepressants** are sometimes used as an alternative to benzodiazepines or benzodiazepine receptor agonists. Amitriptyline (Elavil), 25-50 mg at bedtime, or trazodone (Desyrel), 50-100 mg, are common choices.

References, see page 268.

Nicotine Withdrawal

Smoking causes approximately 430,000 smoking deaths each year, accounting for 19.5% of all deaths. Daily use of nicotine for several weeks results in physical dependence. Abrupt discontinuation of smoking leads to nicotine withdrawal within 24 hours. The symptoms include craving for nicotine, irritability, frustration, anger, anxiety, restlessness, difficulty in concentrating, and mood swings. Symptoms usually last about 4 weeks.

Behavioral counseling, either group or individual, can raise the rate of abstinence to 20%-25%. The primary goals are to change the mental processes of smoking, reinforce the benefits of nonsmoking, and teach skills to help the smoker avoid high-risk situations.

Drugs for Treatment of Nicotine Addiction

A. Treatment with nicotine is the only method that produces significant withdrawal rates. Nicotine replacement comes in three forms: nicotine polacrilex gum (Nicorette), nicotine transdermal patches (Habitrol, Nicoderm, Nicotrol), and nicotine nasal spray (Nicotrol NS) and inhaler (Nicotrol). Nicotine patches provide steady-state nicotine levels, but do not provide a bolus of nicotine on demand as do sprays and gum.

B. Bupropion (Zyban) is an antidepressant shown to be effective in treating the craving for nicotine. The symptoms of nicotine craving and withdrawal are reduced with the use of bupropion, making it a useful adjunct to nicotine replacement systems.

Treatments for smoking cessation		
Drug	**Dosage**	**Comments**
Nicotine gum (Nicorette)	2- or 4-mg piece/30 min	Available OTC; poor compliance
Nicotine patch (Habitrol, Nicoderm CQ)	1 patch/d for 6-12 wk, then taper for 4 wk	Available OTC; local skin reactions
Nicotine nasal spray (Nicotrol NS)	1-2 doses/h for 6-8 wk	Rapid nicotine delivery; nasal irritation initially
Nicotine inhaler (Nicotrol Inhaler)	6-16 cartridges/d for 12 wk	Mimics smoking behavior; provides low doses of nicotine
Bupropion (Zyban)	150 mg/day for 3 d, then titrate to 300 mg	Treatment initiated 1 wk before quit day; contraindicated with seizures, anorexia, heavy alcohol use

C. **Nicotine polacrilex (Nicorette)** is available OTC. The patient should use 1-2 pieces per hour. A 2-mg dose is recommended for those who smoke fewer than 25 cigarettes per day, and 4 mg for heavier smokers. It is used for 6 weeks, followed by 6 weeks of tapering. Nicotine gum improves smoking cessation rates by about 40%-60%. Drawbacks include poor compliance and unpleasant taste.

D. **Transdermal nicotine (Habitrol, Nicoderm, Nicotrol)** doubles abstinence rates compared with placebo. The patch is available OTC and is easier to use than the gum. It provides a plateau level of nicotine at about half that of what a pack-a-day smoker would normally obtain. The higher dose should be used for 6-12 weeks followed by 4 weeks of tapering.

E. **Nicotine nasal spray (Nicotrol NS)** is available by prescription and is a good choice for patients who have not been able to quit with the gum or patch or for heavy smokers. It delivers a high level of nicotine, similar to smoking. Nicotine nasal spray doubles the rates of sustained abstinence. The spray is used 6-8 weeks, at 1-2 doses per hour (one puff in each nostril). Tapering over about 6 weeks. Side effects include nasal and throat irritation, headache, and eye watering.

F. **Nicotine inhaler (Nicotrol Inhaler)** delivers nicotine orally via inhalation from a plastic tube. It is available by prescription and has a success rate of 28%, similar to nicotine gum. The inhaler has the advantage of avoiding some of the adverse effects of nicotine gum, and its mode of delivery more closely resembles the act of smoking.

G. **Bupropion (Zyban)**
1. Bupropion is appropriate for patients who have been unsuccessful using nicotine replacement. Bupropion reduces withdrawal symptoms and can be used in conjunction with nicotine replacement therapy. The treatment is associated with reduced weight gain. Bupropion is contraindicated with a history of seizures, anorexia, heavy alcohol use, or head trauma.
2. Bupropion is started at a dose of 150 mg daily for 3 days and then increased to 300 mg daily for 2 weeks before the patient stops smoking. Bupropion is then continued for 3 months. When a nicotine patch is added to this regimen, the abstinence rates increase to 50% compared with 32% when only the patch is used.

References, see page 268.

Alcohol and Drug Addiction

In primary care outpatients, the prevalence of alcohol disorders is 16-28%, and the prevalence of drug disorders is 7-9%. Alcoholism is characterized by continuous or periodic impaired control over drinking, preoccupation with alcohol, use of alcohol despite adverse consequences, and distortions in thinking, most notably denial. Substance abuse is a pattern of misuse during which the patient maintains control. Addiction or substance dependence, is a pattern of misuse during which the patient has lost control.

I. **Clinical assessment of alcohol use and abuse**
A. The amount and frequency of alcohol use and other drug use in the past month, week, and day should be evaluated. Determine whether the patient ever consumes five or more drinks at a time (binge drinking). Previous abuse of alcohol or other drugs should be assessed.
B. Effects of the alcohol or drug use on the patient's life may include problems with health, family, job or financial status or with the legal system. History of blackouts, motor vehicle crashes, and the effect of alcohol use on family members or friends should be evaluated.

Clinical Clues to Alcohol and Drug Disorders

Social history

Arrest for driving under the influence: one time has a 75% association with alcoholism, two times has a 95% association

Loss of job or sent home from work for alcohol- or drug-related reasons

Domestic violence

Child abuse/neglect

Family instability (divorce, separation)

Frequent, unplanned absences

Personal isolation

Problems at work/school

Mood swings

Medical history

History of addiction to any drug

Withdrawal syndrome

Depression

Anxiety disorder

Recurrent pancreatitis

Recurrent hepatitis

Hepatomegaly

Peripheral neuropathy

Myocardial infarction at less than age 30 (cocaine)

Blood alcohol level greater than 300 mg per dL or greater than 100 mg per dL without impairment

Alcohol smell on breath or intoxicated during office visit

Tremor

Mild hypertension

Estrogen-mediated signs (telangiectasias, spider angiomas, palmar erythema, muscle atrophy) Gastrointestinal complaints

Sleep disturbances

Eating disorders

Sexual dysfunction

II. **Laboratory screening**
   A. **Mean corpuscular volume.** An elevated mean corpuscular volume (MCV) level may result from folic acid deficiency, advanced alcoholic liver disease, or the direct toxic effect of alcohol on red blood cells. MCV has poor sensitivity for predicting addiction.
   B. **Gamma-glutamyltransferase.** The sensitivity of GGT for predicting alcohol addiction is higher than that of MCV, but its specificity is low.
   C. **Other liver function test** results may be elevated because of heavy alcohol consumption, including aspartate aminotransferase (AST) and alanine aminotransferase (ALT). These markers have low sensitivity and specificity. An AST/ALT ratio greater than 2:1 is highly suggestive of alcohol-related liver disease.
   D. **Carbohydrate-deficient transferrin (CDT).** Consumption of 4 to 7 drinks daily for at least 1 week results in a decrease in the carbohydrate content of transferrin. The sensitivity and specificity of CDT are high; it can differentiate patients who drink heavily from those who drink very little or no alcohol.

DSM-IV Diagnostic Criteria for Substance Dependence

A maladaptive pattern of substance use leading to clinically significant impairment or distress as manifested by 3 or more of the following occurring at any time during the same 12-month period.

Tolerance, as defined by one of the following:
- A need for markedly increased amounts of the substance to achieve intoxication of the desired effect.
- Markedly diminished effect with continued use of the same amount of the substance.

Withdrawal, as manifested by one of the following:
- The characteristic withdrawal syndrome for the substance.
- The same, or a closely related, substance is taken to relieve or avoid withdrawal symptoms.
- The substance is often taken in larger amounts or over a longer period than was intended.
- There is a persistent desire or unsuccessful efforts to cut down or control substance use.
- A great deal of time is spent in activities necessary to obtain the substance, use the substance, or recover from its effects.
- Important social, occupational, or recreational activities are given up or reduced because of substance use.
- Substance use is continued despite knowledge of having a persistent or recurrent physical or psychologic problem that is likely caused or exacerbated by the substance.

III. **Alcohol intoxication**
   A. Alcohol is classified as a sedative-hypnotic drug, and alcohol intoxication is similar to intoxication produced by other sedative-hypnotic drugs.
   B. Support is the main treatment for alcohol intoxication. Respiratory depression is frequently the most serious outcome of severe alcohol intoxication. Alcohol can cause hypoglycemia, and the presence of thiamine deficiency may further complicate hypoglycemia. Thus, unconscious patients should receive thiamine intravenously before receiving glucose.

IV. **Alcohol withdrawal**
   A. Withdrawal seizures are a common symptom of sedative-hypnotic withdrawal. Seizures occur in 11% to 33% of patients withdrawing from alcohol.
   B. Treatment consists of four doses of chlordiazepoxide, 50 mg every 6 hours, followed by 3 doses of 50 mg every 8 hours, followed by 2 doses of 50 mg every 12 hours, and finally 1 dose of 50 mg at bedtime.

Signs and Symptoms of Alcohol Withdrawal

Withdrawal is characterized by the development of a combination of any of the following signs and symptoms several hours after stopping a prolonged period of heavy drinking:

1. Autonomic hyperactivity: diaphoresis, tachycardia, elevated blood pressure
2. Tremor
3. Insomnia
4. Nausea or vomiting
5. Transient visual, tactile, or auditory hallucinations or illusions
6. Psychomotor agitation
7. Anxiety
8. Generalized seizure activity

Signs and Symptoms of Cocaine or Stimulant Withdrawal

1. Dysphoric mood
2. Fatigue, malaise
3. Vivid, unpleasant dreams
4. Sleep disturbance
5. Increased appetite
6. Psychomotor retardation or agitation

Signs and Symptoms of Opiate Withdrawal

1. Mild elevation of pulse and respiratory rates, blood pressure, and temperature
2. Piloerection (gooseflesh)
3. Dysphoric mood and drug craving
4. Lacrimation and/or rhinorrhea
5. Mydriasis, yawning, and diaphoresis
6. Anorexia, abdominal cramps, vomiting, and diarrhea
7. Insomnia
8. Weakness

Agents Used to Treat Opiate Withdrawal

Methadone (Dolophine) is a pure opioid agonist restricted to inpatient treatment or specialized outpatient drug treatment programs. Treatment is a 15- to 20-mg daily dose for 2 to 3 days, followed by a 10 to 15 percent reduction in daily dose, guided by patient symptoms and clinical findings.

Clonidine (Catapres) is an alpha-adrenergic blocker. One 0.2-mg dose every 4 hours to relieve symptoms of withdrawal may be effective. Hypotension is a risk. It may be continued for 10 to 14 days, followed by tapering to 0.2 mg daily starting on day 3.

Buprenorphine (Buprenex) is a partial mu-receptor agonist which can be administered sublingually in doses of 2, 4, or 8 mg every 4 hours for the management of opiate withdrawal symptoms.

Naltrexone (ReVia, Trexan)/clonidine is a rapid form of opiate detoxification involves pretreatment with 0,2 to 0.3 mg of clonidine, followed by 12.5 mg of naltrexone (a pure opioid antagonist). Naltrexone is increased to 25 mg on day 2, 50 mg on day 3, and 100 mg on day 4, with clonidine doses of 0.1 to 0.3 mg 3 times daily.

V. Sedative-hypnotic withdrawal is similar for all drugs in this class. Establishment of physical dependence usually requires daily use of therapeutic doses of these drugs for 6 months or higher doses for 3 months. Treatment of withdrawal from sedative-hypnotics is similar to that of withdrawal from alcohol; long-acting benzodiazepines are the drugs of choice.

VI. Maintenance treatment

  A. Twelve-step programs make a significant contribution to recovery. Alcoholics Anonymous (AA) is the root of 12-step programs.

  B. Drugs for treatment of alcohol addiction

  1. **Disulfiram** inhibits aldehyde dehydrogenase, the enzyme that catalyzes the oxidation of acetaldehyde to acetic acid. On ingesting alcohol, patients taking disulfiram experience the disulfiram-ethanol reaction, an increase in the acetaldehyde level that manifests as flushing of the skin, palpitations,

decreased blood pressure, nausea, vomiting, shortness of breath, blurred vision, and confusion. Death has been reported. Common side effects include drowsiness, lethargy, peripheral neuropathy, hepatotoxicity, and hypertension. The usual dose of disulfiram is 250 to 500 mg daily.

2. **Naltrexone,** an opioid antagonist, reduces drinking. It has diminished effectiveness over time and does not reduce relapse rates of heavy drinkers.

3. **Serotonergic drugs** reduce drinking in heavy-drinking, nondepressed alcoholic patients, but only 15% to 20% from pretreatment levels.

4. **Acamprosate (calcium acetylhomotaurinate)** reduces the craving for alcohol. Acamprosate appears to result in more frequent and longer-lasting periods of abstinence than does naltrexone.

Management of Alcohol Withdrawal

Clinical Disorder	Mild/Moderate AWS, able to take oral	Mild/Moderate AWS, unable to take oral	Severe AWS
Adrenergic Hyper-activity	Lorazepam (Ativan) 2 mg po q2h or Chlordiazepoxide (Librium) 25-100 mg po q6h	Lorazepam 1-2 mg IM/IV q1-2h as needed	Lorazepam 1-2 mg IV q 5-10 min
Dehydration	Water or juice po	NS 1 liter bolus, then D5NS 150-200 mL/h	Aggressive hydration with NS /D5NS
Nutritional Deficiency	Thiamine 100 mg po Multivitamins Folate 1 mg po	Thiamine 100 mg IV Multivitamins 1 amp in first liter of IV fluids Folate 1 mg IV in first liter of IV fluids	Thiamine 100 mg IV Multivitamins 1 amp in first liter of IV fluids Folate 1 mg IV in first liter of IV fluids
Hypoglycemia	High fructose solution po	25 mL D50 IV (repeat as necessary)	25 mL D50 IV (repeat as necessary)
Hyperthermia			Cooling blankets
Seizures	Lorazepam (Ativan) 2 mg IV	Lorazepam 2 mg IV	Lorazepam 2 mg IV

References, see page 268.

Anorexia Nervosa

Anorexia nervosa is a psychologic illness characterized by marked weight loss, an intense fear of gaining weight even though the patient is underweight, a distorted body image and amenorrhea. Anorexia primarily affects adolescent girls and occurs in ap proximately 0.2 to 1.3 percent of the general population.

I. Diagnosis and Clinical Features

A. The typical patient with anorexia nervosa is an adolescent female who is a high achiever. She usually has successful parents and feels compelled to excel. She is a perfectionist and a good student, involved in many school and community activities.

DSM-IV Diagnostic Criteria for Anorexia Nervosa

- Refusal to maintain body weight at or above a minimally normal weight for age and height (eg, weight loss leading to maintenance of body weight less than 85 percent of that expected; or failure to make expected weight gain during a period of growth, leading to body weight less than 85 percent of that expected).
- Intense fear of gaining weight or becoming fat, even though underweight.
- Disturbance in the way in which one's body weight or shape is experienced, undue influence of body weight or shape on self-evaluation, or denial of the seriousness of the current low body weight.
- In postmenarchal females, amenorrhea, ie, the absence of at least three consecutive menstrual cycles. (A woman is considered to have amenorrhea if her periods occur only following hormone, eg, estrogen, administration.)

Specify type:
- Restricting type: During the current episode of anorexia nervosa, the person has not regularly engaged in binge-eating or purging behavior (ie, self-induced vomiting or the misuse of laxatives, diuretics or enemas).
- Binge-eating/purging type: During the current episode of anorexia nervosa, the person has regularly engaged in binge-eating or purging behavior (ie, self-induced vomiting or the misuse of laxatives, diuretics or enemas).

B. Persons with anorexia nervosa have a disturbed perception of their own weight and body shape. Individuals perceive themselves as overweight even though they are emaciated.

Features Associated with Anorexia Nervosa

Bulimic episodes	Edema
Preparation of elaborate meals for others but self-limitation to a narrow selection of low-calorie foods Obsessive-compulsive, behaviors	Lanugo
	Overactivity, exercise
	Early satiety
Denial or minimization of illness	Constipation
Delayed psychosexual development	Skin dryness
Hypothermia	Hypercarotenemia
Bradycardia	Hair loss
Hypotension	Dehydration

Assessment of Eating Disorders

History
Eating habits and rituals
Body image
Weight, minimum and maximum weights, desired weight
Menstrual pattern
Use of laxatives, diuretics or diet pills
Exercise participation
Binging and purging behaviors
Substance abuse, personality, mood and anxiety
disorders, and suicidal thoughts
Past medical history
Family history of medical and psychiatric disorders

Physical examination
Vital signs, and standard weight and height
Mental status
Complete physical examination

Laboratory: Complete blood count, electrolytes, blood urea nitrogen, creatinine, calcium, magnesium, phosphate, cholesterol, lipids, amylase, total protein, albumin, liver function tests, thyroid function tests, urinalysis, electrocardiogram

Complications of Anorexia Nervosa

Metabolic Hypothermia Dehydration Electrolyte abnormalities: hypokalemia, hyponatremia, hypochloremic alkalosis, hypocalcemia, metabolic acidosis secondary to keto- sis, hypercholesterolemia, hypercarotenemia, hypoglycemia	**Hematologic** Pancytopenia Hypocellular bone marrow Decreased plasma proteins	**Gastrointestinal** Swollen salivary glands, dental caries, erosion of tooth enamel (with vomit- ing) Delayed gastric emptying, constipation, bowel ob- struction Early satiety
Cardiovascular Bradycardia, hypotension, decreased heart size Arrhythmias (atrial flutter, atrial fibrillation, premature ventricular contractions, right bundle branch block) Superior mesenteric artery syndrome Pericardial effusion	**Renal** Prerenal azotemia Chronic renal failure	**Dermatologic** Dry, pale skin

Endocrine	Musculoskeletal	Cognitive and behavior
Decreased gonadotropins, estrogens, testosterone Sick euthyroid syndrome Increased cortisol and growth hormone Amenorrhea, infertility, impotence Thinning hair Lanugo	Cramps, tetany, weakness Osteopenia, stress fractures	Depression Poor concentration Food preoccupation Impaired sleep Decreased libido

II. **Treatment**
   A. A trial of outpatient treatment may be attempted if the patient is not severely emaciated, has had the illness for less than six months, has no serious medical complications, is accepting her illness and is motivated to change, and has supportive and cooperative family and friends.
   B. The first step in the treatment of anorexia nervosa is correction of the starvation state. A goal weight should be set and the patient's weight should be monitored once or twice a week in the office. A caloric intake to provide a weight gain of 1 to 3 lb per week should be instituted. Initially, weight gain should be gradual to prevent gastric dilation, pedal edema and congestive heart failure. Often, a nutritional supplement is added to the regimen to augment dietary intake.
   C. During the process of refeeding, weight gain as well as electrolyte levels should be strictly monitored. The disturbed eating behavior must be addressed in specific counseling sessions.
   D. Inpatient treatment is indicated if weight loss exceeds 30 percent of ideal weight; patient is having suicidal thoughts; patient is abusing laxatives, diuretics or diet pills, or outpatient treatment has failed.
   E. The drug of choice for the treatment of anorexia nervosa is food. Depression, a common finding in anorexia nervosa, is usually alleviated with renourishment. In cases of depression refractory to proper nutrition, an antidepressant may be helpful. Tricyclic antidepressants have been used with success but cause sedation and anticholinergic and alpha-adrenergic side effects, which may limit effectiveness. The use of serotonin-specific reuptake inhibitors (SSRIs) is common and has proved to alleviate the depressed mood and moderate obsessive-compulsive behaviors occurring in some individuals. Fluoxetine (Prozac) has been used successfully in the therapy of anorexia and bulimia; 20-40 mg PO qAM.
   F. Behavior therapies are commonly used in the treatment of anorexia nervosa, using a system of positive and negative reinforcements based on weight gain or loss. Weight gain is rewarded by attainment of desired activities such as participation in recreational activities, television privileges and home visits. Conversely, weight loss results in loss of privileges or confinement to bed rest.

References, see page 268.

Bulimia Nervosa

Bulimia nervosa is characterized by binge eating and inappropriate vomiting, fasting, excessive exercise and the misuse of diuretics, laxatives or enemas. Bulimia nervosa is 10 times more common in females than in males and affects up to 3 percent of young women. The condition usually becomes symptomatic between the ages of 13 and 20 years.

There may be a genetic predisposition to bulimia nervosa. Predisposing factors include psychologic and personality factors, such as perfectionism, impaired self-concept, affective instability, and poor impulse control.

I. **Diagnostic Criteria**
   A. The diagnostic criteria for bulimia nervosa now include subtypes to distinguish patients who compensate for binge eating by purging (vomiting and/or the abuse of laxatives and diuretics) from those who use nonpurging behaviors (eg, fasting or excessive exercising).

DSM IV Diagnostic Criteria for Bulimia Nervosa

- Recurrent episodes of binge eating. An episode of binge eating is characterized by both of the following:
- Eating, in a discrete period of time (eg, within a two-hour period), an amount of food that is definitely larger than most people would eat during a similar period of time and under similar circumstances.
- A sense of lack of control over eating during the episode (eg, a feeling that one cannot stop eating or control what or how much one is eating).
- Recurrent inappropriate compensatory behavior in order to prevent weight gain, such as self-induced vomiting; misuse of laxatives, diuretics, enemas, or other medications; fasting or excessive exercise.
- The binge eating and inappropriate compensatory behaviors both occur, on average, at least twice a week for three months.
- Self-evaluation is unduly influenced by body shape and weight.
- The disturbance does not occur exclusively during episodes of anorexia nervosa.

Specify type:
- **Purging type:** during the current episode of bulimia nervosa, the person has regularly engaged in self-induced vomiting or the misuse of laxatives, diuretics, or enemas.
- **Nonpurging type:** during the current episode of bulimia nervosa, the person has used other inappropriate compensatory behaviors, such as fasting or excessive exercise, but has not regularly engaged in self-induced vomiting or the misuse of laxatives, diuretics, or enemas.

Psychiatric Conditions Commonly Coexisting with Bulimia Nervosa

Mood disorders	**Anxiety disorders**
Major depression	Panic disorder
Dysthymic disorder	Obsessive-compulsive disorder
Bipolar disorder	Generalized anxiety disorder
Substance-related disorders	Post-traumatic stress disorder
Alcohol abuse	**Personality disorders**
Stimulant abuse	Borderline personality disorder
Polysubstance abuse	Histrionic personality disorder
	Narcissistic personality disorder
	Antisocial personality disorder

Medical Complications of Bulimia Nervosa	
Gastric rupture Nausea Abdominal pain and distention Prolonged digestion Weight gain Dental erosion Enlarged salivary glands Oral/hand trauma Esophageal/pharyngeal damage Irritation of esophagus and/or pharynx due to contact with gastric acids Heart- burn and sore throat Upper gastrointestinal tears	Perforation of upper digestive tract, esoph- agus or stomach Excessive blood in vomitus and gastric pain Electrolyte imbalances Hypokalemia Fatigue Muscle spasms Heart palpitations Paresthesias Tetany Seizures Cardiac arrhythmias

II. Medical complications

A. The medical complications of bulimia nervosa range from fatigue, bloating and constipation to hypokalemia, cathartic colon, impaired renal function and cardiac arrest.

B. **Gastric rupture**, the most serious complication of binge eating, is uncommon. Nausea, abdominal pain and distention, prolonged digestion and weight gain are common.

C. **Self-induced vomiting**, the most common means of purging, is used by more than 75 percent of patients with bulimia nervosa.

D. **Dental erosion.** Gastric acids may cause deterioration of tooth enamel.

E. **Enlarged salivary glands.** Frequent vomiting causes swelling of the salivary glands in approximately 8 percent of patients with bulimia.

F. **Oral and hand trauma.** The induction of vomiting with a finger or an object can cause lacerations of the mouth and throat. Bleeding lacerations can also occur on the knuckles because of repeated contact with the front teeth.

G. **Esophageal and pharyngeal complications.** Because of repeated contact with gastric acids, the esophagus or pharynx may become irritated.

H. **Blood in the vomitus** is an indication of upper gastrointestinal tears, which are a more serious complication of purging. Most tears heal well with cessation of vomiting.

I. **Electrolyte imbalances.** Serious depletions of hydrogen chloride, potassium, sodium and magnesium can occur because of the excessive loss of fluids during vomiting.

III. Patient evaluation

A. Physical examination should include vital signs and an evaluation of height and weight relative to age. General hair loss, lanugo, abdominal tenderness, acrocyanosis (cyanosis of the extremities), jaundice, edema, parotid gland tenderness or enlargement, and scars on the dorsum of the hand should be sought.

B. **Laboratory tests** include a complete blood count with differential, serum chemistry and thyroid profiles, and urine chemistry microscopy testing. A chest radiograph and electrocardiogram may be indicated in some cases.

C. **Psychiatric assessment**
   1. Standardized testing should document the patient's general personality features, characterologic disturbance and attitudes about eating, body size and weight.
   2. A complete history should document the patient's body weight, eating

patterns and attempts at weight loss, including typical daily food intake, methods of purging and perceived ideal weight.
3. The patient's interpersonal history and functioning, including family dynamics, peer relationships, and present or past physical, sexual or emotional abuse should be assessed.
4. An evaluation of medical and psychiatric comorbidity, as well as documentation of previous attempts at treatment.

IV. Treatment

A. Tricyclic antidepressants. Desipramine, 150 to 300 mg per day, is superior to placebo in the treatment of bulimia nervosa. Imipramine, 176 to 300 mg per day, is also more beneficial than placebo. Amitriptyline, 150 mg per day, is more effective than placebo in reducing binge eating (72 percent versus 52 percent).

B. Selective serotonin reuptake inhibitors. Fluoxetine (Prozac), 20-mg dosage, results in a 45 percent reduction in binge eating. Fluoxetine in a dosage of 60 mg per day produces the best treatment response, demonstrating a 67 percent reduction in binge eating.

C. Psychotherapy. Cognitive-behavioral therapy has resulted in the most significant reductions of binge eating and/or purging. Cognitive-behavioral therapy principally involves interventions aimed at addressing preoccupation with body, weight and food, perfectionism, dichotomous thinking and low self-esteem. The initial goal of cognitive-behavioral therapy is to restore control over dietary intake.

References

References are available at www.ccspublishing.com/ccs.

Index